Free Video  **Free Video**

Essential Test Tips Video from Trivium Test Prep

Dear Customer,

Thank you for purchasing from Trivium Test Prep! We're honored to help you prepare for your CEN exam.

To show our appreciation, we're offering a **FREE CEN *Essential Test Tips* Video by Trivium Test Prep.*** Our video includes 35 test preparation strategies that will make you successful on the CEN. All we ask is that you email us your feedback and describe your experience with our product. Amazing, awful, or just so-so: we want to hear what you have to say!

To receive your **FREE CEN *Essential Test Tips* Video**, please email us at 5star@triviumtestprep.com. Include "Free 5 Star" in the subject line and the following information in your email:

1. The title of the product you purchased.

2. Your rating from 1 – 5 (with 5 being the best).

3. Your feedback about the product, including how our materials helped you meet your goals and ways in which we can improve our products.

4. Your full name and shipping address so we can send your **FREE CEN *Essential Test Tips* Video.**

If you have any questions or concerns please feel free to contact us directly at 5star@triviumtestprep.com.

Thank you!

- Trivium Test Prep Team

*To get access to the free video please email us at 5star@triviumtestprep.com, and please follow the instructions above.

CEN REVIEW BOOK AND STUDY GUIDE 2019–2020

Comprehensive Certified Emergency Nursing
Exam Prep and Practice Test Questions

Contributors

Kylee Cisneros, MSN-Ed., RN, CEN, TCRN, has been a registered nurse for eight years and specializes in emergency and trauma nursing. She served in the United States Navy Nurse Corps for five years. Since leaving the US Navy, she has worked in nursing education and in management of the emergency department of a level three trauma center.

Amanda Constantino, MSN, RN, CEN, has been a registered nurse for over ten years with experience in medical, surgical, telemetry, oncology, and emergency departments. She received her BSN and MSN from the University of Central Florida. In addition, she teaches BLS, ACLS, and PALS courses.

Roma Lightsey, MSN, RN, has been a registered nurse since 2003, with thirteen years of ICU, ED, and critical care experience. She was a national clinical nurse educator for two years for a medical device company and has been a medical writer since 2005. She has contributed to NCLEX case studies and item-writing development, as well as content creation for online BSN programs.

Rochelle Santopoalo, Ph.D., RN, has a rich history in health care including clinical, administration, research, and education. Her clinical specialty is geriatric rehabilitation. While serving as a nursing administrator, she became fascinated with organizational behavior, finding the principles directly applicable to health care. Her passion led to the pursuit of a doctorate in Human and Organizational Systems from Fielding Graduate University in Santa Barbara, CA. She resides in central Florida, providing health care to geriatric clients in long-term care.

Carla J. Smith, MSN, RN, CEN, NCSN, is a registered nurse with sixteen years of experience in nursing education, public health, school nursing, emergency nursing, cardiovascular nursing, and critical care. Carla currently teaches Advanced Health Caring Concepts for NCLEX prelicensure at St. Joseph School of Nursing in Nashua, NH. She serves on the New Hampshire Nurses Association Government Affairs Commission and has worked closely with the New Hampshire School Nurses Association and state Department of Education. She was a CEN at Portsmouth Regional Hospital of Portsmouth, NH and a National Certified School Nurse (NCSN) at Ellis School of Fremont, NH. She received the New Hampshire PTA Outstanding Partnership Award in 2014 and the National Healthy Schools Campaign School Nurse Leadership Award in 2015. She served for five years as the Deputy Health Officer for the Town of Fremont, NH and is a former member of the Medical Reserves Corp.

Carolyn Tinsley, MSN, RN, APRN, ACNS-BC, has worked in critical care for over thirty years. She is currently nursing faculty at Murray State University in Murray, KY. She has taught Adult Health III (critical care). She also teaches pathophysiology.

Marna Watson, MSN, RN, is a registered nurse in Cincinnati, OH. Following eighteen years in clinical research, she received her BSN at University of Cincinnati, and her MSN at South University. After several years focusing on acute care, wound care and the geriatric population, she has spent the past nine years teaching in higher education at Galen College of Nursing in Cincinnati. She feels being an educator is very rewarding, and she has played an integral part in bringing the next generation of nurses into the workforce. She is studying to obtain her NP license.

TABLE OF CONTENTS

ONLINE RESOURCES

To help you fully prepare for your Certified Emergency Nurse (CEN) Exam, Ascencia includes online resources with the purchase of this study guide.

Practice Test

In addition to the practice test included in this book, we also offer an online exam. Since many exams today are computer based, getting to practice your test-taking skills on the computer is a great way to prepare.

Flash Cards

A convenient supplement to this study guide, Ascencia's flash cards enable you to review important terms easily on your computer or smartphone.

Cheat Sheets

Review the core skills you need to master the exam with easy-to-read Cheat Sheets.

From Stress to Success

Watch "From Stress to Success," a brief but insightful YouTube video that offers the tips, tricks, and secrets experts use to score higher on the exam.

Reviews

Leave a review, send us helpful feedback, or sign up for Ascencia promotions—including free books!

Access these materials at: **www.ascenciatestprep.com/cen-online-resources**

INTRODUCTION

Congratulations on choosing to take the Certified Emergency Nurse (CEN) Exam! Passing the CEN is an important step forward in your nursing career.

In the following pages, you will find information about the CEN, what to expect on test day, how to use this book, and the content covered on the exam. We also encourage you to visit the website of the Board of Certification for Emergency Nursing (https://bcen.org) to register for the exam and find the most current information on the CEN.

The BCEN Certification Process

The **Certified Emergency Nurse (CEN) Exam** is developed by the **Board of Certification for Emergency Nursing (BCEN)** as part of its certification program for emergency nurses. The CEN measures the nursing skills necessary to excel as a nurse in an emergency department. To qualify for the exam, you must have a current Registered Nurse license in the United States or its territories. The BCEN also recommends that you have at least two years of nursing experience in an emergency department. There's no level of experience that's *required* for the exam, but many nurses find that the practical knowledge they have acquired while working in the ED is vital to passing the exam.

Once you have met the qualifications and passed the exam, you will have your CEN certification, and you may use the credentials as long as your certification is valid. You will need to recertify every four years. You can earn your recertification by taking continuing education courses or by retaking the exam. If you are taking the exam for recertification, you must submit your application 91 days before your certification lapses. You must then pass the exam within the 90-day testing window.

CEN Questions and Timing

The CEN consists of **175 questions**. Only 150 of these questions are scored; 25 are unscored, or *pretest* questions. These questions are included by the BCEN to test their suitability for inclusion in future tests. You'll have no way of knowing which questions are unscored, so treat every question like it counts.

The questions on the CEN are multiple-choice with four answer choices. Some questions will include exhibits such as ECG reading strips or laboratory results. The CEN has **no guess penalty**. That is, if you answer a question incorrectly, no points are deducted from your score; you simply do not get credit for that question. Therefore, you should always guess if you do not know the answer to a question.

You will have **3 hours** to complete the test. During this time you will also need to complete the BCEN Examination Rules and Regulations Agreement. You may take breaks at any point during the exam, but you will not be given extra time, and you cannot access personal items (other than medications).

CEN Content Areas

The BCEN develops its exams based on feedback from emergency nursing professionals about the nursing concepts and skills that are most important to their work. This feedback has been used to develop an exam framework that emphasizes the assessment, diagnosis, and treatment of conditions emergency nurses are likely to encounter in the ED.

The framework is broken down into seven sections loosely based on human body systems and one section devoted to professional issues. The table below gives the breakdown of the questions on the exam, and the content outline objectives are listed below the table.

Quick Summary of CEN Test Sections

Section		Approx. No. of Questions
1.	Cardiovascular Emergencies	23
2.	Respiratory Emergencies	19
3.	Neurological Emergencies	19
4.	Gastrointestinal, Genitourinary, Gynecology, and Obstetrical Emergencies	24
5.	Psychosocial and Medical Emergencies	29
6.	Maxillofacial, Ocular, Orthopedic, and Wound Emergencies	24
7.	Environment and Toxicology Emergencies, and Communicable Diseases	18
8.	Professional Issues	19
Total		175 questions

CEN CONTENT OUTLINE
Cardiovascular Emergencies

- Acute coronary syndrome
- Aneurysm/dissection
- Cardiopulmonary arrest
- Dysrhythmias
- Endocarditis
- Heart failure
- Hypertension
- Pericardial tamponade
- Pericarditis
- Peripheral vascular disease
- Thromboembolic disease
- Trauma
- Shock (cardiogenic and obstructive)

Respiratory Emergencies

+ Aspiration
+ Asthma
+ Chronic obstructive pulmonary disease (COPD)
+ Infections
+ Inhalation injuries
+ Obstruction
+ Pleural effusion
+ Pneumothorax
+ Pulmonary edema, noncardiac
+ Pulmonary embolus
+ Respiratory distress syndrome
+ Trauma

Neurological Emergencies

+ Alzheimer's disease/dementia
+ Chronic neurological disorders
+ Guillain-Barré syndrome
+ Headache
+ Increased intracranial pressure (ICP)
+ Meningitis
+ Seizure disorders
+ Shunt dysfunctions
+ Spinal cord injuries, including neurogenic shock
+ Stroke (ischemic or hemorrhagic)
+ Transient ischemic attack (TIA)
+ Trauma

Gastrointestinal Emergencies

+ Acute abdomen
+ Bleeding
+ Cholecystitis
+ Cirrhosis
+ Diverticulitis
+ Esophageal varices
+ Esophagitis
+ Foreign bodies
+ Gastritis
+ Gastroenteritis
+ Hepatitis
+ Hernia
+ Inflammatory bowel disease
+ Intussusception
+ Obstructions
+ Pancreatitis
+ Trauma
+ Ulcers

Genitourinary Emergencies

+ Foreign bodies
+ Infection
+ Priapism
+ Renal calculi
+ Testicular torsion
+ Trauma
+ Urinary retention

Gynecology Emergencies

+ Bleeding/dysfunction (vaginal)
+ Foreign bodies
+ Hemorrhage
+ Infection
+ Ovarian cyst
+ Sexual assault/battery
+ Trauma

Obstetrical Emergencies

+ Abruptio placenta
+ Ectopic pregnancy
+ Emergent delivery
+ Hemorrhage
+ Hyperemesis gravidarum
+ Neonatal resuscitation
+ Placenta previa
+ Postpartum infection
+ Preeclampsia, eclampsia, HELLP syndrome
+ Preterm labor
+ Threatened/spontaneous abortion
+ Trauma

Psychosocial Emergencies

+ Abuse and neglect
+ Aggressive/violent behavior
+ Anxiety/panic
+ Bipolar disorder
+ Depression
+ Homicidal ideation
+ Psychosis
+ Situational crisis
+ Suicidal ideation

Medical Emergencies

+ Allergic reactions and anaphylaxis
+ Blood dyscrasias
+ Disseminated intravascular coagulation (DIC)
+ Electrolyte/fluid imbalance
+ Endocrine conditions
+ Fever
+ Immunocompromise
+ Renal failure
+ Sepsis and septic shock

Maxillofacial Emergencies

+ Abscess
+ Acute vestibular dysfunction
+ Dental conditions
+ Epistaxis
+ Facial nerve disorders
+ Foreign bodies
+ Infections
+ Ruptured tympanic membrane
+ Temporomandibular joint (TMJ) dislocation
+ Trauma

Ocular Emergencies

+ Abrasions
+ Burns
+ Foreign bodies
+ Glaucoma
+ Infections

+ Retinal artery occlusion
+ Retinal detachment
+ Trauma
+ Ulcerations/keratitis

Orthopedic Emergencies

+ Amputation
+ Compartment syndrome
+ Contusions
+ Costochondritis
+ Foreign bodies
+ Fractures/dislocations

+ Inflammatory conditions
+ Joint effusion
+ Low back pain
+ Osteomyelitis
+ Strains/sprains
+ Trauma

Wound Emergencies

+ Abrasions
+ Avulsions
+ Foreign bodies
+ Infections
+ Injection injuries

+ Lacerations
+ Missile injuries
+ Pressure ulcers
+ Puncture wounds
+ Trauma

Environment Emergencies

+ Burns
+ Chemical exposure
+ Electrical injuries
+ Envenomation emergencies
+ Food poisoning

+ Parasite and fungal infestations
+ Radiation exposure
+ Submersion injury
+ Temperature-related emergencies
+ Vector-borne illnesses

Toxicology Emergencies

+ Acids and alkalis
+ Carbon monoxide
+ Cyanide
+ Drug interactions (including alternative therapies)

+ Overdose and ingestions
+ Substance abuse
+ Withdrawal syndrome

Communicable Diseases

- C. Difficile
- Childhood diseases
- Herpes zoster
- Mononucleosis
- Multidrug-resistant organisms
- Tuberculosis

Professional Issues

- Nurse
  - Critical Incident Stress Management
  - Ethical dilemmas
  - Evidence-based practice
  - Lifelong learning
  - Research

- Patient
  - Cultural considerations
  - Discharge planning
  - End-of-life issues
  - Forensic evidence collection
  - Pain management and procedural sedation
  - Patient safety
  - Patient satisfaction
  - Transfer and stabilization
  - Transitions of care

- System
  - Delegation of tasks to assistive personnel
  - Disaster management
  - Federal regulations
  - Patient consent for treatment
  - Performance improvement
  - Risk management
  - Symptom surveillance
  - Triage

Exam Administration

To register for the exam, you must first apply through the BCEN website (https://bcen.org/cen/apply-schedule). After your application is accepted, you will receive an email with instructions on how to register for the exam.

The CEN is administered at Pearson VUE testing centers around the nation. Plan to arrive at least **30 minutes before the exam**; if you arrive more than 15 minutes after the test starts, you will not be admitted. Bring **two forms of ID** and be prepared to be photographed and have a palm vein scan. Your primary ID must be government issued, include a recent photograph and signature, and match the name under which you registered to take the test. You secondary ID must include your name and signature or name and photograph. If you do not have proper ID, you will not be allowed to take the test.

You will not be allowed to bring any personal items into the testing room, such as calculators or phones. You may not bring pens, pencils, or scratch paper. Other prohibited items include hats, scarves, and coats. You may wear religious garments, however. Most testing centers provide lockers for valuables.

Exam Results

Once you have completed your test, the staff at the Pearson VUE testing center will give you a score report; you can also request to receive the report via email. The score report will include your raw score (the number of questions you answered correctly) for the whole test and for each content area.

The report will also include a pass/fail designation. The number of correct answers needed to pass the exam will vary slightly depending on the questions included in your version of the test (i.e., if you took a version of the test with harder questions, the passing score will be lower). For most test takers, **a passing score will be between 105 and 110** questions answered correctly.

If you do not pass the exam, you will be able to reapply and retake the test after 90 days.

Using This Book

This book is divided into two sections. In the content area review, you will find the pathophysiology, risk factors, signs and symptoms, diagnostic findings, and treatment protocols for the conditions included in the CEN framework. Throughout the chapter you'll also see Quick Review Questions that will help reinforce important concepts and skills.

The book also includes two full-length practice tests (one in the book and one online) with answer rationales. You can use these tests to gauge your readiness for the test and determine which content areas you may need to review more thoroughly.

Ascencia Test Prep

With health care fields such as nursing, pharmacy, emergency care, and physical therapy becoming the fastest-growing industries in the United States, individuals looking to enter the health care industry or rise in their field need high-quality, reliable resources. Ascencia Test Prep's study guides and test preparation materials are developed by credentialed industry professionals with years of experience in their respective fields. Ascencia recognizes that health care professionals nurture bodies and spirits, and save lives. Ascencia Test Prep's mission is to help health care workers grow.

ONE: CARDIOVASCULAR EMERGENCIES

Physiology and Terminology Review

+ The heart has 4 chambers: the left atrium, right atrium, left ventricle, and right ventricle.
  ⬦ The **left and right atria** receive blood returning to the heart from other locations in the body.
  ⬦ The **left and right ventricles** receive blood from the atria and then push blood out of the heart into the vessels.

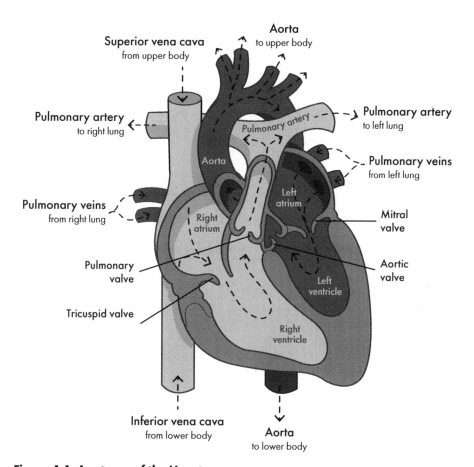

Figure 1.1. Anatomy of the Heart

- The **atrioventricular valves** (tricuspid and mitral valves) are located between the atria and ventricles and cause the first heart sounds (S1) when they close.

- **Semilunar valves** (aortic and pulmonic valves) are located between the ventricles and great vessels and cause the second heart sound (S2) when they close.

- Blood flows through the cardiac valves in the following order: tricuspid → pulmonic → mitral → aortic (use the mnemonic **Tissue Paper My Assets**).

- The cardiac wall has 3 layers: the **epicardium**, **myocardium**, and **endocardium**.

- The **pericardium** is the sac surrounding the heart. It is divided into 2 layers: the fibrous pericardium and the serous pericardium. The serous pericardium is further divided into the visceral and parietal layers. The space between these 2 layers is the pericardial space, which contains pericardial fluid.

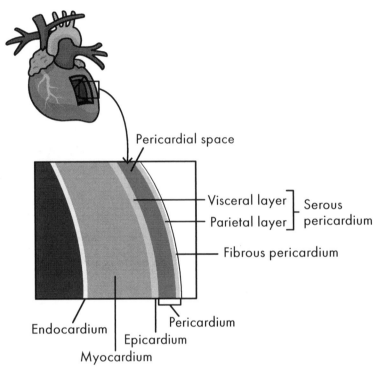

Figure 1.2. Layers of the Heart

- **Stroke volume (SV)**, the volume of blood pumped from the left ventricle during one contraction, depends on several conditions:
    - **preload**: how much the ventricles stretch at the end of diastole
    - **afterload**: the amount of resistance needed for the heart to open the aortic valve and force blood volume into circulation
    - **contractility**: the force of the heart, independent of preload and afterload

- Normal SV is 60 – 130 mL per contraction.

- **Heart rate (HR)** is how many times the ventricles contract each minute.

- **Cardiac output (CO)** is the volume of blood that the heart pumps every minute.
    - To calculate CO, multiply SV by HR.
    - Normal CO is 4 – 8 L per minute.

- Normal **central venous pressure (CVP)**, the blood pressure in the venae cavae, is 2 – 6 mm Hg.
- **Mean arterial pressure (MAP)** is the average pressure within the arteries during a single cardiac cycle.
  - MAP is the most accurate indicator of perfusion, as compared to blood pressure alone.
  - Calculate MAP by multiplying the diastolic blood pressure (DBP) by 2, adding the sum of the systolic blood pressure (SBP) and then dividing by 3: MAP = [SBP + 2 (DBP)] ÷ 3.
- **Pulse pressure** is the difference between the systolic pressure (the highest value during a heartbeat) and diastolic pressure (the low value found between beats).
- Tachycardia is common in pediatrics due to children's cardiovascular physiology.
- As adults age, changes occur in all bodily systems, including the cardiovascular system.
  - Cardiac output decreases with age, and cardiac reserve is reduced. Consequently, older adults are less able to respond to cardiac stressors.
  - Vascular changes also occur with age and may increase blood pressure.
  - Pulses on the older adult may be difficult to palpate.
  - Because other organs, such as the liver and kidneys, also change with age, drugs are metabolized more slowly. Caution should be taken with drug administration in older adults, who typically should be started with lower doses of medications new to them.

Table 1.1. Normal Heart and Respiratory Rates

Age	Normal Heart Rate: Awake (bpm)	Normal Heart Rate: Sleeping (bpm)	Normal Respiratory Rate (breaths per minute)
Newborn to 3 months	85 – 205	80 – 160	30 – 60
3 months to 2 years	100 – 180	75 – 160	24 – 40
2 – 10 years	60 – 140	60 – 90	18 – 30
> 10 years	60 – 100	50 – 90	12 – 20

Cardiovascular Assessment

GENERAL SURVEY

- Cardiovascular assessment should include monitoring of the following:
  - LOC: should be baseline for patient, typically alert and responsive
  - color of skin: should be appropriate for ethnicity
  - moisture of skin: should be dry
  - temperature: should be warm
  - edema: should not normally be present; check for pitting and if edema is unilateral or generalized to a specific area
  - capillary refill: should be less than 2 seconds
  - pulses: should be strong and regular
- Women, people with diabetes, and adults over 65 often have atypical cardiac signs and symptoms. Complaints of upper abdominal pain, back pain, heartburn, or reflux should have a cardiac workup to rule out a potential cardiac origin of their symptoms.

+ **Chest pain** is one of the most common complaints among patients presenting to the ED. Some patients may instead describe pressure, tightness, indigestion, or burning in the chest, back, or upper abdomen. The mnemonic **PQRST** (Table 1.2.) is helpful to assess chest pain.

Table 1.2. Assessing Chest Pain	
P	What **provokes** or **palliates** the pain? (What makes it better or worse? Was anything tried to relieve the pain at home before arrival at the ED?)
Q	What is the **quality** of the pain? (What does it feel like? Is it sharp, throbbing, aching?)
R	What is the **region** of the pain, and where does the pain radiate? (Where is the pain? Does the pain go anywhere else?)
S	What is the **severity** of the pain (on a scale from 1 to 10)?
T	What **time** did the pain begin? (When did the pain start, and has it been constant or intermittent? What were you doing when the pain first began?)

+ Monitor for orthostatic changes in cardiac patients.
    ⬦ To measure orthostatic blood pressure, take the patient's baseline blood pressure from a lying position, have the patient stand, measure blood pressure again after 1 minute and again at 3 minutes, and then compare readings for significant drops.
    ⬦ A drop of 20 mm Hg in systolic blood pressure or 10 mm Hg in diastolic blood pressure when standing (at 1 or 3 minutes) is considered abnormal and can indicate a cardiac problem.

ECG

+ A 12-lead **electrocardiogram (ECG)** is a noninvasive diagnostic tool that records the heart's electrical activity. This diagnostic test can help determine a patient's cardiac rhythm and rate. It can also help diagnose electrolyte imbalances, hypertrophy, ischemia, injury, and infarction.

+ Any patient complaining of chest pain should have an ECG performed within 10 minutes of arrival.

+ A patient's heart rhythm can be continuously assessed with a 3- or 5-lead ECG by remote telemetry.

+ Patients with any cardiac complaint or electrolyte imbalance should remain on continuous telemetry monitoring to observe for rhythm changes.

+ Waveforms
    ⬦ **P wave**: represents atrial depolarization
    ⬦ **QRS complex**: represents ventricular depolarization; consists of 3 waves: Q wave (initial negative deflection), R wave (positive deflection), and S wave (subsequent negative deflection); duration is normally less than 0.10 seconds
    ⬦ **T wave**: represents ventricular repolarization

+ Intervals between waveforms

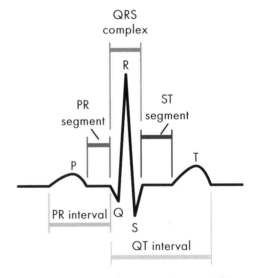

Figure 1.3. Waveforms and Intervals on an ECG

- ❖ **PR interval**: measured from the beginning of the P wave to the beginning of the QRS complex; normal range is between 0.12 and 0.20 seconds
- ❖ **ST segment**: portion of the wave that extends from the end of the QRS complex to the beginning of the T wave; shape and location are evaluated instead of duration; normally flat and at the same level as the isoelectric line (the flat line that occurs when no electrical activity is occurring)
- ❖ **QT interval**: measured from the beginning of the QRS complex to the end of the T wave; indicates total time interval from onset of depolarization to the completion of repolarization; normal duration of 0.36 – 0.44 seconds

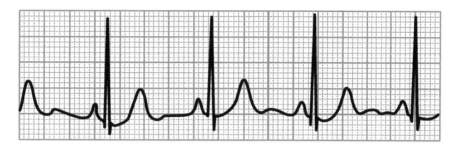

Figure 1.4. ECG: Normal Sinus Rhythm

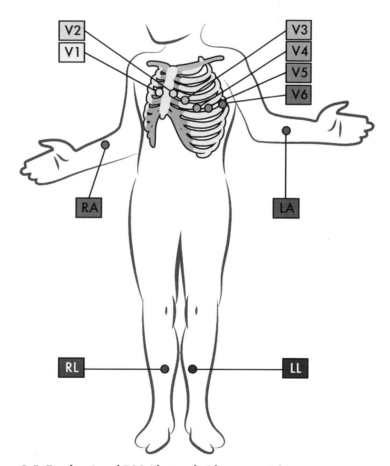

Figure 1.5. Twelve-Lead ECG Electrode Placement Diagram

The most significant finding of an ECG is the presence of ST elevation.

+ A physician should sign any ECG performed in the ED to ensure the patient is not experiencing a STEMI (ST-elevation myocardial infarction).

Table 1.3. Twelve-Lead ECG Electrode Placement

Electrode	Placement
V1	Fourth intercostal space to the right of the sternum
V2	Fourth intercostal space to the left of the sternum
V3	Midway between V2 and V4
V4	Fifth intercostal space at the midclavicular line
V5	Anterior axillary line at the same level as V4
V6	Midaxillary line at the same level as V4 and V5
RA	Between right shoulder and right wrist
LA	Between left shoulder and left wrist
RL	Above right ankle and below the torso
LL	Above left ankle and below the torso

HEART SOUNDS

+ Using a stethoscope, auscultate for heart sounds. Use the diaphragm for high-pitched sounds such as murmurs or friction rubs and the bell for low-pitched sounds such as valve stenosis. The following areas should be auscultated:
    ◇ mitral valve: found at the fifth left intercostal space at the midclavicular line
    ◇ tricuspid valve: found at the fifth left intercostal space at the left sternal border
    ◇ Erb's point: found at the third left intercostal space at the left sternal border
    ◇ pulmonic valve: found at the second left intercostal space at the left sternal border
    ◇ aortic valve: found at the second right intercostal space at the right sternal border

+ S1 is the heart sound caused by the closure of the atrioventricular (AV) valves.
    ◇ indicates the end of diastole and beginning of systole
    ◇ heard best at the apex

+ S2 is the heart sound caused by the closure of the semilunar valves.
    ◇ indicates the end of systole and beginning of diastole
    ◇ heard best at the base

+ S3, an extra heart sound sometimes referred to as a ventricular gallop, is caused by a rush of blood into a dilated ventricle.
    ◇ sounds dull and low-pitched and occurs during the early part of diastole
    ◇ sounds similar to "Ken-tuc-ky," with S3 being the "ky"
    ◇ usually indicative of heart failure, fluid overload, or cardiomyopathy
    ◇ normal in children but associated with ventricular systolic failure in adults

+ S4, an extra heart sound sometimes referred to as an atrial gallop, is caused by the atrial contraction of blood into a ventricle.

- ⬦ sounds dull and low-pitched and occurs during the late part of diastole
- ⬦ sounds similar to "*Ten-nes-see*," with S4 being the "ten"
- ⬦ usually indicative of MI, hypertension, or ventricular hypertrophy
+ **Pericardial friction rub**, a high-pitched, leathery sound heard characteristically in pericarditis, is caused by inflammation.
  - ⬦ heard loudest at the fourth and fifth intercostal spaces, with patient leaning forward
  - ⬦ will continue even if patient is holding breath
+ **Murmurs** are the sounds made by turbulent blood flow in and around the heart.
  - ⬦ can be systolic (occurring during ventricular contraction) or diastolic (occurring during ventricular filling)
  - ⬦ murmurs caused by increased blood flow across a normal valve:
    - ✦ usually soft and systolic
    - ✦ commonly caused by anemia, pregnancy, hyperthyroidism, fever, or exercise
  - ⬦ abnormal murmurs
    - ✦ can be caused by septal defects such as holes in the heart, infections, or structural damage such as stenosis, endocarditis, or rheumatic fever
  - ⬦ normal murmurs
    - ✦ typically disappear over time; of little concern
    - ✦ common in pediatrics

Cardiac Medications

ANGIOTENSIN-CONVERTING ENZYME (ACE) INHIBITORS

+ used to treat hypertension and heart failure
+ improve survival after MI
+ reduce infarct size
+ improve ventricular remodeling
+ decrease preload *HOW MUCH THE VENTRICLES STRETCH @ END OF DIASTOLE.*
+ should not be used in patients with:
  - ⬦ hypotension
  - ⬦ bradycardia
  - ⬦ renal failure
  - ⬦ hyperkalemia

+ can cause life-threatening angioedema in some patients
+ commonly used ACE inhibitors:
  - ⬦ benazepril (Lotensin)
  - ⬦ captopril (Capoten)
  - ⬦ enalapril (Vasotec)
  - ⬦ lisinopril (Zestril)

ANGIOTENSIN II RECEPTOR BLOCKERS (ARBS)

+ used to treat hypertension
+ used for heart failure patients to improve symptoms
+ block stress hormones
+ make the heart pump easier

+ should not be used in patients with:
  - ⬦ hypotension
  - ⬦ pregnancy
  - ⬦ kidney failure
  - ⬦ hyperkalemia

+ commonly used ARBs:
  ⋄ irbesartan (Avapro)
  ⋄ losartan (Cozaar)
  ⋄ telmisartan (Micardis)
  ⋄ valsartan (Diovan)

ANTIDYSRHYTHMICS

+ used to control irregular heart rhythms
+ restore or control normal rhythms and heart conduction
+ may be used to prevent dysrhythmias
+ some antidysrhythmics should not be used in patients with:
  ⋄ heart failure
  ⋄ long QT syndrome
  ⋄ heart blocks

+ commonly used antidysrhythmics:
  ⋄ amiodarone (Cordarone)
  ⋄ disopyramide (Norpace)
  ⋄ flecainide (Tambocor)
  ⋄ procainamide (Procan)

ANTICOAGULANTS

+ prevent blood from coagulating to reduce the risk of clot formation
+ should not be used in patients with:
  ⋄ bleeding problems
  ⋄ pregnancy
  ⋄ trauma

+ Commonly used anticoagulants:
  ⋄ enoxaparin (Lovenox)
  ⋄ fondaparinux (Arixtra)
  ⋄ heparin
  ⋄ warfarin (Coumadin)

ANTIPLATELETS

+ decrease platelet aggregation to reduce clot formation
+ should not be used in patients with:
  ⋄ bleeding disorders
  ⋄ liver disease
  ⋄ thrombocytopenia

+ commonly used antiplatelets:
  ⋄ aspirin
  ⋄ cilostazol (Pletal)
  ⋄ clopidogrel (Plavix)
  ⋄ ticlopidine (Ticlid)

THROMBOLYTICS

+ help dissolve blood clots
+ activate plasminogen, which forms plasmin, an enzyme that can break down fibrin, which forms clots
+ should not be used in patients with:
  ⋄ bleeding problems
  ⋄ pregnancy
  ⋄ trauma

+ commonly used thrombolytics:
  ⋄ reteplase (Retavase)
  ⋄ tenecteplase (TNKase)
  ⋄ tPA
  ⋄ streptokinase (Streptase)

ANTI-HYPERTENSIVES

+ treat hypertension
+ reduce systemic vascular resistance
+ should not be used in patients with hypotension
+ may be contraindicated in patients who are pregnant or patients with bradycardia

+ commonly used anti-hypertensives:
    ✧ doxazosin (Cardura)
    ✧ clonidine (Catapres)
    ✧ hydralazine (Apresoline)
    ✧ minoxidil
    ✧ terazosin (Hytrin)

BETA BLOCKERS

+ lower blood pressure and heart rate
+ decrease myocardial oxygen demand by decreasing heart rate, contractility, and blood pressure
+ should not be used in patients with:
    ✧ hypotension
    ✧ bradycardia
    ✧ asthma
    ✧ recent cocaine use

+ commonly used beta blockers:
    ✧ atenolol (Tenormin)
    ✧ bisoprolol (Zebeta)
    ✧ carvedilol (Coreg)
    ✧ labetalol (Trandate)
    ✧ metoprolol (Lopressor)

NITRATES

+ relieve anginal chest pain
+ vasodilate blood vessels, increasing blood supply and oxygen to the heart
+ should not be used in patients who
    ✧ have taken phosphodiasterase medications in last 24 – 48 hours (can cause severe hypotension)
    ✧ are hypotensive or bradycardic
    ✧ have been diagnosed with right ventricular infarctions
+ commonly used nitrates:
    ✧ nitroglycerin (administered orally or as an ointment, a patch, a spray, or a sublingual tablet)

CALCIUM CHANNEL BLOCKERS

+ treat hypertension and dysrhythmias
+ restrict the regular flow of calcium into heart and blood vessels
+ reduce workload of the heart and oxygenation need
+ should not be used in patients with:
    ✧ hypotension
    ✧ bradycardia

+ commonly used calcium channel blockers:
    ✧ amlodipine (Norvasc)
    ✧ diltiazem (Cardizem)
    ✧ felodipine (Plendil)
    ✧ verapamil (Calan)

VASOPRESSORS

+ treat hypotension
+ cause constriction of blood vessels
+ increase MAP
+ should not be used in patients with hypertension

+ commonly used vasopressors:
    ✧ epinephrine
    ✧ dobutamine
    ✧ dopamine
    ✧ norepinephrine (Levophed)

DIURETICS

+ treat hypertension and to reduce fluid accumulation
+ pull excess fluid and salt from body
+ decrease electrolytes
+ should not be used in patients with:
    ✧ kidney failure
    ✧ dehydration
    ✧ pregnancy
    ✧ hypotension
    ✧ gout
    ✧ hypokalemia

+ commonly used diuretics:
    ✧ bumetanide (Bumex)
    ✧ cholothiazide
    ✧ furosemide (Lasix)
    ✧ hydrocholorothiazide

Acute Coronary Syndrome

Acute coronary syndrome (ACS) is an umbrella term for cardiac conditions in which blood flow to the heart is impaired. ACS includes unstable angina, non-ST-elevation myocardial infarction (NSTEMI), and ST-elevation myocardial infarction (STEMI).

UNSTABLE ANGINA PECTORIS

Pathophysiology

Unstable angina pectoris, also known simply as **angina**, is typically caused by atherosclerosis (plaque buildup that clogs arteries). Pieces of the built-up plaque can block blood flow or break off into the bloodstream and injure the vessels and cause clotting. When these plaques or clots impede blood flow to the heart muscle, oxygen availability is reduced, causing pain.

Risk Factors

+ blood clots
+ smoking
+ chronic illnesses
    ✧ diabetes
    ✧ hypertension
    ✧ high cholesterol

+ family history of heart disease
+ obesity
+ stress
+ intense exercise or exertion

Signs and Symptoms

+ sudden chest pain
  ◇ at rest
  ◇ lasts more than 20 minutes
  ◇ not relieved by rest or medicine
+ pain in arms, neck, jaw, or upper back or abdominal pain

+ nausea
+ dyspnea
+ dizziness
+ diaphoresis
+ Levine's sign (clenched fist to chest)

Diagnostic Tests and Findings

+ troponin or CK-MB labs negative
+ ECG may show ST depression

+ pathologic Q waves may be present, indicating a previous MI

Treatment and Management

+ Conduct an ECG to rule out STEMI.
+ Administer oxygen if oxygen saturation is less than 94%.
+ Obtain CBC, CMP, troponin, PT/PTT, and INR labs.
+ PCI may be needed for stents if coronary artery is blocked.
+ Coronary artery bypass grafts may be needed to redirect blood flow from the impaired artery.

+ Administer aspirin and clopidogrel for platelet aggregation.
+ Administer heparin as an anticoagulant.
+ Admit patient to cardiac unit.
+ At discharge, teach lifestyle changes such as losing weight, improving diet, and smoking cessation.

Table 1.4. The 2 Types of Unstable Angina Pectoris

	Pathophysiology	Signs and Symptoms	Diagnostic Tests and Findings	Treatment and Management
Wellen's syndrome	Proximal stenosis of the left anterior descending coronary artery.	Characteristic T-wave changes, with a history of anginal chest pain *without* elevated troponin.	Must be diagnosed through cardiac catheterization.	Similar to MI: Administer antiplatelets, anticoagulants, and nitrates.
Prinzmetal angina (variant angina)	Spasms within the coronary arteries. Can be caused by smoking, cocaine, stress, cold weather.	Occurs at rest. Typically occurs in younger individuals. Pain is cyclic.	Made through history. ECG findings may show peaked T waves and transient ST elevation. Angiogram that shows spasms.	Administer nitrates to relieve chest pain. Administer calcium channel blockers to relax blood vessels. Administer statins to reduce cholesterol and spasms.

NON-ST-ELEVATION MYOCARDIAL INFARCTION (NSTEMI)

Pathophysiology

A **non–ST-elevation myocardial infarction (NSTEMI)** includes an ST depression, which reflects ischemia resulting from a partial blockage of the coronary artery. The priority goal is to prevent a complete occlusion, which would be reflected by elevated ST segments of the ECG.

Risk Factors

+ chronic diseases
  + diabetes
  + hypertension
  + high cholesterol
+ family history of heart disease

+ smoking
+ physical inactivity
+ obesity
+ stress
+ oral contraceptive use

Signs and Symptoms

+ chest pain
  + continuous
  + may radiate to jaw, neck, or back
+ nausea and vomiting

+ dyspnea
+ dizziness
+ weakness
+ syncope

Diagnostic Tests and Findings

+ elevated troponin (> 0.05) without ST elevation
+ ECG shows ST depression and T-wave abnormalities
+ cardiac catheterization may show a blocked artery or arteries

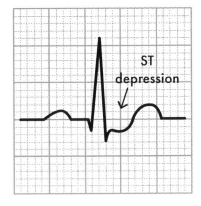

Figure 1.6. ECG: NSTEMI

Treatment and Management

+ Check serial cardiac enzymes every 3 hours to monitor for increase in heart damage.
+ Administer aspirin and clopidogrel for platelet aggregation.
+ Administer anticoagulants (heparin or enoxaparin [Lovenox]), usually as weight-based dosing.
+ Administer morphine.

+ Administer oxygen.
+ Administer nitrates.
+ Admit patient to cardiac unit.
+ Cardiac catheterization may be necessary.

2. A patient is found to have an elevated troponin level with no evidence of ST elevation on the ECG. Initial interventions for this patient should include what? *ADMIN ANTIPLATELETS + ANTICOAGS.*

MONA | morphine / oxygen / nitro / aspirin

ST-ELEVATION MYOCARDIAL INFARCTION (STEMI)

Pathophysiology

An **ST-elevation myocardial infarction (STEMI)** indicates a complete occlusion of a coronary artery. This life-threatening emergency requires immediate intervention and early reperfusion.

Risk Factors

+ smoking
+ chronic diseases
    + diabetes
    + hypertension
    + high cholesterol
+ physical inactivity
+ obesity
+ family history of heart disease
+ cocaine use

Signs and Symptoms

+ chest pain
    + continuous
    + may radiate to back, arm, jaw
+ upper abdominal pain more common in people over 65, people with diabetes, and women
+ dyspnea
+ nausea, vomiting
+ dizziness, syncope
+ diaphoresis
+ palpitations
+ anxiety or feeling of impending doom

Diagnostic Tests and Findings

+ ST elevation (defined as 1 mm in 2 or more leads or a new left bundle branch block)
+ elevated troponin (> 0.05 ng/mL)
+ cardiac catheterization showing blocked artery or arteries

Table 1.5. Heart Wall Affected and Related ECG Leads in STEMI

Wall	Lead
Inferior	II, III, aVF
Lateral	I, aVL, V5, V6
Septal	V1, aVR
Anterior	V2, V3, V4
Posterior	ST depression in V1, V2 and tall R waves

+ ECG should be completed to determine if ST elevation is present.

+ Establish 2 large-bore IVs in the antecubital veins.

+ Apply oxygen if patient is dyspneic or hypoxemic, shows signs of heart failure, or has an oxygen saturation of less than 90%.

+ Administer:

  ⋄ aspirin: have patient chew and do not give coated aspirin

  ⋄ nitroglycerin

  ⋄ morphine as needed for pain

  ⋄ fibrinolytic therapy such rTPA, reteplase, and tenecteplase

  ⋄ heparin IV

  ⋄ bivalirudin (Angiomax)

  ⋄ glycoprotein IIb/IIIa inhibitors such as abciximab (ReoPro), eptifibatide (Integrilin), or tirofiban (Aggrastat)

+ NSAIDs (other than aspirin) are contraindicated in acute phase of MI.

+ Troponin should be repeated every 3 hours twice after initial draw to monitor for continued elevation.

+ Goal is early reperfusion by PCI in the cardiac catheterization lab:

  ⋄ ED door to needle (fibrinolytic) goal time is 30 minutes.

  ⋄ ED door to PCI goal time is 90 minutes.

+ Admit patient to cardiac unit.

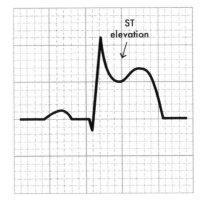

Figure 1.7. ECG: STEMI

QUICK REVIEW QUESTION

3. A patient arrives at the ED with complaints of severe chest pressure and dyspnea and appears diaphoretic. The patient appears anxious and has his hand clenched over his chest. An ECG confirms ST elevation. What are the priority interventions for the nurse?

2 x LG IV, O2, LABS, ASPIRIN + HEPARIN IV, CATH LAB

Aneurysm and Dissection

An **aneurysm** is a bulge within the wall of a blood vessel. Aneurysms can occur in any artery but most commonly occur in the abdominal aorta, the thoracoabdominal aorta, the thoracic aorta, the popliteal artery (behind the knee), the cerebral artery (in the brain), the mesenteric artery (in the intestine), or the splenic artery.

A **dissection** is when the aneurysm becomes so large that it dissects (bursts), leading to blood loss and possibly death. A dissection is considered an emergent medical condition that requires immediate care.

Some aneurysms are not considered immediately dangerous but will need continual follow-up to ensure their stability. Activities or conditions that cause excessive pressure or stress on the blood vessels, such as smoking or hypertension, can cause aneurysms to dissect, so treatment is focused on medical management to reduce pressure (usually with medications). In some cases, surgical intervention may be needed.

Risk Factors for Aneurysms

+ occurs more often in men than women

+ family history

+ genetic syndromes such as Marfan syndrome, in which connective tissues are weakened

+ heart disease

+ smoking

+ lack of exercise

+ trauma

Treatment and Management of Aneurysms

+ Maintain normotensive blood pressure to reduce pressure on the aortic walls.

+ Surgery is usually not recommended until the aneurysm is larger than 5 cm or if it enlarges rapidly.

+ Follow-up CT scans at 3- or 6-month intervals are typically recommended to monitor the growth of the aneurysm.

+ Treatment is focused on preventing the aneurysm from rupturing:
  ⬦ encouraging smoking cessation
  ⬦ lowering blood pressure
  ⬦ lowering cholesterol

ABDOMINAL AORTIC ANEURYSM

Pathophysiology

An **abdominal aortic aneurysm**, often called a *triple A*, occurs when the lower aorta is enlarged. The size of the aneurysm determines the immediacy of treatment. Once an aneurysm is identified, periodic imaging exams and follow-ups are required so that action can be taken if the aneurysm becomes too large. The abdominal aortic aneurysm is the most common type of aneurysm.

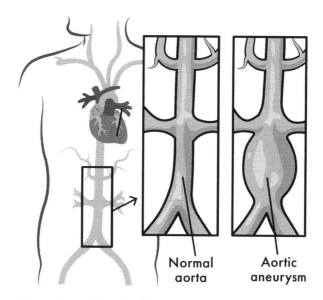

Figure 1.8. Abdominal Aortic Aneurysm (Triple A)

Signs and Symptoms

+ usually asymptomatic

+ abdominal pain

+ back pain

+ a pulsating feeling by the umbilicus

Diagnostic Tests and Findings

+ CT scan to show size and location of aneurysm

+ abdominal ultrasound to show structures of heart and presence of aneurysm

QUICK REVIEW QUESTION

4. A patient with complaints of abdominal pain that radiates to the back is found to have an abdominal aortic aneurysm. What priority assessment should the nurse perform to prevent dissection?

MAINTAIN NORMOTENSIVE BP.

THORACIC ANEURYSM

Pathophysiology

A **thoracic aneurysm** is a rare condition that occurs when the upper part of the aorta (located in the thorax) balloons or widens. The aneurysm can weaken the artery, putting it at risk of tears or dissection.

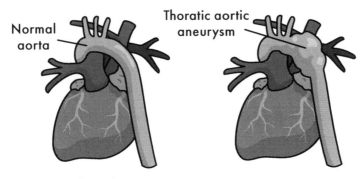

Figure 1.9. Thoracic Aneurysm

Signs and Symptoms

+ chest pain
    ◇ may present as vague pain
    ◇ may present as sudden, sharp pain if tear or dissection occurs

+ back pain

+ jaw or neck pain

+ coughing (due to pressure on the trachea)

+ hoarseness (due to pressure placed on the vocal cords)

+ dyspnea

+ difficulty swallowing (due to pressure on the esophagus)

Diagnostic Tests and Findings

+ chest X-ray showing widened mediastinum

+ CT angiography of the chest necessary to show aneurysm and approximate size

5. A patient presents to the ED, and the nurse suspects a thoracic aneurysm. What assessments can confirm this diagnosis?

CXR + CTA chest / pain (location), difficulty swallowing, hoarseness, @ cough

THORACOABDOMINAL ANEURYSM

Pathophysiology

A **thoracoabdominal aortic aneurysm** occurs when both the upper and the lower portions of the aorta balloon or widen, weakening the aorta and causing a risk of dissection. This type of aneurysm extends from the chest down to the abdomen.

Signs and Symptoms

+ usually asymptomatic
+ pain (dependent on location of aneurysm)
  ⋄ abdominal
  ⋄ back
  ⋄ chest
  ⋄ groin
+ hoarseness
+ cough
+ dyspnea
+ hypotension
+ dizziness or syncope
+ difficulty swallowing

Diagnostic Tests and Findings

+ CT scan to show size and location of aneurysm
+ abdominal ultrasound to show structures of heart and presence of aneurysm

6. The ED nurse is caring for a patient suspected of having a thoracoabdominal aneurysm. What definitive tests can be done to make this diagnosis?

CT, U/S

AORTIC DISSECTION

Pathophysiology

An **aortic dissection** is a tear in the innermost layer of the aorta; the tear allows blood to enter the aortic media. When the pressure compresses the aortic lumen, blood flow through the vessels is reduced, leading to ischemia of distal tissues and organs. Patient decline is rapid, and death ensues quickly without immediate surgical intervention.

Risk Factors

+ hypertension
+ atherosclerosis

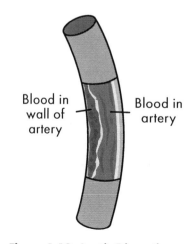

Blood in wall of artery

Blood in artery

Figure 1.10. Aortic Dissection

- genetic diseases in which connective tissues are weakened (e.g., Marfan syndrome)
- smoking

Signs and Symptoms

- acute onset of severe sharp, ripping, tearing pain in the chest and/or abdomen
    - can radiate to the back, flank, or shoulders
- blood pressure difference of 20 mm Hg between left and right arms
- weak, unequal pulses
- dyspnea
- anxiety
- hypertension
- diaphoresis
- headache
- deviated trachea
- blurred vision
- dizziness, syncope
- altered LOC

Diagnostic Tests and Findings

- CT scan showing dissection
- chest X-ray may show a widened mediastinum
- TEE to visualize extent of dissection
- 12-lead ECG may show MI if dissection affects coronary blood flow
- occurs rapidly; laboratory values of little diagnostic value

Treatment and Management

- Blood pressure should be maintained between 100 and 120 mm Hg systolic.
- Assess vital signs frequently.
- Administer beta blockers such as labetalol, esmolol, or propranolol via IV. *to control HR.*
- Administer nitroglycerin.
- Opioids can be given for pain and to decrease blood pressure.
- Immediate surgical intervention is needed to repair dissection.

QUICK REVIEW QUESTION

7. A patient presents to the ED with a known history of an abdominal aortic aneurysm. He complains of a sudden onset of severe chest pain and dyspnea. Blood pressure comparisons in both arms reveal a significant discrepancy. What priority assessment findings would the nurse expect to confirm a dissection?

BP difference of 10 mmHg between R + L arms; CT/CXR

Cardiopulmonary Arrest

Pathophysiology

Cardiopulmonary arrest occurs when the heart stops beating, which causes blood flow to stop. The patient will have no pulse and either will not be breathing or will display agonal gasps. Immediate CPR should be started for any patient in arrest. Four rhythms can cause cardiopulmonary arrest:

- ventricular fibrillation (V-fib)
- pulseless ventricular tachycardia (V-tach)
- pulseless electrical activity
- ventricular asystole

Risk Factors

- previous MI
- coronary artery disease
- heart failure
- electrolyte imbalances
- family history of cardiac arrest
- drowning
- electrical shock
- asphyxiation
- hypothermia
- substance abuse

Signs and Symptoms

- no pulse
- no breathing, or agonal breathing (intermittent gasps)

Diagnostic Tests and Findings

- absence of heart activity confirmed by FAST (Focused Assessment of Sonography in Trauma) ultrasound exam

Treatment and Management

- Check pulse and breathing to confirm their absence.
    - Current guidelines:
        - C-A-B (compression, airway, breathing) instead of A-B-C, so circulation (pulse) should always be checked first before airway.
    - If possible, check both pulse and breathing simultaneously.
- Call for help, and activate code team.
- Immediately begin high-quality CPR at a rate of 100 – 120 compressions per minute for any patient without a pulse.
- Use defibrillation as soon as possible if patient is in a shockable rhythm (V-fib or pulseless V-tach).
    - Immediately after defibrillation, always resume compressions.
    - If the patient has an ICD, pads should be placed to the side of ICD or directly below it.
    - Shave any hair off the patient's chest.
- Aim for the priority goal of as few interruptions in chest compressions as possible:
    - Take less than 10 seconds to switch compressors.
    - Take less than 10 seconds to check a pulse.
    - Continue to provide compressions while the defibrillator is charging.
- Ensure that the chest rises and falls with each ventilation, but avoid excessive ventilation, which can increase intrathoracic pressure and subsequently decrease cardiac output.
- Adhere to these guidelines for pregnant women in cardiac arrest:

- Patient should have the uterus manually displaced to the left or a wedge placed under the pelvis and chest at a 30-degree left lateral tilt to avoid compressing the inferior vena cava.
- Chest compressions should be performed higher on the chest, because of the elevated diaphragm in pregnancy.
- Priority goal is always to save the mother first.
- Use mnemonic **BEAU CHOPS** for possible causes of cardiac arrest in pregnancy:
  - Bleeding or DIC
  - Embolism: either coronary, pulmonary, or amniotic fluid
  - Anesthetic complications
  - Uterine atony: uterus does not contract after delivery; can lead to hemorrhage
  - Cardiac disease: MI, aortic dissections, cardiomyopathy
  - Hypertension: preeclampsia and eclampsia
  - Other causes: consider so-called H's and T's (see table 1.6)
  - Placental abruption or placenta previa
  - Sepsis

Summary of Current American Heart Association (AHA) 2015 Basic Life Support Guidelines

- Compression rate is 100 – 120 per minute (infants, children, and adults).
- Depth of compressions for adults is 2 – 2.4 inches (5.1 – 6.1 cm).
- Depth for children and infants is 1/3 of the chest depth (approximately 2 inches in children and 1.5 inches in infants).
- Ensure a complete chest recoil to allow the heart to refill with blood after each compression.
- Check pulse and breathing for no more than 10 seconds.
- Switch compressors every 2 minutes or every 5 cycles.
- For 1 rescuer, the compression-to-ventilation ratio for adults, children, and infants is 30:2.
- For 2 rescuers, the compression-to-ventilation ratio for adults is also 30:2, but for infants and children is 15:2.
- Cardiopulmonary arrest in infants and children is most commonly caused by hypoxia. The priority intervention for pediatrics should always be focused on respiratory interventions, whereas priority interventions for adults should be focused on cardiac interventions.

Summary of Current AHA 2015 Advanced Cardiac Life Support Guidelines

- Advanced guidelines follow changes in Basic Life Support guidelines, including compressions at a rate of 100 – 120 per minute and depth of chest compressions of 2 – 2.4 inches.
- Emphasis is on high-quality CPR with as few interruptions as possible.
- Quantitative waveform capnography is described as the most reliable indicator for compression quality, ET tube placement, and return of spontaneous circulation (ROSC).
  - The normal range for end-tidal CO_2 ($PetCO_2$) is 35 – 45 mm Hg.
  - The $PetCO_2$ range during cardiac arrest while compressions are being performed should ideally be between 10 and 20 mm Hg.

- A PetCO$_2$ of less than 10 indicates ineffective CPR.
- When circulation spontaneously returns, the PetCO$_2$ will rise suddenly because the patient is perfusing on his or her own and therefore CO$_2$ is pushed into the lungs, causing levels to increase.
+ Vasopressin was removed from the cardiac arrest algorithm and is no longer indicated.
+ Epinephrine 1 mg every 3 – 5 minutes by IV or IO is the first drug of choice for cardiac arrest.
+ Amiodarone and lidocaine are the 2 anti-dysrhythmics preferred for shock-refractory V-fib or pulseless V-tach.
+ Patients with an advanced airway have ventilations performed at a rate of 1 breath every 5 – 6 seconds, or 10 – 12 breaths per minute.
+ Post–cardiac-arrest interventions should be focused on ensuring adequate oxygenation and ventilation and TTM. — TARGETED TEMP. MNGMT.
  - TTM should be performed per hospital policy, most often done in witnessed cardiac arrests.
  - The targeted temperature range is 32° – 36°C (89.6° – 96.8°F).
  - TTM should be performed for at least 24 hours.
  - The main purpose of TTM is to preserve neurological function.
+ Team dynamics is an important component of a cardiac arrest resuscitation attempt.
  - Closed-loop communication is the preferred type of communication during a resuscitation attempt. It involves the "repeat back" method of confirming orders.

QUICK REVIEW QUESTION

8. Upon entering an exam room, the ED nurse finds a patient unresponsive in bed. What priority interventions should the nurse take?

CHECK PULSE, C-A-B, CALL CODE
① ③ ②

Dysrhythmias

A cardiac **dysrhythmia** is an abnormal heartbeat or rhythm. The disruption in the rate is typically due to a malfunction in the heart's electrical system. Treatment is based on patient stability. Stable patients can receive noninvasive interventions or drugs to correct an abnormal rhythm as a priority intervention. Unstable patients should receive the appropriate electrical treatment (i.e., synchronized cardioversion for tachycardias and transcutaneous pacing for bradycardias) as a priority intervention. A hypotensive patient should always be considered unstable.

BRADYCARDIA

Pathophysiology

Bradycardia is defined as a heart rate less than 60 bpm. It results from a decrease in the sinus node impulse formation (automaticity). Bradycardia is normal in certain individuals and does not always require an intervention other than observation if the patient is stable (asymptomatic). Symptomatic patients, however, need immediate treatment to address the cause of bradycardia and correct the dysrhythmia.

Risk Factors

+ athletes (typically lower resting heart rates because structural changes in the heart allow for greater efficiency in pumping blood)

- medications (beta blockers)
- heart failure
- infection of heart tissue
- hypothyroidism
- inflammatory diseases
- congenital disorder

Signs and Symptoms

- dizziness, syncope
- confusion
- hypotension
- dyspnea

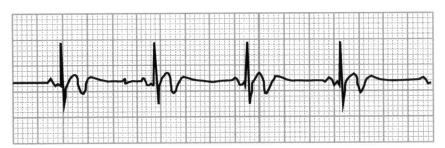

Figure 1.11. ECG: Bradycardia

Treatment and Management

- Conduct a 12-lead ECG.
- Stable patients may not need any treatment if bradycardia is normal for them.
  - Monitor these patients for any changes and treat if they become symptomatic.
- Bradycardia may also occur in sleeping patients, because of the reduced workload of the heart.
- Provide oxygen.
- Follow these guidelines for stable patients who need treatment:
  - The first-line drug is atropine.
  - If atropine fails or if the maximum dose has already been given and the patient is still stable, administer dopamine or epinephrine.
  - Patients with bradycardia who have had a heart transplant should be administered isoproterenol (Isuprel), as atropine is ineffective for these patients.
- Unstable patients need cardiology consultation and TCP.
  - Do not use carotid pulse to confirm mechanical capture as the electrical impulses can be mistaken for the pulse.
  - Consider sedation before TCP if the patient has stable vital signs.
  - The TCP device's rate should be set at 70 bpm, and milliamps (mA) should be slowly increased until electrical capture is achieved.
- Bradycardia in children is considered a worrisome sign.
  - Any pediatric patient in bradycardia should immediately be ventilated with 100% oxygen.
  - If adequate oxygenation and ventilation is not achieved and the patient remains bradycardic and hypoxic, chest compressions should be started at a rate of 100 – 120 compressions per minute.
  - Epinephrine 0.01 mg/kg is the first-line drug for bradycardia in children.
  - Atropine may also be given in certain cases.

9. A long-distance runner is a patient in the ED. His heart rate is 49 in sinus bradycardia on the monitor. What interventions should the ED nurse take?

MONITOR FOR D'S; TREAT IF THEY BECOME SYMPTOMATIC.

TACHYCARDIA

Pathophysiology

Tachycardia is a heart rate greater than 100 bpm and typically less than 150 bpm. This condition results from an impulse originating in the sinus node.

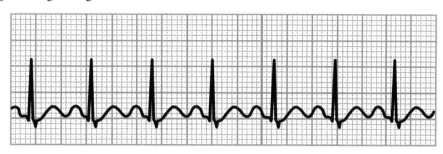

Figure 1.12. ECG: Tachycardia

Risk Factors

+ fever
+ anxiety
+ stimulant drug use (e.g., cocaine, methamphetamines)

+ heart failure
+ stress
+ caffeine
+ anemia/blood loss

Signs and Symptoms

+ palpitations
+ dizziness

+ dyspnea
+ chest pain

Treatment and Management

+ Address underlying cause of the tachycardia.
+ Obtain CBC, CMP, troponin, and thyroid levels to monitor for infection, electrolyte imbalances, cardiac ischemia, or hormone imbalances.

10. A patient in the ED diagnosed with influenza shows a sinus tachycardia on the monitor at a rate of 115. The patient has a fever (temperature 39.5°C [103.1°F]), blood pressure of 135/80 mm Hg, and oxygen saturation of 97% on room air. What is the most likely cause of the tachycardia, and what would the treatment be?

FEVER → TYLENOL/ FLUIDS

VENTRICULAR FIBRILLATION (V-FIB)

Pathophysiology

Ventricular fibrillation (V-fib) occurs when the lower chambers of the heart quiver and the heart cannot effectively pump blood, leading to cardiac arrest. It is characterized by chaotic, irregular depolarizations with no cardiac output. This is a shockable rhythm. The quicker a patient in V-fib can be defibrillated, the better the person's chance of survival.

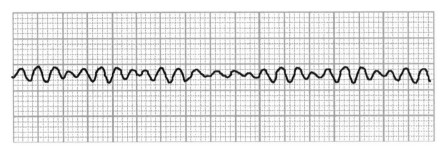

Figure 1.13. ECG: Ventricular Fibrillation (V-Fib)

Risk Factors

+ STEMI or NSTEMI
+ cardiomyopathy
+ coronary artery disease
+ previous cardiac arrest

+ drug toxicity
+ electrolyte imbalances
+ sepsis

Signs and Symptoms

+ often preceded by V-tach
+ cardiac arrest may be preceded by
  ⬦ dizziness, syncope
  ⬦ chest pain
  ⬦ dyspnea

+ patient unresponsiveness
+ lack of pulse; no breathing

Treatment and Management

+ Immediately initiate high-quality CPR at a rate of 100 – 120 compressions per minute.
+ In V-fib, defibrillation should occur ASAP before the administration of any drugs.
  ⬦ Remember this mnemonic: In **V-fib**, you always **de-fib**.
  ⬦ Defibrillation doses are as follows: 200 J → 300 J → 360 J (biphasic).
+ Ensure at least 2 defibrillation attempts before giving any medications.
+ Prepare patient for IV or IO placement.
+ First-line drug to give is epinephrine.
+ For shock-refractory V-fib (V-fib that is unresponsive to shocks), administer amiodarone.

11. A patient is found unresponsive with no pulse and is not breathing. The cardiac monitor displays V-fib. What initial actions should the nurse take?

ADMIN COMPRESSIONS WHILE YOU GET READY TO SHOCK.

VENTRICULAR TACHYCARDIA (V-TACH)

Pathophysiology

Ventricular tachycardia (V-tach) occurs when there are 3 or more premature ventricular complexes in a row and the rate is over 100 bpm. The QRS complex in this type of tachycardia is wide, with the tachycardia originating in the ventricles. Patients in this rhythm may have reduced cardiac output, resulting in hypotension. The accelerated heart rates and lack of coordinated atrial contraction are often referred to as loss of atrial kick. V-tach is often described as a wide-complex tachycardia because of the width of the QRS complex. Monomorphic V-tach (pictured below) occurs when all the QRS complexes are symmetrical.

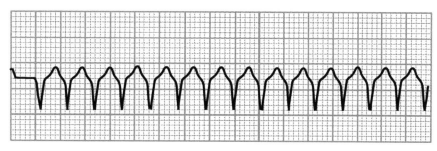

Figure 1.14. ECG: Ventricular Tachycardia (V-Tach)

Risk Factors

+ previous MI
+ hypertension

+ heart failure
+ cardiomyopathy

Signs and Symptoms

+ dizziness, syncope
+ palpitations
+ dyspnea

+ fatigue
+ chest pain

Treatment and Management

+ The priority intervention for a patient who displays a rhythm of V-tach is to check for a pulse.
+ Follow these procedures for pulseless V-tach:
    ⬦ Begin immediate CPR and defibrillation.
    ⬦ Follow V-fib algorithm.
+ For V-tach with a pulse in a stable patient, administer one of the following:
    ⬦ amiodarone
    ⬦ procainamide (contraindicated in prolonged QT and congestive heart failure)
    ⬦ sotalol (contraindicated in prolonged QT)

- For V-tach with a pulse in an unstable (hypotensive) patient, treat patient with synchronized cardioversion:
  - If QRS complex is narrow, regular, cardiovert at 50 – 100 J.
  - If QRS is narrow, irregular, cardiovert at 120 – 200 J.
  - If QRS is wide, regular, cardiovert at 100 J.

QUICK REVIEW QUESTION

12. A patient is brought in by EMS in V-tach with no pulse. What immediate actions should the ED nurse take?

CPR + DEFIB.

ASYSTOLE

Pathophysiology

Asystole, also called "flatlining," occurs when there is no electrical or mechanical activity within the heart. There are no QRS complexes or P waves. The survival rate for patients in asystole is very low. Asystole is a nonshockable rhythm.

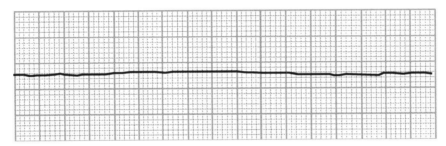

Figure 1.15. ECG: Asystole

Risk Factors

- can occur after prolonged V-fib arrest
- MI
- dysrhythmias
- congestive heart failure
- pulmonary embolism
- trauma

Signs and Symptoms

- no pulse
- no breathing, or agonal breathing

Treatment and Management

- Immediately administer high-quality CPR at a rate of 100 – 120 compressions per minute.
- Administer epinephrine.
- Consider H's and T's to determine an underlying cause.

Table 1.6. H's and T's Summary

	Pathophysiology	Signs and Symptoms	Treatment and Management
Hypovolemia	Loss of fluid volume	+ Blood loss + Signs of dehydration	Administer IV fluids or blood.
Hypoxia	Lack of adequate oxygen supply	+ Inadequate breathing + Agonal gasps + Cyanosis	+ Maintain airway patency. + Provide adequate oxygenation and ventilation.
Hydrogen ion (acidosis)	Occurs when body fluids or tissues accumulate an excess of acid	+ Prolonged downtime can cause acidosis. + Arterial blood gas may reflect respiratory acidosis.	Administer sodium bicarbonate.
Hyperkalemia/ hypokalemia	+ Hyperkalemia: elevated potassium (K+) level, typically > 5.2 mEq/ L + Hypokalemia: low potassium level, typically, < 3.0 mEq/L	+ Hyperkalemia usually causes tall and peaked T waves and a widened QRS complex on the ECG. + Hypokalemia usually causes flattened T waves and U waves and may cause a widened QRS complex on the ECG.	+ Replace electrolytes if low levels present. + Dilute and administer IV potassium as a drip. + Hyperkalemia can be treated with IV insulin and dextrose.
Hypothermia	Low body temperature, typically below 35°C (95°F)	+ Shivering + Lethargy + Hypotension	+ Patient should be warmed. + Cardiac arrest interventions may be unsuccessful in hypothermic patients.
Toxins	May be due to overdose of prescribed medications such as beta blockers or calcium channel blockers, or may be due to street drug use such as cocaine	+ Bradycardia + Pupils may be pinpoint or dilated, depending on toxin.	Contact poison control center to obtain information about how to treat specific overdoses.
Tamponade	Fluid buildup in the pericardium; can impair the heart's ability to pump and can cause cardiac arrest	+ ECG may show a narrow QRS complex and a rapid heartbeat. + Patient may have JVD, low blood pressure, muffled heart tones.	Perform pericardiocentesis to remove fluid.

Table 1.6. H's and T's Summary (continued)

	Pathophysiology	Signs and Symptoms	Treatment and Management
Tension pneumothorax	Occurs when there is a shift in intrathoracic pressure; can cause cardiovascular collapse	+ JVD + tracheal deviation to one side + decreased breath sounds on affected side	Use needle decompression.
Thrombosis (coronary or pulmonary)	Can be due to a coronary blockage such as an MI or a pulmonary blockage such as a PE	+ 12-lead ECG will show ST elevation in STEMI. + Also may show T-wave inversions or pathological Q waves. + ECG may show a narrow QRS complex and tachycardia in a PE. + D-dimer will be elevated in PE. + Troponin will be elevated in MI.	+ PCI is needed for MI. + Thrombectomy and/or fibrinolytic therapy is needed to treat PE.

QUICK REVIEW QUESTION

13. A patient is found to be in asystole and a 10-second pulse check reveals the absence of a pulse. Aside from chest compressions, what other intervention should be a priority?

EPI —> THEN H + Ts.

PULSELESS ELECTRICAL ACTIVITY

Pathophysiology

Pulseless electrical activity (PEA) is an organized rhythm without a pulse. The monitor shows an electrical rhythm, but the heart is not functioning. The result is the absence of a pulse. PEA is a nonshockable rhythm and has a poor survival rate.

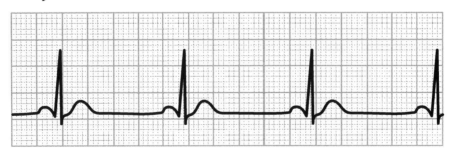

Figure 1.16. ECG: Pulseless Electrical Activity (PEA)

Risk Factors

- MI
- trauma
- dysrhythmias

- congestive heart failure
- pulmonary embolism
- H's and T's, the most common risk factors

Signs and Symptoms

- organized rhythm on the monitor but with no pulse

- no breathing, or agonal breathing

Treatment and Management

- Immediately administer high-quality CPR at a rate of 100 – 120 compressions per minute.

- Administer epinephrine.
- Use the mnemonic **PEA: push epi always.**
- Consider H's and T's for underlying cause.

QUICK REVIEW QUESTION

14. During CPR, the team leader calls for a rhythm check. After holding compressions to analyze the rhythm, the nurse sees an organized rhythm on the monitor. What is the priority intervention the nurse should take?

CHECK FOR A PULSE

SUPRAVENTRICULAR TACHYCARDIA

Pathophysiology

Supraventricular tachycardia (SVT) is an umbrella term for rhythms that are more than 150 beats per minute. Because the heart is beating so fast, it is impossible to determine the actual underlying rhythm. Therefore, the goal of treating SVT is to slow the rhythm down enough to be able to read the underlying rhythm. SVT is often referred to as a narrow complex tachycardia because of the narrow width of the QRS complex (< 0.12 seconds).

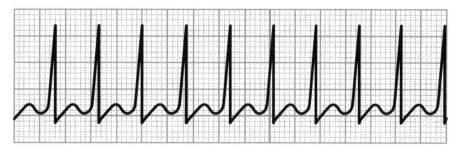

Figure 1.17. Supraventricular Tachycardia (SVT)

Patients with SVT are classified as stable if they show few or minimal symptoms related to tachycardia. Unstable SVT patients will show symptoms related to tachycardia, including hypotension, syncope, or chest pain.

Risk Factors

+ anxiety
+ stress
+ thyroid problems
+ smoking
+ substance abuse

+ excess caffeine use
+ surgery
+ pregnancy
+ chronic heart or lung diseases

Signs and Symptoms

+ ventricular rate is usually between 150 and 300 bpm
+ P waves difficult to recognize and often hidden in the preceding QRS complex
+ palpitations

+ dizziness, syncope
+ dyspnea
+ fatigue
+ diaphoresis

Treatment and Management

+ For stable SVT:
    ⋄ Initiate vagal maneuvers: ask patients to bear down as if they were having a bowel movement, or have them blow through a straw.
    ⋄ Administer adenosine.
+ For unstable SVT:
    ⋄ Priority intervention should be synchronized cardioversion (50 – 150 J).
    ⋄ No drugs or vagal maneuver for a patient that is unstable.
+ For pediatric SVT (heart rate > 180 bpm):
    ⋄ Apply ice to the face to stimulate the vagal nerve.
    ⋄ Older children may blow through a straw.
    ⋄ If unsuccessful, administer adenosine.
    ⋄ Synchronized cardioversion in pediatrics is 0.5 – 1 J/kg.

QUICK REVIEW QUESTION

15. A 55-year-old patient presents to the ED with complaints of dyspnea and dizziness. His heart rate is 216 bpm, and the monitor displays a narrow complex tachycardia. His blood pressure is 68/40 mm Hg. What is the priority intervention for this patient?

UNSTABLE – SYNCHRONIZED CARDIOVERSION

Conduction Defects

The **cardiac conduction system** generates impulses to make the heart contract and controls the heart rhythm and rate. Under certain conditions, the impulses do not occur regularly or are blocked. These conduction defects include bundle branch blocks, AV blocks, long QT syndrome, Brugada syndrome, and Wolfe-Parkinson-White syndrome.

Table 1.7. Summary of Conduction Defects

Conduction Defect	Pathophysiology	Risk Factors	Signs and Symptoms	Treatment and Management
Bundle branch block (BBB)	+ First division of the ventricle conduction system after the bundle of His + Two types: left and right bundle branches + Causes a delay or blockage of electrical impulses, resulting in the heart's pumping blood less efficiently	+ MI + Infections + Hypertension + PE	+ Usually asymptomatic + Dizziness, syncope	+ Treatment is usually not needed. + Regular follow-ups to monitor for changes is encouraged.
AV block	Occurs when the electrical conduction between the atria and the ventricles is delayed or blocked	+ Heart disease + Certain medications such as beta blockers and calcium channel blockers + Congenital heart disease	+ May be asymptomatic + Dizziness, syncope + Dyspnea + Chest pain	+ First degree and second degree, type 1, are usually asymptomatic and only need monitoring. + Second degree, type 2, and third degree are typically unstable and need TCP. — *pacing*
Long QT syndrome	+ The QT interval is measured from the start of the QRS complex until the end of the T wave and is usually 0.36 – 0.44 seconds; an interval > 0.50 seconds is a cause for concern + Susceptible to rapid ventricular rhythms	+ Hereditary + Certain medications, including antibiotics, antidepressants, antihistamines, diuretics, and anti-emetics	+ Syncope + Seizure + Weakness	+ Administer beta blockers. + Administer anti-arrhythmics. + Surgery may be necessary. + ICD may be necessary.

Table 1.7. Summary of Conduction Defects (continued)

Conduction Defect	Pathophysiology	Risk Factors	Signs and Symptoms	Treatment and Management
Brugada syndrome	+ Characterized by right BBB with ST elevation in leads V1 – V3 + Can cause sudden cardiac arrest + Usually occurs in individuals with no cardiac disease	+ Hereditary + Structural abnormalities of the heart + Electrolyte imbalances + Cocaine use	+ Palpitations + Syncope + Seizures + Dyspnea	ICD may be necessary.
Wolfe-Parkinson-White syndrome	Extra connection between upper and lower heart chambers, resulting in tachycardia	+ Congenital + Idiopathic cause	+ Palpitations + Dizziness, syncope + Dyspnea	Ablation may be performed to fix the extra connection in the heart causing the tachycardia.

QUICK REVIEW QUESTION

16. A patient presents to the ED with a second-degree AV block, type 2. What priority intervention is necessary by the nurse?

GET READY FOR TRANSCUTANEOUS PACING.

Acute Cardiac Inflammatory Diseases

Inflammation of the heart can be caused by viruses, bacteria, or environmental agents. When inflammation occurs within the heart muscle, its ability to pump blood is compromised. Acute cardiac inflammatory diseases include myocarditis, pericarditis, and endocarditis.

MYOCARDITIS

Pathophysiology

Myocarditis, or inflammation of the myocardium, can cause problems with the heart muscle itself or the electrical system. Both types of problems could lead to dysrhythmias.

Risk Factors

+ most often caused by viral infections such as those caused by coxsackievirus, Epstein-Barr virus, HIV, hepatitis viruses, and varicella viruses

+ bacterial infections such as those caused by *Corynebacterium diphtheriae*, *Staphylococcus*, and *Streptococcus*

+ inflammatory diseases such as lupus and sarcoidosis

ENDOCARDIUM → MYOCARDIUM → EPICARDIUM → PERICARDIUM
(INNER ✓) *(OUTSIDE) ✓*

Signs and Symptoms

+ chest pain
+ tachycardia
+ dyspnea
+ fever

+ joint pain
+ crackles
+ distant heart sounds; S3 or S4 sounds may be heard

Diagnostic Tests and Findings

+ elevated WBC possible
+ elevated CK-MB and troponin possible
+ elevated sedimentation rate possible

+ chest X-ray may show cardiomegaly or pulmonary congestion
+ dysrhythmias possible

Treatment and Management

+ Prepare blood cultures to determine if infectious bacteria are present in the bloodstream.
+ Administer antibiotics for bacterial infections.
+ ACE inhibitors, beta blockers, or diuretics may be used.
+ Steroids may be indicated to treat inflammation.
+ Admit patient to cardiac unit.

QUICK REVIEW QUESTION

17. The ED nurse who is caring for a patient diagnosed with myocarditis knows that the patient will probably exhibit what symptoms?

CHEST PAIN / TACHY ✓ / DYSPNEA / FEVER / JOINT PAIN / CRACKLES / DISTANT ✓ SOUNDS (MAYBE S3, S4)

PERICARDITIS

Pathophysiology

Pericarditis is the inflammation of the pericardium. When inflammation occurs, fluid can accumulate and impair the ability of the heart to pump blood sufficiently, a condition called pericardial tamponade. Medical professionals can perform a pericardiocentesis by using a needle to withdraw the fluid.

Risk Factors

+ mostly idiopathic causes
+ viral illness
+ inflammatory diseases
+ MI

+ cardiac surgery
+ trauma
+ renal failure

Signs and Symptoms

+ chest pain
  ⬦ increases with movement, lying flat, and inspiration
  ⬦ decreases by sitting up or leaning forward
  ⬦ sudden and severe
+ tachycardia (earliest sign)

+ pericardial friction rub
+ tachypnea
+ dyspnea
+ fever
+ chills
+ cough

Diagnostic Tests and Findings

+ elevated troponin
+ elevated WBC
+ elevated sedimentation rate
+ elevated C-reactive protein
+ if caused by a connective-tissue disorder, antinuclear antibodies may be elevated
+ positive blood culture if infection present

+ ST elevation possible, usually in all leads except AVR and V1
+ tall, peaked T waves
+ chest X-ray showing "water bottle" silhouette in pericardial effusion
+ echocardiogram may show pericardial effusion, thickening, or calcifications

Treatment and Management

+ Allow patient to remain in a comfortable position, such as leaning over a bedside table.
+ Pain is not relieved by nitroglycerin or rest.
+ Administer anti-inflammatories such as ibuprofen or indomethacin (Indocin).
+ Administer antibiotics if bacterial infection is present.
+ Administer steroids if a connective-tissue disorder is the cause.
+ Pericardiocentesis is appropriate if large effusion is present.
+ Prescribe bed rest.
+ Administer oxygen.
+ Monitor for complications such as dysrhythmias, cardiac tamponade, or heart failure.
+ Admit patient to cardiac unit.

QUICK REVIEW QUESTION

18. A patient with a significant cardiac history is being seen in the ED. The nurse knows that the hallmark signs of pericarditis include which symptoms?

ENDOCARDITIS

Pathophysiology

Endocarditis occurs when some type of bacteria causes inflammation of the endocardium. This inflammation of the heart structures, muscles, and linings can impair cardiac function. The most common bacterial infections are caused by *Staphylococcus aureus*, *Streptococcus*, and *Pseudomonas*. Viruses such as the coxsackievirus and adenovirus may also be contributing agents. Left untreated, endocarditis can be fatal.

Risk Factors

+ more common in women
+ immunocompromised individuals
+ heart valve problems or surgery involving heart valves
+ poor dental health or recent dental work

+ central venous line access
+ rheumatic heart disease
+ body piercings
+ IV substance abuse

Signs and Symptoms

+ chest pain
+ flulike symptoms (chills, fatigue)
+ fever
+ petechiae
+ Janeway lesions
+ Osler's nodes
+ Roth's spots

+ joint pain
+ dyspnea
+ splinter hemorrhages under fingernails
+ hematuria
+ night sweats
+ weight loss

Diagnostic Tests and Findings

+ blood cultures showing bacteria present in the bloodstream
+ WBC may be elevated because of infection
+ C-reactive protein and sedimentation rate may be elevated because of inflammation
+ echocardiogram and TEE showing any possible heart valve damage and vegetations

Treatment and Management

+ Conduct a full lab panel, including blood cultures, WBC, C-reactive protein, and sedimentation rate.
+ Administer IV antibiotics, typically for several weeks.
+ In some cases, heart surgery to repair the valve may be necessary.
+ Admit patient to cardiac unit.

QUICK REVIEW QUESTION

19. The ED nurse is told that a patient is suspected of having endocarditis. What signs would the nurse expect to be present?

Heart Failure

Heart failure occurs when either one of both of the ventricles in the heart is unable to efficiently pump blood. The condition is typically due to another disease or illness, most commonly coronary artery disease. Because the heart is unable to pump effectively, blood and fluid back up into the lungs (causing pulmonary congestion), or the fluid builds up peripherally (causing edema of the lower extremities). Heart failure is most commonly categorized into left ventricular heart failure or right ventricular heart failure, although it is possible for both sides of the heart to fail at the same time.

Stages of Heart Failure

+ **Stage A**: high risk of developing heart failure
    ◇ considered pre-heart-failure for individuals with risk factors
    ◇ treatment includes these:
        + smoking cessation
        + maintaining normotensive blood pressure
        + maintaining normal cholesterol levels
+ **Stage B**: diagnosis of left systolic ventricular failure with no symptoms
    ◇ in addition to treatment from stage A, patients may also be started on medications, including these:
        + ACE inhibitors or angiotensin II receptor blockers
        + beta blockers
        + aldosterone antagonist
+ **Stage C**: diagnosis of heart failure, with symptoms
    ◇ in addition to treatment from stages A and B, these treatments are initiated:
        + diuretics
        + possible fluid restriction
        + sodium restriction
        + daily weights to monitor for fluid imbalances
        + an implantable cardiac defibrillator may be necessary
+ **Stage D**: advanced symptoms that have not improved with treatment
    ◇ pacemaker most likely required
    ◇ last treatment options available include the following:
        + heart surgery
        + heart transplant
        + palliative care

Causes of Heart Failure

+ volume overload
+ hypertension
+ cardiomyopathy
+ coronary artery disease
+ dysrhythmias
+ congenital heart defects
+ diabetes
+ chronic illnesses such as AIDS
+ certain chemotherapy drugs

Risk Factors

+ coronary artery disease
+ history of MI
+ hypertension
+ smoking

- diabetes
- obesity
- poor diet
- lack of exercise
- congenital heart disease

Precipitating Factors

- medication noncompliance
- infection
- increased salt intake
- increased fluid intake
- anemia
- uncontrolled hypertension

Signs and Symptoms

- left-sided heart failure: symptoms more pulmonary, such as dyspnea and cough
- right-sided heart failure: symptoms more related to systemic circulation (e.g., edema or swelling in lower legs and abdomen)
- left ventricular heart failure
  - dyspnea or orthopnea
  - tachycardia
  - crackles
  - cough, frothy sputum, hemoptysis
  - weakness, fatigue
  - left-sided S3 sound
  - diaphoresis
  - pulsus alternans (alternating pulse waves, where every other beat is weaker than the one before)
  - oliguria
- right ventricular heart failure
  - JVD
  - dependent edema usually in lower legs
  - hepatomegaly
  - ascites
  - weakness, fatigue
  - right-sided S3 sound
  - weight gain
  - nausea, vomiting, abdominal pain
  - nocturia

Diagnostic Tests and Findings

- BNP: main laboratory value to measure heart failure levels
  - More than 100 pg/mL is indicative of heart failure.
- electrolyte imbalances
  - hypokalemia
  - hyponatremia
- chest X-ray may show cardiomegaly or pulmonary congestion
- echocardiogram may show abnormalities in the chambers, valve motion, and wall thickness

Treatment and Management

- Provide oxygen.
- Position patient with head elevated 30 – 45 degrees.
- Employ continuous positive airway pressure.

- Administer diuretics to reduce fluid buildup.

- Administer morphine to reduce preload.

QUICK REVIEW QUESTION

20. The ED nurse suspects that a patient has left ventricular heart failure. What signs and symptoms would be consistent with this diagnosis?

Hypertension

Hypertension is an elevated blood pressure over 120/80 mm Hg. At least 2 readings on separate days must be conducted to diagnose hypertension. Hypertension occurs when the arterioles narrow, causing more pressure against the vessels. This increased pressure can eventually cause the heart muscles and vessels to weaken.

HYPERTENSIVE CRISES

Pathophysiology

Hypertensive crises include hypertensive urgency and hypertensive emergencies. **Hypertensive urgency** is a blood pressure greater than 180/110 mm Hg without evidence of organ dysfunction. A **hypertensive emergency** is a systolic blood pressure greater than 180 mm Hg or diastolic blood pressure greater than 120 mm Hg accompanied by evidence of impending or progressive organ dysfunction. Hypertensive crises increase the risk of stroke because of the damage they can cause in blood vessels in the brain. Additionally, prolonged hypertension can lead to renal failure.

Risk Factors

- older adults more susceptible because of decreased elasticity of blood vessels
- African Americans more likely to develop hypertension
- family history
- kidney disease
- obesity
- sedentary lifestyle
- tobacco use
- poor diet
- noncompliance with medications

Signs and Symptoms

- usually asymptomatic
- headache
- blurred vision
- dizziness
- dyspnea
- retinal hemorrhages
- epistaxis
- chest pain

Diagnostic Tests and Findings

- systolic blood pressure greater than 180 mm Hg
- diastolic blood pressure greater than 120 mm Hg

+ chest X-ray may show left ventricular enlargement

+ BUN/creatinine may be elevated because of kidney damage caused by hypertension

Treatment and Management

+ Always double-check that the blood pressure is accurate by taking a second reading in the opposite arm and ensuring that cuff size is appropriate. A manual blood pressure reading should also be taken to confirm the automated reading.

    ⬧ A blood pressure cuff that is too small can cause a falsely high reading.

    ⬧ A blood pressure cuff that is too large can cause a falsely low reading.

+ Blood pressure reduction should be limited to a decrease of no more than 25% within the first 2 hours to maintain cerebral perfusion.

+ Administer one of the following first-line drugs:

    ⬧ labetalol

    ⬧ hydralazine

    ⬧ clonidine

    ⬧ metoprolol

+ Provide a quiet, non-stimulating environment for relaxation.

+ Administer oxygen.

QUICK REVIEW QUESTION

21. A patient is found to be alert and oriented with a blood pressure of 200/100 mm Hg and is asymptomatic. What priority intervention should the nurse take?

PULMONARY HYPERTENSION

Pathophysiology

Pulmonary hypertension, elevated blood pressure in the arteries to the lungs (> 20 mm Hg), is caused by occlusions or narrowing of the arteries. Because blood cannot pass through the arteries, extra strain is placed on the heart, reducing its ability to pump effectively.

Risk Factors

+ can be idiopathic

+ hereditary

+ chronic conditions

    ⬧ lupus

    ⬧ liver disease

    ⬧ obesity

    ⬧ presence of HIV

+ stimulant drug use (e.g., cocaine, methamphetamines)

Signs and Symptoms

+ dyspnea

+ JVD

- lower-extremity edema
- irregular heart sounds
- ascites
- fatigue
- dizziness
- decreased appetite
- upper right-sided abdominal pain
- difficulty completing activities as normal

Diagnostic Tests and Findings

- echocardiogram necessary to ascertain pressures within the pulmonary arteries
- CT scan of the chest may show pulmonary hypertension
- chest X-ray may show enlarged arteries or ventricles
- ECG may show enlarged ventricles or dysrhythmia
- heart catheterization may show blockages and problems with heart valves and can measure pressures within the pulmonary arteries and right ventricle
- heart sounds may include
    - a loud pulmonic valve sound
    - systolic murmur from tricuspid regurgitation
    - a gallop from ventricular failure

Treatment and Management

- There is currently no cure for pulmonary hypertension; treatment is focused on reducing symptoms through medications.
- Administer oxygen.
- Administer medications:
    - vasodilators:
        - epoprostenol (Flolan)
        - iloprost (Ventavis)
        - bosentan (Tracleer)
        - macitentan (Opsumit)
        - sildenafil
        - tadalafil
    - diuretics
    - anticoagulants
- Lung replacement may be necessary for patients who do not respond to medication therapy.

QUICK REVIEW QUESTION

22. A patient with a history of pulmonary hypertension presents to the ED and has not taken her medications for a month. Which types of intervention and medications will this patient probably need?

Pericardial Tamponade

Pathophysiology

Pericardial tamponade is a buildup of fluid in the pericardial space. The pressure from the fluid prevents the ventricles from functioning properly, compromising cardiac filling and cardiac output. This is a life-threatening condition.

Risk Factors

+ trauma, most common cause of pericardial tamponade
+ rib fractures
+ MI
+ inflammation such as in pericarditis
+ anticoagulant therapy due to bleeding risk
+ dissecting aneurysms
+ connective-tissue disorders (e.g., lupus, rheumatoid arthritis, and scleroderma)

Signs and Symptoms

+ Beck's triad:
    ⋄ hypotension
    ⋄ JVD
    ⋄ muffled heart tones
+ pulsus paradoxus
+ Kussmaul's sign
+ chest pain
+ dizziness
+ dyspnea
+ penetrating chest wound
+ hypotension
+ weakness
+ cyanosis
+ signs of shock

Diagnostic Tests and Findings

+ chest X-ray may show a globe-shaped heart
+ echocardiogram showing collapsed ventricles during diastole
+ CT scan of chest may show excess fluid in the pericardial sac
+ ECG may show ST elevation

Treatment and Management

+ Perform pericardiocentesis to remove fluid from heart.
+ Pericardial window to remove the pericardium may be necessary.
+ Administer inotropic drugs.
+ Administer vasopressors for hypotension.

QUICK REVIEW QUESTION

23. A patient presents to the ED with the 3 main signs of pericardial tamponade, often referred to as Beck's triad. What are these 3 signs?

Thromboembolic Diseases

Thromboembolic diseases involve a thromboembolism, a blood clot or thrombus that breaks off and travels through the bloodstream and blocks a vessel in another area such as the lung or brain.

DEEP VEIN THROMBOSIS

Pathophysiology

A **deep vein thrombosis (DVT)** occurs when a blood clot forms within a deep vein, typically in the legs. Left untreated, these blood clots can dislodge, causing a pulmonary embolism. Certain individuals are more prone to developing blood clots, but these clots can occur in anyone, especially after any period when the blood flow to the legs is diminished because of inactivity.

Risk Factors

+ Virchow's triad: the 3 main conditions that predispose individuals to clot formation
    ✧ hypercoagulability (e.g., estrogen or contraceptive use or malignancy)
    ✧ venous stasis (any activity that results in decreased physical movement or bed rest)
    ✧ endothelial damage (damage to the vessel wall such as trauma, drug use, and inflammatory processes)
+ sedentary lifestyle
+ long trips where mobility is limited (e.g., airplane travel or car rides)
+ pregnancy
+ hormone replacement therapy
+ oral contraceptives
+ smoking
+ sickle cell disease
+ recent surgery
+ obesity

Signs and Symptoms

+ pain that is localized to a specific area, usually the foot, ankle, calf, or behind the knee
+ unilateral edema
+ erythema in area
+ warmth in area
+ positive Homan's sign
+ other signs, including those related to a pulmonary embolism, as this is the main adverse event associated with DVTs:
    ✧ dyspnea, usually occurs suddenly
    ✧ chest pain
    ✧ dizziness, syncope
    ✧ tachycardia
    ✧ hemoptysis
    ✧ cough

Diagnostic Tests and Findings

+ D-dimer elevated
+ coagulation studies may be abnormal
+ Doppler ultrasound showing thrombus

Treatment and Management

+ Maintain frequent neurovascular checks to area.

+ Administer anticoagulants:
  ⬧ heparin or enoxaparin injections
  ⬧ warfarin

+ Do not massage the area.

+ Perform a CT scan of the chest to rule out a pulmonary embolism.

+ Monitor the patient for respiratory complications that could indicate a pulmonary embolism.

+ An inferior vena cava filter may be placed to avoid a pulmonary embolism.

QUICK REVIEW QUESTION

24. A pregnant patient presents to the ED after returning from vacation with complaints of right leg pain. On inspection, the nurse notes that the area is red and warm. What does the nurse anticipate as priority interventions for this patient?

ACUTE ARTERIAL OCCLUSION

Pathophysiology

An **acute arterial occlusion** most often occurs from a thrombosis and prevents blood from reaching the affected tissue, resulting in ischemia and the possible loss of a limb. The most commonly affected arteries are the femoral, popliteal, and aortoiliac; however, an arterial occlusion can occur in any artery within the upper or lower extremity.

Risk Factors

+ smoking

+ valvular heart disease

+ PVD

+ hypertension

+ trauma

+ fractures and subsequent compartment syndrome

+ circumferential burns

+ A-fib

+ heart failure

Signs and Symptoms

+ 6 P's (hallmark signs of an arterial occlusion):
  ⬧ pain
  ⬧ pallor
  ⬧ pulselessness
  ⬧ paresthesia
  ⬧ paralysis

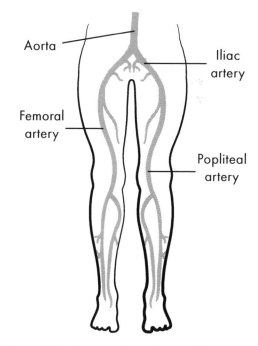

Figure 1.18. Common Locations of Acute Arterial Occlusion

- ✧ poikilothermia
- ✦ petechiae can be seen with microemboli

Diagnostic Tests and Findings

- ✦ Doppler ultrasound showing occlusion and lack of blood flow
- ✦ ankle-brachial index below 0.30 indicates poor outcome of limb survivability
- ✦ coagulation studies may show abnormalities

Treatment and Management

- ✦ Administer IV anticoagulants such as heparin.
- ✦ Administer pain medication.
- ✦ Patient needs immediate surgical intervention to remove thrombosis (embolectomy).
- ✦ In severe cases if ischemia is prolonged, amputation of limb may be required.
- ✦ Elevate head of bed to encourage blood flow to limb.
- ✦ Do not apply heat.
- ✦ Do not elevate the extremity.

QUICK REVIEW QUESTION

25. A patient presents to the ED complaining of left foot and leg pain. He is found to have no left pedal pulse. A Doppler exam reveals an acute arterial occlusion. What priority intervention should the nurse prepare for?

CAROTID ARTERY STENOSIS

Pathophysiology

Carotid artery stenosis, a narrowing or hardening of the carotid arteries, is usually caused by atherosclerosis. The artery may be occluded, or plaque may break off and travel to the brain, causing a TIA or an ischemic stroke.

Risk Factors

- ✦ hypertension
- ✦ smoking
- ✦ diabetes
- ✦ obesity
- ✦ sedentary lifestyle

Signs and Symptoms

- ✦ can be asymptomatic
- ✦ dizziness
- ✦ blurred vision
- ✦ usually found after a TIA or stroke
- ✦ signs of stroke include:
  - ✧ weakness or numbness in face or arms
  - ✧ difficulty speaking or slurred speech
  - ✧ sudden, severe headaches

Diagnostic Tests and Findings

+ Carotid ultrasound may show areas of blocked blood flow within artery.

+ CT angiography may show blocked arteries.

Treatment and Management

+ Carotid artery angioplasty is typically needed to open the blocked artery.

+ A stent may be placed to keep the artery open.

+ Carotid endarterectomy may be required to remove the buildup of plaque on the artery.

QUICK REVIEW QUESTION

26. Which common signs and symptoms does the ED nurse know are associated with carotid artery stenosis?

Cardiac Trauma

Cardiac trauma can occur when an outside force causes injury to the heart. Cardiac trauma can cause rupture of heart chambers, dysrhythmias, damage to the heart valves, or cardiac arrest. Blunt cardiac trauma and penetrating cardiac trauma can both be fatal.

BLUNT TRAUMA

Pathophysiology

Blunt cardiac trauma occurs when an object forcefully strikes the chest. Because the atria and right ventricle are anteriorly positioned, they are typically the most affected. Blunt trauma to the heart causes a decrease in the right ventricle contractility and ejection fraction. In blunt cardiac trauma, the heart is compressed between the sternum and the spine. Sudden cardiac death can also occur from blunt trauma.

Risk Factors

+ MVC (e.g., the impact of a car steering wheel against the chest or injury from the shoulder strap of a seatbelt)

+ assault

+ projectile objects

+ being kicked in chest by large animal

Signs and Symptoms

+ chest pain that worsens with inspiration

+ dyspnea

+ cough

+ tachycardia

+ ecchymosis to affected area of chest

+ Signs of right ventricular failure
  ⬦ JVD
  ⬦ hepatomegaly
  ⬦ edema

Diagnostic Tests and Findings

+ CK-MB and troponin may be elevated.
+ ECG may show dysrhythmias:
    ⋄ AV blocks
    ⋄ bundle branch blocks
    ⋄ A-fib or atrial flutter
    ⋄ V-tach
    ⋄ premature ventricular complexes
    ⋄ T waves to indicate changes
+ echocardiogram showing reduced heart wall motion and decreased right ventricular ejection fraction

Treatment and Management

+ Administer inotropes (e.g., dobutamine).
+ Administer anti-inflammatories.
+ Administer oxygen.
+ Administer opioid pain medications.
+ Treat dysrhythmias if they are present.
+ Monitor for complications:
    ⋄ cardiac tamponade
    ⋄ valve or ventricular rupture
    ⋄ heart failure
    ⋄ cardiogenic shock

QUICK REVIEW QUESTION

27. The ED is caring for a patient who has been hit in the chest with a baseball. What diagnostic exams should be ordered as priorities?

PENETRATING TRAUMA

Pathophysiology

Penetrating cardiac trauma involves the puncture of the heart by a sharp object or by a broken rib. The most frequently affected area is the right ventricle. The penetration causes blood to leak into the pericardial space or mediastinum; the leakage can result in cardiac tamponade. Fluid or blood loss from penetrating injuries can also result in shock.

Risk Factors

+ workplace accidents
+ assaults (e.g., gunshot or knife wounds)
+ explosions

Signs and Symptoms

+ chest pain
+ object may be visible
+ hypotension
+ tachycardia

Diagnostic Tests and Findings

+ decreased hemoglobin and hematocrit
+ chest X-ray may show visible object

Treatment and Management

+ Control bleeding.
+ Maintain oxygenation.
+ Do not remove object.
+ Prepare 2 large-bore IVs.
+ Administer IV fluid and/or blood replacement.
+ Provide pain control with NSAIDs or opioids.

+ Patient should be prepared for surgery to have object removed.
+ Monitor for complications:
  ⋄ shock
  ⋄ cardiac tamponade
  ⋄ hemothorax
  ⋄ pneumothorax

QUICK REVIEW QUESTION

28. A patient arrives at the ED with a knife impaled in the chest. The patient is awake and alert but anxious and appears pale. What priority interventions should the nurse perform?

Shock

Shock occurs when there is inadequate tissue perfusion. The resulting lack of oxygen circulating to major organs can lead to organ failure and death.

CARDIOGENIC SHOCK

Pathophysiology

Cardiogenic shock occurs when the heart can no longer pump effectively, reducing blood flow and available oxygen throughout the body. This type of shock is most commonly seen in individuals having an MI.

Risk Factors

+ myocarditis
+ cardiac history
  ⋄ CAD
  ⋄ heart failure
  ⋄ MI
+ diabetes

+ hypertension
+ endocarditis
+ chest trauma
+ drug overdoses

Signs and Symptoms

+ hypotension
+ oliguria
+ tachycardia
+ dyspnea
+ crackles
+ tachypnea
+ dizziness

+ diaphoresis
+ pallor
+ JVD
+ altered level of consciousness
+ cool, clammy skin
+ S3 heart sound may be present

Diagnostic Tests and Findings

+ ECG may show ischemia, injury, or infarction

+ troponin levels to monitor for MI

+ CBC to monitor for infection, blood loss, and platelets

+ CMP to monitor for electrolyte imbalances and kidney function

+ lactate level to assess tissue perfusion

+ arterial blood gas to monitor for hypoxia or acidosis

+ chest X-ray to rule out other causes such as aortic dissection or tension pneumothorax

+ echocardiogram may show structural or valve problems, wall rupture, or pericardial tamponade

+ cardiac catheterization may show blockages in the coronary arteries (stents can be placed to keep artery open)

Treatment and Management

+ The main treatment goal is to identify the underlying cause.

+ Treatment should focus on reducing cardiac workload and improving myocardial contractility.

+ Manage patient's airways.

+ Administer the following:
  ✧ antiplatelets (aspirin or clopidogrel)
  ✧ thrombolytics (alteplase [Activase] or reteplase)
  ✧ morphine
  ✧ nitroprusside (Nipride)
  ✧ dobutamine

+ Place patient in Fowler's position or semi-Fowler's position to decrease preload.

+ Patient may need to have an intra-aortic balloon pump placed.

+ Cardiac catheterization may be needed to improve myocardial perfusion and increase contractility.

+ Monitor patient for cardiac dysrhythmias.

QUICK REVIEW QUESTION

29. The most common cause of cardiogenic shock is an MI. What interventions should the ED nurse perform as a priority?

HYPOVOLEMIC SHOCK

Pathophysiology

Hypovolemic shock (hypovolemia) occurs when rapid fluid loss decreases circulating blood volume and cardiac output, resulting in inadequate tissue perfusion.

Risk Factors

+ excessive vomiting or diarrhea

+ bleeding from injuries/trauma

+ GI bleeding

+ placenta previa

- abruption of placenta
- aortic dissection
- burns
- trauma

Signs and Symptoms

- tachycardia
- hypotension
- tachypnea
- oliguria
- dizziness
- confusion
- weakness
- headache
- nausea
- diaphoresis
- cool, clammy skin

Diagnostic Tests and Findings

- electrolyte imbalances
  - hyperkalemia
  - increased magnesium
  - hypernatremia
- increased BUN/creatinine
- increased lactate
- increased urine specific gravity and urine osmolality

Treatment and Management

- Conduct volume resuscitation with an isotonic crystalloid (i.e., normal saline or lactated Ringer's).
- Administer oxygen.
- If hypotension persists, medication infusions such as dopamine, epinephrine, norepinephrine, or dobutamine may be used to increase blood pressure and cardiac output.
- Perform a blood transfusion if needed.
- Monitor patient for cardiac dysrhythmias.
  - Patients who take beta blockers may not have tachycardia as it is masked by the effects of the medication.
- Blood pressure is not always a reliable indicator of shock.
  - A lower pulse pressure indicates the patient's level of shock.

QUICK REVIEW QUESTION

30. A patient presents to the ED with tachycardia, hypotension, and confusion. The family reports that the patient has been having frequent episodes of bloody stools. The patient is diagnosed with hypovolemic shock. What priority interventions should the ED nurse perform?

ANSWER KEY

1. Any patient with chest pain should immediately have an ECG to rule out any STEMI. Secondary interventions include establishing IV access, placing hypoxic patients on oxygen, and obtaining a full panel of bloodwork, including troponin to monitor for NSTEMI.

2. Remember the acronym MONA for initial interventions for NSTEMI: **M**orphine, **O**xygen, **N**itroglycerin, and **A**spirin.

3. Prepare the patient for immediate transfer to the cardiac catheterization lab for PCI for early reperfusion within 90 minutes. Establish 2 large-bore IVs to administer appropriate medications. Initial medications should always include aspirin, nitroglycerin, and morphine. Apply oxygen for any patient with low oxygen saturation, dyspnea, or signs of heart failure.

4. A patient with an abdominal aortic aneurysm should have his or her blood pressure closely monitored. Higher blood pressure places tension on the vessels and aortic walls and can increase the chances of aneurysm dissection.

5. A CT scan can definitively confirm the presence of a thoracic aneurysm. Other assessment findings that would be present are chest or back pain, coughing, and hoarseness. A full patient history would also be helpful in the diagnosis, as family history, genetic conditions affecting connective tissue, and poor lifestyle habits are risk factors.

6. A CT scan is the fastest way to show the presence of a thoracoabdominal aneurysm. An abdominal ultrasound will also show blood flow and structures within the abdominal cavity.

7. A patient with an abdominal aortic aneurysm dissection may have a blood pressure difference of about 20 mm Hg between the left and right arms, in addition to the complaint of severe ripping or tearing pain. A chest X-ray would show a widened mediastinum, and a CT scan would confirm dissection. The patient should be prepped for the operating room immediately to have dissection repaired.

8. The priority intervention is to check the patient's pulse and breathing for no more than 10 seconds. If the patient does not have a pulse, the code team should be activated and the nurse should immediately begin high-quality CPR at a rate of 100 – 120 compressions per minute at a depth of 2 – 2.4 inches.

9. The nurse should take the patient's blood pressure and ask him how he feels to determine whether he is stable or unstable. A patient with a normotensive blood pressure that is asymptomatic is stable and does not need intervention. He can be safely monitored by telemetry. Athletes tend to have lower resting pulse rates, so a heart rate of 49 is not unusual.

10. The patient has a viral infection (influenza), which can cause a fever and tachycardia. The infection puts extra stress on the heart, causing it to beat faster to circulate oxygen. Treatment for this patient would include acetaminophen or ibuprofen to fix the underlying cause of the tachycardia (fever from influenza) and IV placement with IV fluids to help rehydrate, which will also help lower the heart rate.

11. Immediate chest compressions and defibrillation should be the first 2 priority interventions. Also ensure that these interventions are done before administering any drugs. Current AHA Advanced Cardiac Life Support guidelines should be followed, including compressions at a rate of 100 – 120 per minute and initial defibrillation dose of 200 J. Defibrillation should be attempted at least twice before administering epinephrine.

12. A patient in pulseless V-tach should have chest compressions started at a rate of 100 – 120 per minute, and preparations to defibrillate should be started immediately. These priority interventions should be performed before the administration of any medication.

13. The 2 main interventions for a patient in asystole are chest compressions and administration of epinephrine 1 mg IV or IO every 3 – 5 minutes. The nurse could try to determine a cause for the patient's asystole by considering the H's and T's.

14. The only way to tell whether the rhythm on the monitor is a sinus rhythm, which would indicate ROSC, is to check for a pulse. If there is no pulse associated with the organized rhythm on the monitor, then the rhythm is PEA. Interventions for PEA include high-quality CPR and the administration of epinephrine 1 mg IV or IO every 3 – 5 minutes.

15. The patient is in unstable SVT because of hypotension, dyspnea, and dizziness. The priority intervention for an unstable patient in SVT is to immediately prepare for synchronized cardioversion.

16. A patient with a second-degree AV block, type 2, is at high risk of progressing to a third-degree block and is considered unstable. The patient should be connected to the TCP pads, and the nurse should be prepared to initiate TCP if the patient is symptomatic or hypotensive or exhibits signs of deterioration.

17. A patient with myocarditis will most likely have chest pain, tachycardia, dyspnea, fever, and joint pain. The patient's lung sounds may reveal crackles. The patient's heart sounds may sound distant, and S3 or S4 may be heard.

18. Hallmark signs indicating pericarditis include sudden, severe chest pain that is worsened with movement and lessened by sitting up or leaning forward, as well as tachycardia and a pericardial friction rub heard on auscultation. Other signs include tachypnea, dyspnea, fever, chills, and cough.

19. The patient with endocarditis would be likely to exhibit flulike symptoms, including petechiae, joint pain, chest pain, Janeway lesions, and Osler's nodes.

20. Left-sided heart failure signs involve the pulmonary system and include dyspnea, orthopnea, cough, frothy sputum, hemoptysis, and crackles.

21. After confirming that the blood pressure reflects a hypertensive crisis, the nurse should administer an antihypertensive medication but should aim for a reduction of no more than 25% within the first 2 hours.

22. Patients with pulmonary hypertension who have been off their medications may experience dyspnea, edema, and fatigue. This patient may need oxygenation and vasodilators and may need to continue the medication she was previously prescribed.

23. Hypotension, JVD, and muffled heart tones are the hallmark signs of pericardial tamponade; these 3 signs are known as Beck's triad.

24. This patient has risk factors (recent travel and pregnancy) as well as symptoms that indicate a possible DVT. The nurse should assess for pulses and insert an IV to prepare the patient for a CT scan to rule out a pulmonary embolism. The patient should be monitored for respiratory symptoms that may indicate dislodgement of the DVT.

25. The patient with an acute arterial occlusion needs immediate surgical intervention to remove the thrombosis causing the occlusion. The nurse should prepare to give an IV anticoagulant such as heparin while awaiting transfer of the patient to surgery.

26. Carotid artery stenosis may have no symptoms at all or may include dizziness or blurred vision. If the carotid artery stenosis has blocked the blood flow to the brain, then the signs and symptoms most commonly found would be those of a TIA or stroke and would include weakness, slurred speech or difficulty speaking, and a sudden, severe headache.

27. An ECG should be performed to monitor for dysrhythmias that may have been caused by the blunt trauma. Labs, including troponin and CK-MB, should be drawn to measure cardiac muscle damage. An echocardiogram should be done to look for injury to the ventricles and heart wall.

28. Any patient with a penetrating object injury should have the nurse ensure that the object is stabilized but not removed. Bleeding should be controlled, and 2 large-bore IVs should be placed for the administration of IV fluids and blood if needed. The patient should be prepped for surgery to have the object removed and to be assessed for underlying damage to organs and surrounding areas.

29. An immediate ECG should be performed to assess for ST segment elevation. An IV should be placed, and full lab work conducted, to include troponin, CMP, and CBC.

30. The patient in hypovolemic shock should immediately have an IV placed and be administered at least 2 boluses of an isotonic crystalloid, typically normal saline. If the patient remains hypotensive, vasopressors should be considered. If hypovolemic shock is due to blood loss, a blood transfusion is indicated.

TWO 2: RESPIRATORY EMERGENCIES

Respiratory Assessments

LUNG SOUNDS

+ Lung sounds should be assessed after confirmation of airway patency.

+ Auscultate each lung field bilaterally to determine the nature and characteristic of function of the lungs.

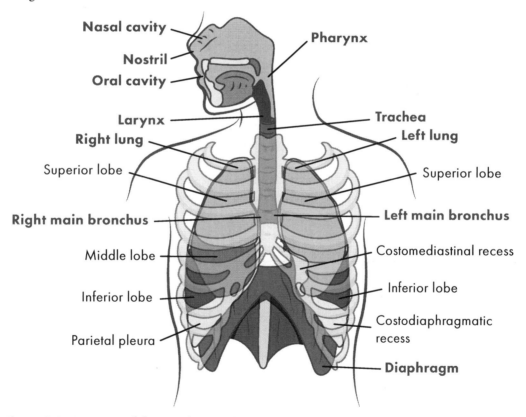

Figure 2.1. Anatomy of the Respiratory System

+ To perform the assessment:
  ◇ Begin at the apex of the lung, and assess from side to side at each point.
  ◇ Proceed down the anterior chest wall, listening to several points symmetrically (on both the right and left sides) throughout the lung fields.
  ◇ Repeat this assessment posteriorly and medially.
+ Abnormal breath sounds:
  ◇ **wheezes**: can occur on inspiration or expiration, continuous musical-like sound from air being forced through narrowed passages in the airway
  ◇ **rhonchi**: low-pitched, coarse rattling lung sounds caused by secretions in the airway
  ◇ **stridor**: typically found with upper airway obstruction; characterized by high-pitched wheezing sound
  ◇ **rales**: also called **crackles**, sound can be coarse or fine; related to fluid in the small airways of the lung
  ◇ **pleural friction rub**: characterized by a grating, creaking sound due to inflamed pleural tissue

ARTERIAL BLOOD GASES

+ An **arterial blood gas (ABG) test** measures the pH and amount of dissolved carbon dioxide and oxygen in the blood.
+ ABGs provide information on the function of the respiratory system, specifically acid-base balance and pulmonary gas exchange.
+ Arterial blood is collected from either the radial or the ulnar artery; if an arterial line is already placed, it can be drawn from that access.

Table 2.1. Normal Values for ABG

Elements of an ABG	Normal Value
pH	7.35 – 7.45
Partial pressure of oxygen (PaO_2)	75 – 100 mm Hg
Partial pressure of carbon dioxide ($PaCO_2$)	35 – 45 mm Hg
Bicarbonate (HCO_3)	22 – 26 mEq/L
Oxygen saturation	94 – 100%

Table 2.2. Common Causes of Changes in ABG Values

Abnormality	pH	ABG	Cause
Respiratory acidosis	Decreased	$PaCO_2$ increased	Asthma, COPD
Respiratory alkalosis	Increased	$PaCO_2$ decreased	Hyperventilation
Metabolic alkalosis	Increased	HCO_3 increased	Overabundance of bicarbonate, loss of lactic acid in the blood because of kidney dysfunction or diabetic disorders
Metabolic acidosis	Decreased	HCO_3 decreased	Diarrhea, vomiting (prolonged), kidney dysfunction; occurs because decreased bicarbonate in blood cannot neutralize acids

CAPNOGRAPHY (PetCO$_2$)

+ **Capnography** is used to monitor the concentration of carbon dioxide in respiratory gases.

+ PetCO$_2$ is the measure of **end-tidal carbon dioxide** (partial pressure of CO$_2$ at the end of exhalation) and is often displayed graphically as a waveform.

  ⋄ EtCO$_2$ refers to end-tidal carbon dioxide; PetCO$_2$ refers to the *measurement* of end-tidal carbon dioxide.

    ‣ P = pressure; et = end-tidal; CO$_2$ = carbon dioxide

+ Normal PetCO$_2$ in adult patients is between 35 and 45 mm Hg.

+ If a patient is in cardiac arrest and CPR is in progress, high-quality chest compressions will result in PetCO$_2$ between 10 and 20 mm Hg.

Rapid Sequence Intubation

+ **Rapid sequence intubation (RSI)** is used in emergency settings when there is a risk of, or a concern for, aspiration.

+ The nurse assists the provider with equipment, medication administration, and management of the airway before and after intubation.

EQUIPMENT NEEDED

+ cardiac monitor
+ pulse oximeter
+ blood pressure cuff
+ arterial line
+ bag-valve mask with oxygen
+ EtCO$_2$ detector
+ laryngoscope and blade
+ ET tube and stylet

+ suction
+ 10 mL syringe
+ airway adjuncts
+ percutaneous tracheostomy kit in case of failed intubation
+ ACLS crash cart in case of respiratory or cardiac arrest

COMMON DRUGS

+ pretreatment drugs:
  ⋄ lidocaine
  ⋄ fentanyl
  ⋄ vecuronium
  ⋄ atropine
+ paralytics
  ⋄ rocuronium
  ⋄ succinylcholine
  ⋄ vecuronium

+ sedatives/hypnotics (induction)
  ⋄ midazolam
  ⋄ fentanyl
  ⋄ propofol
  ⋄ etomidate
  ⋄ ketamine
+ pressors
  ⋄ phenylephrine
  ⋄ ephedrine

STEPS FOR RSI

1. **Prepare:** Establish IV access, measure vital signs, gather equipment, prepare medications, assess for potential difficult airway.

2. **Pre-oxygenate:** Pre-oxygenate the patient with 100% oxygen for at least 3 minutes before intubation to prevent desaturation during the procedure.

3. **Pretreatment:** Administer pretreatment medications as ordered by provider.

4. **Paralysis:** Administer induction agent via rapid IV push as ordered by provider, followed by paralytic agent immediately after.

5. **Protection:** If indicated, perform the Sellick maneuver (cricoid cartilage pressure).

6. **Placement:** The ET tube is placed by provider, the cuff is inflated, and placement is confirmed with an $EtCO_2$ detector and bilateral lung sound auscultation. Secure the tube and release cricoid pressure if it has been applied.

7. **Post-intubation management:** The patient's chest is X-rayed to confirm the correct placement of the ET. The patient receives long-acting sedation or paralytics, and mechanical ventilation is initiated.

Acute Respiratory Infections

COMMUNITY-ACQUIRED PNEUMONIA (CAP)

Pathophysiology

Pneumonia is a lower respiratory tract infection that can be caused by bacteria, fungi, protozoa, or parasites. The infection causes inflammation in the alveoli and can cause them to fill with fluid. CAP is contracted in the community (as opposed to hospital-acquired pneumonia (HAP)). Causative organisms include:

+ *Streptococcus pneumoniae*
+ *Mycoplasma pneumoniae*
+ *Haemophilus pneumoniae*
+ *Legionella pneumoniae*

Aspiration pneumonia is most often caused by ingestion of oropharyngeal secretions via the trachea and into the lungs. Risk factors, signs and symptoms, and treatment of CAP, HAP, and aspiration pneumonia are similar.

Risk Factors

+ age > 65 years
+ immunodeficiency
+ lung disease (COPD)
+ smoking
+ intubation
+ residence in nursing home or other long-term care facility
+ neurologic dysfunction
+ difficulty swallowing

Signs and Symptoms

+ cough
+ pleuritic chest pain
+ fever
+ dyspnea
+ hemoptysis

- abnormal lung sounds in the affected lung/lobe
  - decreased lung sounds
  - inspiratory crackles

Diagnostic Tests and Findings

- elevated white blood cell count
- chest X-ray showing infiltrates
- positive blood cultures or sputum cultures

Treatment and Management

- Support adequate ventilation and oxygenation through oxygen adjuncts or mechanical ventilation where necessary.
- Administer antibiotics, using broad-spectrum ones until cultures are made for sensitivity.
- Ensure adequate hydration.
- Practice pulmonary hygiene:
  - Have patient do deep breathing.
  - Encourage coughing to clear the lungs.
  - Chest physiotherapy can help relieve congestion in the lungs.

QUICK REVIEW QUESTION

1. A 70-year-old patient is transported from a nursing home to the ED with complaints of shortness of breath, fever, chills, and a productive cough with thick, brown sputum. His pulse oximetry reading is 86% on room air. What are the first actions the nurse should take?

CROUP
Pathophysiology

Croup is an upper airway obstruction caused by subglottic inflammation that results from viral illness (although rarely it can be caused by bacterial infection). The inflammation results in edema in the trachea and adjacent structures. Additionally, thick, tenacious mucus further obstructs the airway. Croup is associated with a characteristic high-pitched stridor.

Risk Factors

- age 6 months to 3 years old
- slightly more prevalent in male patients
- cooler weather
- respiratory infection

Signs and Symptoms

- barking cough
- hoarse cry
- high-pitched, inspiratory stridor
- tachypnea
- anxiety
- symptoms of viral infection:
  - fever
  - fatigue
  - dehydration

Diagnostic Tests and Findings

+ soft-tissue X-ray to rule out epiglottitis

Treatment and Management

+ Provide oxygen support as needed.
+ Administer cool mist therapy.
+ Administer corticosteroids.
+ Administer dexamethasone.

+ Administer nebulized racemic epinephrine for moderate to severe croup.
  ◇ Patient should be monitored 2 – 3 hours after the dose.
+ Take measures to reduce patient's anxiety.

QUICK REVIEW QUESTION

2. A 1-year-old patient arrives at triage with her mother. The mother says that the child has had a barking cough and seems to have difficulty breathing. The nurse notes a hoarse cry and notes that the child seems to be fatigued. What should the nurse prepare to do for this patient?

BRONCHITIS

Pathophysiology

Bronchitis is inflammation of the bronchi. Most cases (> 90%) are caused by a viral infection, but bronchitis can also result from bacterial infection or environmental irritants. Bronchitis is classified as acute or chronic. Symptoms of acute bronchitis typically last for 3 weeks; chronic bronchitis is associated with other chronic conditions, such as COPD.

Risk Factors

+ smoking
+ pediatrics and adults > 65

+ higher risk during winter months

Signs and Symptoms

+ nonproductive cough that evolves into a productive cough
+ sore throat
+ congestion

+ fever
+ chest discomfort
+ fatigue

Diagnostic Tests and Findings

+ diagnosis based on signs and symptoms

+ chest X-ray to rule out pneumonia

Treatment and Management

+ Acute bronchitis will usually spontaneously resolve without intervention.

- Recommend supportive treatment for symptoms:
    - fluids
    - antitussives
    - analgesics
- Antibiotics are given if:
    - The underlying infection is bacterial.
    - Secondary bacterial infections develop.

- At discharge, teach the following practices to alleviate symptoms:
    - Drink adequate fluids.
    - Avoid irritants (such as smoke).
    - Use a humidifier.
    - Use OTC antitussives and NSAIDs.

QUICK REVIEW QUESTION

3. A patient complains of chest discomfort, fatigue, and a productive cough that has lasted for 10 days. The ED physician determines that the patient has bronchitis. What should the nurse recommend to the patient upon discharge to assist with symptom management?

BRONCHIOLITIS

Pathophysiology

Bronchiolitis is inflammation of the bronchioles, usually because of infection by RSV or human rhinovirus. The inflammation and congestion lead to a narrowing of the airway, resulting in dyspnea. Bronchiolitis is seen in children younger than 2 years and will usually spontaneously resolve.

Risk Factors

- age < 2 years
- premature birth
- immunosuppression
- chronic heart or lung disease
- exposure to inhaled toxins or chemicals

Signs and Symptoms

- early presentation mimics common cold
    - rhinorrhea
    - congestion
- later symptoms indicate lower respiratory involvement
    - coughing
    - wheezing and crackles
    - increased respiratory effort
    - dyspnea
    - tachypnea

Diagnostic Tests and Findings

- chest X-ray to rule out pneumonia
- sputum culture to identify underlying virus
- CBC: WBC count increased when inflammation is the result of infection

Treatment and Management

+ Supportive treatment is provided for symptoms.
    ⋄ Provide nasal suctioning.
    ⋄ Give fluids.
    ⋄ Administer oxygen.
+ Pharmacological treatments are used only for severe cases.
    ⋄ Have patient use a bronchodilator.
    ⋄ Administer steroids.
    ⋄ Administer NSAIDs.
    ⋄ Administer nebulized albuterol.
+ Antibiotics are only necessary if secondary infection is present.

> ## QUICK REVIEW QUESTION
>
> **4.** The mother of an 18-month-old is concerned that her child has pneumonia. She asks the nurse to describe the difference between a diagnosis of pneumonia and a diagnosis of bronchiolitis. How should the nurse respond?

Chronic Respiratory Condition
CHRONIC OBSTRUCTIVE PULMONARY DISEASE
Pathophysiology

Chronic obstructive pulmonary disease (COPD) is characterized by a breakdown in alveolar tissue (emphysema) and long-term obstruction of the airways by inflammation and edema (chronic bronchitis). The most common cause of COPD is smoking, although the disease can be caused by other inhaled irritants (e.g., smoke, industrial chemicals, air pollution).

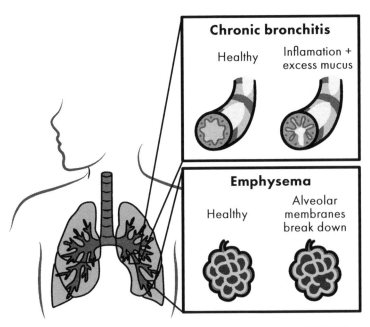

Figure 2.2. Chronic Obstructive Pulmonary Disease (COPD)

Risk Factors

+ smoking (> 30 pack years [pack-years = packs per day × years])
+ passive exposure to cigarette smoke
+ occupational exposure to inhaled chemicals
+ indoor or outdoor pollution
+ severe childhood respiratory illness

Signs and Symptoms

+ chronic, productive cough
+ dyspnea
+ wheezing
+ prolonged expiration
+ cyanosis
+ hypoxemia
+ pulmonary hypertension
+ barrel chest (late sign)

Diagnostic Tests and Findings

+ chest X-ray
  + will have findings demonstrating COPD with advanced disease only
  + may show flattened diaphragm, irregular air pockets (bullae), and enlarged lungs
+ serum WBC to rule out infectious process
+ pulmonary function tests:
  + in the ED, spirometry most often used
  + spirometry demonstrating decreased forced expiratory flow from the lungs

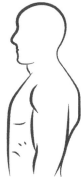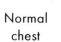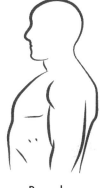

Normal chest   Barrel chest

Figure 2.3. Barrel Chest

+ ABG analysis may be abnormal in acute COPD exacerbation
  + decreased PaO_2 and low-to-normal $PaCO_2$

Treatment and Management

+ Treatment of COPD focuses on reducing symptoms and preventing further lung tissue damage.
+ Chest physiotherapy and placing patients in positions of comfort and maximum expansion of the chest wall can assist with symptom management.
+ Pharmacological treatment includes:
  + expectorants
  + inhaled bronchodilators
  + inhaled corticosteroids
+ At discharge, teach smoking cessation.

QUICK REVIEW QUESTION

5. A 50-year-old patient has been newly diagnosed with COPD and is anxious about the diagnosis. The patient wants to know if there is a cure for COPD. How should the nurse respond?

ASTHMA

Pathophysiology

Asthma, an obstructive disease of the lungs, is characterized by long-term inflammation and constriction of the bronchial airways. Patients with asthma often experience exacerbations triggered by lung irritants, exercise, stress, or allergies. Asthma cannot be cured but can be managed through pharmacological measures and lifestyle changes.

Risk Factors

+ higher rate of diagnosis in childhood
+ male gender
+ family history
+ allergies such as atopic dermatitis or allergic rhinitis
+ occupational exposure
+ smoking, exposure to secondhand cigarette smoke or other smoke
+ obesity

Signs and Symptoms

+ wheezing
+ frequent cough (productive or nonproductive)
+ shortness of breath
+ tightness in the chest
+ severe exacerbations marked by:
  ◇ tachypnea
  ◇ audible wheezing
  ◇ anxiety
  ◇ hypoxia

Diagnostic Tests and Findings

+ chest X-ray to rule out other lung conditions
+ spirometry to measure respiratory function
+ ABG will show decreased PaO_2 and $PaCO_2$

Treatment and Management

+ Asthma is managed with consideration of short-term and long-term needs.
+ Short-term management is appropriate for flare-ups or exacerbation:
  ◇ Bronchodilators such as albuterol or ipratropium are used for acute exacerbations.
  ◇ Oxygen is supplied via a non-rebreather mask.
  ◇ Administer systemic corticosteroids (e.g., prednisone, prednisolone, or methylprednisolone).
  ◇ Conduct continuous pulse oximetry.
  ◇ In severe cases, keep patient under close observation.
+ Long-term treatment of asthma involves a combination of a corticosteroid and a bronchodilator (e.g., fluticasone/salmeterol or mometasone/formoterol).
+ Patients are taught to recognize and manage triggers for asthma exacerbation, including:
  ◇ smoke
  ◇ dust and dust mites
  ◇ pet dander
  ◇ cold air
  ◇ exercise
  ◇ mold
  ◇ air pollution (indoor and outdoor)

STATUS ASTHMATICUS

Pathophysiology

Status asthmaticus is a severe condition in which the patient is experiencing intractable asthma exacerbations with limited pauses or no pause between the exacerbations. The symptoms are unresponsive to initial treatment and can ultimately lead to acute respiratory failure. Status asthmaticus can develop over hours or days.

Risk Factors

+ history of recent intubation/mechanical ventilation

+ recent use of systemic corticosteroids

+ presence of current respiratory illness

+ increased home use of bronchodilator without desired effect

+ O_2 saturation below 94% with supplemental oxygen

Signs and Symptoms

+ dyspnea

+ wheezing (inspiratory and expiratory)

+ crackles

+ tachypnea

+ pulsus paradoxus

+ chest tightness

+ dry, nonproductive cough

+ abdominal pain (from abdominal accessory muscle use)

+ signs and symptoms that are unresponsive to standard asthma treatment

Diagnostic Tests and Findings

+ chest X-ray to rule out pneumonia

+ decreased peak-flow measurements

+ ABGs to inform treatment

Treatment and Management

+ Immediate management of status asthmaticus is pharmacological:
  ⋄ beta-agonists (albuterol, levalbuterol)
  ⋄ corticosteroids
  ⋄ sedatives
  ⋄ anesthetics
  ⋄ anticholinergics
  ⋄ theophylline (given in refractory status asthmaticus)

+ Ensure adequate hydration.

+ Provide oxygen therapy.

+ Intubation and mechanical ventilation are used in severe cases that do not respond to pharmacological intervention.

Hemothorax

Pathophysiology

A **hemothorax** is the collection of blood in the pleural space. This blood displaces lung tissue, subsequently decreasing lung volume and inhibiting inhalation and gas exchange. The most common cause of a hemothorax is chest or thoracic trauma, but a hemothorax can also occur secondary to aortic dissections.

Risk Factors

+   trauma

Signs and Symptoms

+   decreased or absent breath sounds

+   cyanosis

+   unequal chest wall movement

+   hypotension

+   tachycardia

+   tachypnea

+   pale, cool, clammy skin

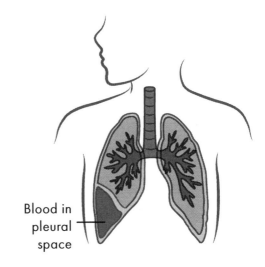

Blood in pleural space

Figure 2.4. Hemothorax

Diagnostic Tests and Findings

+   on chest X-ray, areas of white where the concentration of blood is in the tissue

Treatment and Management

+   Place a chest tube to remove the blood and air from the pleural space; connect it to suction as needed.

+   Identify the source of bleeding, and stop the bleed.

+   Maintain hemodynamic stability of the patient with fluid resuscitation.

Inhalation Injuries

Pathophysiology

Inhalation injuries fall into three categories differentiated by the mechanism of the injury:

+ Exposure to asphyxiants such as carbon monoxide (CO) can cause injuries. In the case of CO poisoning, the CO displaces the oxygen on the hemoglobin molecule, leading to hypoxia and eventual death of tissue.

+ Thermal or heat inhalation injuries can be caused by steam, heat from explosions, or the consumption of very hot liquids. The resulting edema and blistering of the airway mucosa lead to airway obstruction.

+ Smoke exposure, from fire or toxic gases causes damage to pulmonary tissue and causes mucosal edema and the destruction of epithelia cilia. Pulmonary edema is a late development, one to two days after the injury.

Risk Factors

+ occupational exposure to asphyxiants or toxic gases

+ proximity to fire

+ intentional inhalation of toxic gases

Signs and Symptoms

+ depend on what irritant the patient is exposed to

+ mucosal and pulmonary edema possible up to 48 hours after exposure

+ general signs and symptoms:
  ⋄ hypoxia
  ⋄ dyspnea
  ⋄ altered level of consciousness
  ⋄ cardiac dysrhythmias
  ⋄ wheezing
  ⋄ restlessness

+ for airway edema:
  ⋄ hoarse voice
  ⋄ muffled speech
  ⋄ stridor

+ may be signs of injury at mouth, nose, or oral mucosa

Diagnostic Tests and Findings

+ detailed history of the events leading up to and following the exposure or injury, to understand the depth of exposure

+ smokers may have higher baseline of CO (10% – 15%)

+ carboxyhemoglobin (COHb) levels above 60% incompatible with life
  ⋄ COHb measured with CO-oximeter in the ED
  ⋄ serum tests to measure CO levels

+ pulse oximetry reading may be deceiving; does not differentiate between CO and O_2 loading on hemoglobin

Treatment and Management

+ Protect and maintain the patient's airway:
    - Use airway adjuncts as appropriate.
    - Early intubation and ventilation may be necessary.
+ Provide oxygen therapy (humidified).

+ Administer antidotes if they are available:
    - Examples include the cyanide antidote hydroxocobalamin (Cyanokit).
+ Practice vigorous pulmonary hygiene with patient (including suctioning of airways, blow bottles, and nasotracheal suction).

QUICK REVIEW QUESTION

9. EMS arrives with a patient who was rescued from a home fire. The patient is unconscious, but the airway is currently clear and intact. Assessment of the airway reveals black soot at the opening of the mouth and at the nares. What is the next nursing consideration for this patient?

Obstruction

Pathophysiology

Airway **obstruction**, or blockage of the upper airway, can be caused by a foreign body (e.g., teeth, food, marbles), the tongue, vomit, blood, or other secretions. Possible causes of airway obstruction include traumatic injuries to the face, edema in the airway, peritonsillar abscess, and burns to the airway. Small children may also place foreign bodies in their mouths or obstruct their airway with food.

Risk Factors

+ age < 2 years and > 65 years
+ upper airway burn or inhalation injury
+ severe facial trauma
+ seizures
+ infections or inflammation of the upper airway
+ difficulty swallowing
+ croup

Signs and Symptoms

+ visually observed obstruction in airway
+ dyspnea
+ gasping for air
+ stridor
+ excessive drooling in infants
+ agitation or panic
+ loss of consciousness or altered LOC
+ respiratory arrest

Diagnostic Tests and Findings

+ diagnosis based on signs and symptoms

Treatment and Management

+ Acute airway obstruction requires suctioning of the mouth and upper airway and rapid intubation where appropriate.

+ When ET tube is contraindicated or not possible because of the obstruction, cricothyrotomy is indicated.

  ✧ Cricothyrotomy must be done quickly to reestablish a patent airway.

+ Mechanical ventilation is indicated in situations where the airway will remain obstructed for an extended period.

QUICK REVIEW QUESTION

10. In what order should the nurse perform an airway assessment in a patient with a suspected foreign body obstruction?

Pleural Effusion

Pathophysiology

A **pleural effusion** is the buildup of fluid around the lungs in the pleural space. This fluid buildup can displace lung tissue and inhibit adequate ventilation and lung expansion. There are two types of pleural effusions:

+ **Transudative pleural effusions** occur when fluid leaks into the pleural space. They can be caused by low serum protein levels or increased systemic pressure in the vessels.

+ **Exudative pleural effusions** are due to blockage of blood or lymph vessels, tumors, lung injury, or inflammation.

Risk Factors

+ preexisting lung injury
+ chronic lung disease
+ heart failure
+ neoplasia (lung cancer)
+ lupus or rheumatoid arthritis
+ hypoalbuminemia
+ trauma
+ smoking
+ alcohol abuse

Signs and Symptoms

+ dyspnea
+ dullness upon percussion of the lung area
+ asymmetrical chest expansion
+ decreased breath sounds on affected side
+ cough (dry or productive)
+ pleuritic chest pain

Diagnostic Tests and Findings

+ chest X-ray showing white areas at the base of the lungs (unilaterally or bilaterally)

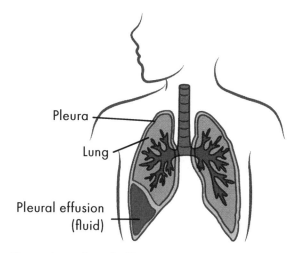

Pleura

Lung

Pleural effusion (fluid)

Figure 2.5. Pleural Effusion

- CT scan to further diagnose the severity of the condition
- thoracentesis to determine the mechanism of effusion

Treatment and Management

- Initial treatment is drainage of excess pleural fluid where appropriate.
- Surgical intervention may be required to address complications of pleural effusion such as tissue adhesion.
- Medications are administered according to the underlying cause.
    - Diuretics are administered to assist with reducing effusion size.
    - Antibiotics are administered when an infectious process is identified as the cause.

QUICK REVIEW QUESTION

11. A nursing student requests assistance with understanding the difference between pulmonary effusion and ARDS. What is your response?

Pneumothorax

Pathophysiology

Pneumothorax is the collection of air between the chest wall and the lung (pleural space). It can occur from blunt chest-wall injury, medical injury, underlying lung tissue disease, or hereditary factors. Pneumothorax is classified according to its underlying cause:

- **Primary spontaneous pneumothorax (PSP)** occurs spontaneously in the absence of lung disease and often presents with only minor symptoms.
- **Secondary spontaneous pneumothorax (SSP)** occurs in patients with an underlying lung disease and presents with more severe symptoms.
- **Traumatic pneumothorax** occurs when the chest wall is penetrated.
- **Tension pneumothorax**, the late progression of a pneumothorax, causes significant respiratory distress in the patient and requires immediate intervention for treatment.

Risk Factors

- for PSP:
    - more common in men
    - 20 – 40 years old
    - tall and underweight
- underlying lung tissue disease
- medical procedures
- blunt chest-wall injuries
- changes in atmospheric pressure
- smoking

Signs and Symptoms

- sudden unilateral chest pain
- dyspnea
- tachycardia
- hypoxia

- cyanosis
- hypotension
- for tension pneumothorax:
  - tracheal deviation away from the side of the tension
  - decreased breath sounds on the affected side
  - increased percussion note
  - distended neck veins

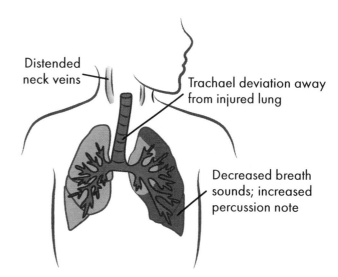

Figure 2.6. Signs and Symptoms of Tension Pneumothorax

Diagnostic Tests and Findings

- chest X-ray
  - showing the lung tissue separated from the chest wall
  - may show decreased or absent lung expansion
  - may show mediastinal shift (for tension pneumothorax)

Treatment and Management

- Interventions are based on the symptoms the patient is experiencing and their severity.
- Patients who are asymptomatic with > 15% pneumothorax may be observed on an inpatient or outpatient basis, with oxygen via non-rebreather mask.
- Patients with larger pneumothoraxes may require needle decompression with the insertion of a chest tube.
- Tension pneumothorax requires immediate decompression, usually via needle thoracostomy.

QUICK REVIEW QUESTION

12. A patient with blunt thoracic trauma has been diagnosed with pneumothorax and was alert and oriented upon arrival via EMS. On reassessment of the patient, the nurse finds the patient restless and anxious. The patient also has tachypnea and tachycardia, with visually distended neck veins. What intervention should the nurse anticipate?

Pulmonary Aspiration

Pathophysiology

Pulmonary aspiration is the entry of foreign bodies, or material from the mouth or gastrointestinal tract, into the upper and/or lower respiratory tract.

Risk Factors

- surgery, or postsurgical patients
- sedation or other altered LOC
- intoxication from alcohol or sedative drugs

Signs and Symptoms

+ coughing

+ dyspnea

+ choking

+ fever and malaise (indicating aspiration pneumonia)

+ lung sounds may be decreased in the lobe in which the aspiration has settled

+ crackles may be heard if fluid was aspirated

Diagnostic Tests and Findings

+ chest X-ray showing infiltrates after the aspiration, depending on the nature, size, and quantity of the aspirated matter

+ serum tests necessary if patient shows signs of infection

  ✧ increased WBC if infection exists

  ✧ blood cultures necessary if sepsis is suspected

Treatment and Management

+ Clear and suction the airway where appropriate.

+ Closely monitor the patient after aspiration.

+ Treat complications secondary to aspiration as necessary:

  ✧ Provide oxygen therapy.

  ✧ Administer antibiotics.

QUICK REVIEW QUESTION

13. A patient presents to the ED with pleuritic chest pain, difficulty breathing, fevers, chills, and an altered LOC. The patient's friend alerts the triage nurse that 3 days ago, the patient was found in a pool of vomit after an overdose. What should the nurse anticipate for this patient?

Pulmonary Edema

NONCARDIAC PULMONARY EDEMA

Pathophysiology

Noncardiac pulmonary edema (NPE) is when fluid collects in the alveoli of the lungs, but the condition is not due to heart failure. This fluid inhibits gas exchange. NPE can be caused by a wide range of injuries and underlying disorders, including:

+ CNS injury (neurogenic pulmonary edema)

+ removal of airway obstruction (postobstructive pulmonary edema)

+ rapid increase in altitude (high-altitude pulmonary edema)

+ reexpansion of the lung (reexpansion pulmonary edema)

+ aspiration

+ inhalation of toxic gases

+ immersion injuries

Risk Factors

+ related to underlying cause of NPE

Signs and Symptoms

+ dyspnea
+ orthopnea
+ cough (dry or productive)
+ chest pain
+ fatigue and weakness

+ tachypnea
+ dizziness
+ hypoxia
+ frothy pink pulmonary secretions
+ crackles

Diagnostic Tests and Findings

+ chest X-ray showing greater white appearance over both lung fields than in a normal X-ray
+ elevated plasma BNP

Treatment and Management

+ Priority treatment is to restore or maintain respiratory function.
    ⬦ Oxygen supplementation is necessary.
    ⬦ Severe cases may require intubation and mechanical ventilation.
+ Secondary treatment to address underlying condition may be necessary.

QUICK REVIEW QUESTION

14. Which is the most effective treatment of high-altitude pulmonary edema?

ACUTE RESPIRATORY DISTRESS SYNDROME

Pathophysiology

Acute respiratory distress syndrome (ARDS) is a sudden and progressive form of NPE in which the alveoli fill with fluid because of damage to the pulmonary endothelium.

There are three stages of ARDS:

1. **Early exudative state** (up to 10 days after injury): There is edema, congestion in the pulmonary capillaries, and atelectasis.

2. **Fibroproliferative stage** (10 days to 3 weeks after injury): Edema is resolved and myofibroblasts (which produce collagen) move into the interstitial space around the alveoli.

3. **Fibrotic stage** (> 3 weeks after injury): This stage is characterized by collagen formation in the alveolar sacs, leading to decreased lung compliance and effectiveness of respiration.

Risk Factors

+ age > 65
+ inhalation injury

+ chronic lung disease
+ sepsis

- blunt trauma to thorax
- smoking
- history of alcohol abuse
- overdose on sedatives or antidepressants

Signs and Symptoms

- dyspnea
- tachypnea
- hypotension
- hypoxia
- crackles in bases of lungs
- dry, hacking cough
- tachycardia
- fever
- fatigue and general weakness
- altered LOC

Diagnostic Tests and Findings

- no definitive diagnostic test for ARDS
- chest X-ray showing white opacities at the base of the lungs where alveolar sacs have filled with fluid
- CT scan of chest to rule out other causes for symptoms

Treatment and Management

- Simultaneously treat underlying cause while managing ARDS symptoms.
- Oxygen supplementation is necessary.
- Intubation and mechanical ventilation are almost always necessary.
- Secondary treatment to address underlying condition if necessary.
- Anticipate starting careful hydration in the presence of hypovolemia.
- Patient will require pulmonary rehabilitation after discharge.

QUICK REVIEW QUESTION

15. A patient presents to the emergency department with hypotension, fever, chills, and an altered LOC. The nurse identifies that the patient is experiencing sepsis. What signs and symptoms should the nurse look for to determine if the patient has ARDS?

Pulmonary Embolism

Pathophysiology

A **pulmonary embolism (PE)** occurs when an embolus occludes an artery of the lungs. The most common embolus is a blood clot caused by deep vein thrombosis (DVT), but tumor emboli, fat emboli, and amniotic fluid emboli can also reach the lungs. PE is an emergent condition that can result in death.

Risk Factors

- history of DVT
- trauma

- prolonged immobilization
- surgery
- birth control
- pregnancy
- polycythemia
- smoking

Signs and Symptoms

- pleuritic chest pain
- dyspnea
- tachypnea
- cough
- hemoptysis
- tachycardia
- hypotension
- anxiety

Diagnostic Tests and Findings

- serum tests considered for patients with suspected PE include:
  - tests to rule out other conditions include:
    - CBC
    - electrolytes
    - BUN and creatinine
  - D-dimer positive (> 500 ng/mL) in patients with PE
- chest X-ray often normal (but collected to rule out other disease processes)
- electrocardiogram often normal, but may show sinus tachycardia
- CTPA showing evidence of PE

Treatment and Management

- Conduct continuous cardiac monitoring.
- Administer IV anticoagulation (heparin) once diagnosis is confirmed.
- Thrombolytic drugs (fibrinolytics) are considered for unstable patients with no contraindications.
- Provide supportive treatment for symptoms.
  - Give oxygen therapy.
  - Administer analgesics.
  - Ensure adequate hydration.
  - Administer vasopressors to manage blood pressure.

QUICK REVIEW QUESTION

16. A pregnant patient presents to the ED complaining of chest pain and shortness of breath. During triage, she mentions having driven 8 hours to visit her sick sister. Which diagnostic tests should the nurse prepare for, given the presentation?

Thoracic Trauma

PENETRATING TRAUMA

Pathophysiology

Penetrating trauma to the thorax comes with high risk of pulmonary injury, because of the amount of space the lungs occupy in the thoracic cavity. The most common injuries to the lungs resulting from penetrating trauma are pneumothorax and hemothorax, which do not often require intervention beyond placement of a chest tube. Penetrating trauma can also cause pulmonary lacerations and blood loss leading to hypovolemic shock.

Risk Factors

+ workplace accidents

+ assaults (e.g., gunshot or knife wounds)

+ explosions

Signs and Symptoms

+ visible penetration injury

+ dyspnea

+ productive cough

+ bloody sputum

+ tachycardia

+ hypotension

+ hypoxia

Diagnostic Tests and Findings

+ chest X-rays not reliable for diagnosis of pulmonary laceration; other thoracic injuries may mask pulmonary injury

+ CT scans showing air and fluid around laceration

Treatment and Management

+ Administer supplemental oxygen.

+ Ensure adequate hydration.

+ Replace blood volume.

+ Place chest tube.

+ Surgery may be required.

QUICK REVIEW QUESTION

17. A patient with a penetrating injury to the chest has difficulty breathing, shortness of breath, and chest pain. The nurse notices that the patient is becoming more and more uncomfortable and that there is increased dyspnea. What should the nurse assess for?

BLUNT TRAUMA

Pathophysiology

Blunt trauma to the thorax can lead to pulmonary contusion and diaphragmatic injury that in turn disrupt the function of the lungs and other respiratory system anatomy.

Pulmonary contusion is the most common chest injury in trauma and can lead to edema and hemorrhage in the lungs. **Diaphragmatic rupture** can occur as a result of blunt trauma to the thorax. If ruptured, stomach contents can enter the thoracic cavity reducing the ability of the lungs to expand.

Risk Factors

+ MVC (e.g., impact of a car steering wheel against the chest or injury from a seatbelt)

+ assault

+ projectile objects

+ being kicked in chest by large animal

Signs and Symptoms

+ chest wall injury such as abrasion, laceration, or ecchymosis

+ dyspnea

+ hemoptysis

+ hypoxia

+ abnormal chest wall movement

+ abnormal breath sounds or bowel sounds heard in lung fields

Diagnostic Tests and Findings

+ CT scan to diagnose extent of injury

+ chest X-ray not helpful at the time of injury, but changes observable ≥ 8 hours post injury

Treatment and Management

+ Place patient in semi-Fowler position to promote lung expansion.

+ Apply suctioning as needed.

+ Intubation and ventilation may be necessary with larger contusions.

+ Patient should receive chest physiotherapy after acute injury is resolved.

QUICK REVIEW QUESTION

18. A patient presents to the triage area approximately 6 hours after an unrestrained MVC. He reports chest pain, blood in his sputum, and increasing difficulty breathing. What would the nurse anticipate as part of the differential diagnosis of this patient?

TRACHEAL RUPTURE

Pathophysiology

Tracheal rupture (or perforation) occurs when there is injury to the structure of the trachea. The perforation can be caused by forceful or poor intubation efforts or by traumatic injury to the trachea such as in crush injuries or hanging injuries.

Risk Factors

+ penetrating wounds (e.g., gunshots, stabbing)

+ blunt trauma to chest (e.g., MVC)

+ endotracheal intubation

Signs and Symptoms

+ hemoptysis
+ dyspnea
+ diffuse subcutaneous emphysema

Diagnostic Tests and Findings

+ bronchoscopy for definitive method of diagnosis
+ chest X-ray for less obvious tracheal rupture concerns
+ CT scan of the neck if higher sensitivity to tissue injury is needed

Treatment and Management

+ Immediately maintain the patency of the airway.
+ Prepare to suction extra oral or tracheal secretions from the airway.
+ The most common method of treatment is surgical repair.

QUICK REVIEW QUESTION

19. The ED physician is preparing to perform an RSI on a patient who is unconscious. Upon placement of the ET tube, the physician, who has just perforated the trachea, feels a slight pop and a sudden loss of resistance. How would this patient present immediately after this event?

ANSWER KEY

1. The nurse should administer oxygen to the patient, establish IV access, and anticipate drawing blood cultures, collecting sputum culture from the patient, and administering antibiotics.

2. The nurse should prepare to provide oxygen therapy and hydration as needed. The patient is presenting with croup and will be treated with dexamethasone and, in a severe case of croup and airway obstruction, will be treated with racemic epinephrine. The nurse should help reduce the child's anxiety and prevent crying to decrease the likelihood of fatigue.

3. The nurse can offer solutions for symptom management such as adequate hydration, humidification of air in the home, avoidance of irritants that promote cough, and OTC antitussives where appropriate.

4. The nurse should inform the mother that bronchiolitis does not present on X-ray with the same findings as pneumonia. If applicable, the nurse can also tell the mother that the health care team performed labs to rule out common underlying causes of pneumonia and/or to confirm the presence of the viruses that cause bronchiolitis.

5. The nurse should explain that the damage done to the lung tissue of people diagnosed with COPD is often irreversible. However, disease progression can be slowed or halted if the patient stops smoking and adheres to the prescribed regimen of medications and therapy.

6. The nurse should apply oxygen via non-rebreather mask to support the patient's oxygen needs and prepare to administer nebulized albuterol and ipratropium.

7. The nurse should inform the parents that intubation is used as an intervention when pharmacological intervention fails, and it is in the patient's best interest to protect the child's airway and respiratory function.

8. Blood will be aspirated first, followed by any air that is in the chest wall and is displacing lung tissue. Where appropriate and indicated, some hemothorax aspirate can be used for autotransfusion.

9. The nurse should administer oxygen to the patient, place the patient on monitors, and alert the provider of the assessment findings. Soot at mucosal openings is a sign of possible inhalation injury and impeding edema formation in the airway, and early intubation should be considered before the airway closes and a cricothyrotomy is needed.

10. (1) Inspect the airway; (2) suction out any visible foreign bodies; and (3) reassess the patency of the airway. If the airway is still obstructed, the nurse should view directly with a laryngoscope. If all attempts fail, cricothyrotomy must be performed to open the airway.

11. Pulmonary effusion and ARDS differ in which lung structures are affected. In a pulmonary effusion, fluid collects in the pleural space that surrounds the lung and limits the ability of the lungs to expand. In ARDS, pulmonary capillary permeability is compromised, and fluid fills the alveolar sacs within the lungs. The fluid limits the ability of the lungs to exchange oxygen and carbon dioxide.

12. The nurse would suspect tension pneumothorax and should prepare to assist the provider with a needle thoracostomy to relieve the tension and to allow the lung to expand within the thorax.

13. The nurse should be concerned with protecting the patient's airway, but he should also prepare the patient for a chest X-ray to determine if the patient has aspirated after the vomiting. The nurse should also be prepared to suction the patient's airway in case the patient vomits again.

14. The patient should be given oxygen therapy and should be removed to a lower altitude to address the underlying cause of the NPE.

15. The patient with ARDS will have tachycardia, tachypnea, dyspnea, and crackles on auscultation. Measurement of the patient's vital signs will show hypoxia. The nurse should anticipate a chest X-ray to confirm or rule out ARDS.

16. The nurse should strongly suspect possible pulmonary embolism because of the long drive without movement of the lower extremities. As a result, the nurse should prepare for blood tests to include CBC, D-dimer, electrolytes, BUN, and creatinine. The patient will also receive a chest X-ray and CTPA.

17. The nurse should assess for complications related to the penetrating trauma; these complications include pulmonary laceration and hypovolemic shock. At this time the nurse should also be ready to set up a chest tube tray.

18. The health care team should consider several diagnoses for this patient, given his presentation. They should strongly suspect pulmonary contusion, because the patient was unrestrained in an MVC.

19. The patient may have decreased chest rise and fall and may begin coughing and choking on the now-present bloody secretions. Hypoxia will ensue, and other vital signs will also change.

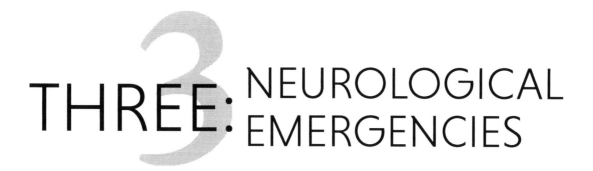

THREE: NEUROLOGICAL EMERGENCIES

Neurological Assessment

PHYSICAL, MENTAL, AND MOTOR ASSESSMENT

+ A short assessment can be done quickly to assess a patient's neurological status. Conduct these assessments for the patient:
  - LOC
  - alertness and orientation
  - PERRLA: pupils equal, round, and reactive to light and accommodation
  - facial symmetry
    + patient's ability to lift eyebrows and smile
  - slurred or incoherent speech
  - muscle tone and coordination
    + bilateral hand squeeze
    + bilateral foot press
    + patient's ability to wiggle fingers and toes
  - response to stimulus (light touch on an area)
    + patient's response or lack of it
    + appropriateness of response
    + patient's ability to name the correct location being touched

+ The **Glasgow Coma Scale (GCS)** is the most commonly used, systematic, objective scoring tool for judging a patient's level of consciousness.

+ Three categories are scored on a numerical scale:
  - eye opening
  - verbal response
  - motor response

+ The sum of the 3 categories is the final GCS score.

+ The lower the patient's score on the GCS, the worse the injury and deficits are:
  - mild: 13 – 15
  - moderate: 9 – 12
  - severe: 8 or less

Table 3.1. Scoring on the Glasgow Coma Scale

Eye Opening (E)	Verbal Response (V)	Motor Response (M)
4 = spontaneous 3 = to sound 2 = to pressure 1 = none NT = not testable	5 = orientated 4 = confused 3 = to words 2 = to sounds 1 = none NT = not testable	6 = obeys command 5 = localizes 4 = normal flexion 3 = abnormal flexion 2 = extension 1 = none NT = not testable

+ The **gag reflex**, controlled by the ninth and tenth cranial nerves, has both a sensory and a motor component.
  ✧ The presence of a gag reflex denotes brain stem function.
  ✧ The nurse should use a tongue depressor or the butt of a long cotton swab to test the gag reflex of a patient.
  ✧ The nurse should never use a finger, as the patient may bite down.

NEURODIAGNOSTIC STUDIES

+ A **lumbar puncture**, also known as a spinal tap, is a diagnostic procedure in which a hollow needle is inserted into the subarachnoid space in the spinal canal between the third and fourth vertebrae and cerebral spinal fluid is aspirated.
  ✧ Encourage the patient to drink water before and after the procedure.
  ✧ Strict aseptic technique and sterile material is required.
  ✧ Support the patient's positioning during the procedure; the patient lies on one side in a curled-spine position with the knees pulled up to the chest and the back exposed.
  ✧ Headache is a common side effect of a lumbar puncture.
  ✧ The patient should remain flat 6 – 12 hours after the procedure; sitting up or standing could induce or exacerbate headache.

+ A **myelogram** is a radiographic diagnostic procedure in which a contrast medium is injected into the spinal column and X-rays or a computed tomography (CT) scan is performed to look for problems such as injury, tumors, and cysts in the spinal cord and connected nerve tissue.
  ✧ The head of the patient's bed should be raised for up to 24 hours after the myelogram.
  ✧ If the contrast medium enters the skull area, it could cause seizures.

+ A **spinal X-ray** uses radiation to allow a view of the bones. It can show if trauma or arthritis is affecting the spinal cord.
  ✧ Make sure the patient has removed any jewelry, eyeglasses, body piercings, or any other metal.
  ✧ Make sure the patient is not pregnant.

+ A **computed tomography (CT or CAT) scan** is a computer-processed combination of many X-rays taken from different angles to produce a cross-sectional view of the body.
  ✧ Make sure the patient has removed any jewelry, eyeglasses, body piercings, or any other metal.
  ✧ Make sure the patient is not pregnant.
  ✧ Make sure the patient has remained NPO for the prescribed amount of time before the procedure.

- If contrast dye is used during the procedure, the nurse assesses the patient for allergic reactions during and after the procedure.
- If contrast dye is used, the nurse alerts the radiologist to any patient history of kidney disease or dialysis, as the contrast dye may cause issues for patients whose kidneys are not functioning properly.

+ **Magnetic resonance imaging (MRI)** is a radiographic diagnostic test that uses strong magnetic fields, electrical field gradients, radio waves, and a computer to produce images of organs, soft tissue, bones, in areas of the body.
    - Make sure the patient has removed any jewelry, eyeglasses, body piercings, or any other metal.
    - Check if the patient has any surgically implanted devices that may contain metal such as pacemakers or heart valves.
    - Make sure the patient is not pregnant.
    - Alert the radiologist to any patient history of kidney disease or dialysis, as the contrast dye may cause issues for patients whose kidneys are not functioning properly.
    - Remind the patient to stay completely still during the entire procedure to obtain the best results.
    - Administer medications (e.g., anti-anxiety medication or pain medication), as prescribed, for patient who might experience difficulty lying on the table for the MRI.
    - Make sure all equipment in the room is MRI compatible; anything that is not may become a projectile as it is magnetized and drawn to the center of the MRI machine.

Altered Level of Consciousness

Pathophysiology

An altered level of consciousness (LOC) is classified as any level or measure of arousal other than a patient's normal baseline. It can be classified as mild, obtunded, stuporous, or comatose. An altered (LOC) can be caused by a variety or a combination of factors that cause chemical alterations in the brain, insufficient oxygen or blood flow to the brain, or excessive pressure in the skull.

Risk Factors

+ cerebral hemorrhage
+ end-stage liver disease
+ hypoglycemia
+ hypoxia
+ playing high-contact sports
+ trauma
+ drug or alcohol use

Signs and Symptoms

+ mild
    - confusion
    - disorientation
    - impaired thinking and responses
    - difficulty following instructions
+ obtunded
    - decreased alertness
    - slowed motor responses
    - lack of awareness of surroundings
    - sleepiness

- stuporous
  - little or no spontaneous activity
  - responses only to painful tactile stimuli
  - sleeplike state, but still conscious
- comatose
  - inability to be aroused by any level of stimulus
  - absent corneal reflex
  - absent gag reflex

Diagnostic Tests and Findings

- CT or MRI to assess for hemorrhage, tumors, or infarcts
- pulse oximetry to test for hypoxemia
- serum glucose levels to test for hypoglycemia
- blood sodium level to assess for hyponatremia, hypernatremia, or dehydration
- CBC to check WBC count to assess for possible infection
- urine drug screen

Treatment and Management

- Treat underlying cause.
  - Administer naloxone (Narcan) if opiate use is suspected.
- Protect patient's airway.
  - Intubation may be necessary if respiratory system is affected.
- Conduct serial neurologic exams to monitor level of consciousness.

QUICK REVIEW QUESTION

1. A patient arrives at the ED by EMS after the family noticed that the patient had begun acting confused. Upon assessment, the nurse notes that the patient has an altered mental status, which the family says is not the person's baseline. What priority interventions should be done for the patient?

Chronic Neurological Disorders
ALZHEIMER'S DISEASE AND DEMENTIA
Pathophysiology

Dementia is a progressive, chronic, irreversible anatomical deterioration of the brain that results in a loss of memory and cognition. Dementia can be classified in several ways, including Alzheimer's versus non-Alzheimer's type. **Alzheimer's disease** is a cognitive deterioration caused by beta-amyloid deposits and neurofibrillary tangles in the cerebral cortex and subcortical gray matter of the brain. Alzheimer's disease is the most common cause of dementia.

Signs and Symptoms

- most notable and first widely recognized sign: loss of short-term memory
- impaired reasoning
- poor judgment

- language dysfunction
    - difficulty recalling commonly used words
    - mixing up words and meanings
- inability to recognize faces and common objects
- behavioral disturbances
    - wandering
    - agitation
    - yelling
    - persecutory ideation

Treatment and Management

- Agitation and aggression are the two most common causes of ED visits for patients with Alzheimer's disease or dementia.
- Aim to identify the underlying cause of the agitation and aggression.
- Assess for the most common causes of agitation and aggression:
    - UTI
    - pain
    - underlying medical condition
    - overload of medications
    - overstimulation
- Antipsychotics or sedatives may be given if patients are seen as a danger to themselves or others.
    - Haloperidol lactate (Haldol) should be used with extreme caution in geriatric patients with Alzheimer's disease.
    - Olanzapine (Zyprexa), administered intramuscularly, is the preferred medication for geriatric patients in acute crises.
    - Lorazepam (Ativan) or diphenhydramine (Benadryl) may be given intramuscularly as well.

QUICK REVIEW QUESTION

2. An elderly patient comes into the ED extremely agitated. The patient's family member says that the patient has been having an increased number of urinary accidents. What specimen should the nurse expect to collect?

AMYOTROPHIC LATERAL SCLEROSIS

Pathophysiology

Amyotrophic lateral sclerosis (ALS), sometimes called Lou Gehrig's disease, is a neurodegenerative disorder that affects the neurons in the brain stem and spinal cord. Symptoms progressively worsen until the respiratory system is affected. ALS is ultimately fatal.

Risk Factors

- most commonly occurs between the ages of 40 and 60 years
- genetic factors
- smoking
- exposure to environmental toxins

Signs and Symptoms

+ progressive asymmetrical weakness
    + can affect both upper and lower extremities
+ difficulty swallowing or eating
+ difficulty walking
+ muscle cramps
+ difficulty speaking or slurred speech

Diagnostic Tests and Findings

+ elevated CPK
+ MRI to rule out spinal cord disease
+ CBC, CMP, and urinalysis to rule out other causes

Treatment and Management

+ ALS has no cure.
+ Treatment is symptomatic.
+ Mechanical ventilation or tracheostomy may be required in later stages.

QUICK REVIEW QUESTION

3. A patient presents to the ED with a recent diagnosis of ALS. What type of weakness would the ED nurse expect the patient to exhibit?

MULTIPLE SCLEROSIS (MS)

Pathophysiology

Multiple sclerosis (MS), a disease of the central nervous system, disrupts the flow of information within the brain, and between the brain and body. Patches of demyelination (the loss of the protective myelin along neurons) in the brain and the spinal cord cause a delay or a failure of signals in the neurological system and lead to neurological deficits. MS has periods of both remission and exacerbation of symptoms, the latter of which leads to gradually growing disability.

Signs and Symptoms

+ paresthesia
    + in one or more extremities
    + in the trunk
    + on one side of the face
    + can occur spontaneously or in reaction to
+ weakness of at least one extremity
+ visual disturbance
    + partial loss of vision and pain in one eye
    + diplopia
+ gait disturbance
+ urinary incontinence
+ vertigo
+ fatigue
+ mild cognitive impairment
+ possible seizures
+ motor disturbances
    + increased deep tendon reflexes
    + positive Babinski sign
    + clonus

Treatment and Management

+ During acute exacerbation, the following medications may be administered:
    ⬧ corticosteroids for inflammation
    ⬧ baclofen (Lioresal) or tizanidine (Zanaflex) for spasticity
    ⬧ gabapentin (Neurontin) or tricyclic antidepressants for pain

QUICK REVIEW QUESTION

4. The nurse is preparing to administer medication to a patient who is in the ED and who has been diagnosed with an acute exacerbation of MS. What medication would the nurse anticipate to administer that will reduce inflammation?

MUSCULAR DYSTROPHY (MD)

Pathophysiology

Muscular dystrophy (MD) is a genetic disorder in which there is a mutation in the recessive dystrophin gene on the X chromosome. MD causes muscle fiber degeneration, which results in progressive proximal muscle weakness.

Signs and Symptoms

+ first noted at 2 – 3 years of age
    ⬧ steady progression of weakness
    ⬧ limb flexion and contraction
    ⬧ scoliosis
+ frequent falls

+ dilated cardiomyopathy
+ conduction abnormalities
+ arrhythmias
+ respiratory insufficiency

Treatment and Management

+ Administer prednisone or deflazacort.
+ Monitor CO_2 levels.
+ Noninvasive ventilator support (e.g., BiPap) may be needed.
+ Elective tracheostomy may be offered.

+ For falls, which are common in children:
    ⬧ Watch for fat embolism if fracture or trauma occurs.
    ⬧ Watch for rapid onset of dyspnea.
    ⬧ Monitor changes in level of consciousness.

QUICK REVIEW QUESTION

5. A patient is being treated for proximal weakness related to MD. The most recent ABG values show a CO_2 level of 32 mmol/L. What intervention should the nurse anticipate?

MYASTHENIA GRAVIS (MG)

Pathophysiology

Myasthenia gravis (MG), an autoimmune disorder that causes cell-mediated destruction of acetylcholine receptors, disrupts neuromuscular transmitters. The disruption results in episodic muscle weakness and fatigue.

A myasthenic crisis is an emergent condition in which MG symptoms rapidly worsen. The weakening of the bulbar and respiratory muscles can cause respiratory failure. Patients with MG are also at risk for a cholinergic crisis if they are given high doses of anticholinesterase medications. The thymus gland is often affected in MG patients.

Risk Factors

+ most common in women aged 20 – 40 years
+ family history of MG
+ excessive stress or fatigue

Signs and Symptoms

+ weakened eye muscles
+ ptosis
+ blurred vision
+ dysphagia
+ myasthenic crisis
    ⋄ dyspnea
    ⋄ pulmonary aspiration
    ⋄ respiratory failure
    ⋄ elevated blood pressure and pulse
    ⋄ no cough or gag reflex
    ⋄ urinary and bowel incontinence

+ dysarthria
+ weakness in arms and legs
+ fatigue
+ cholinergic crisis
    ⋄ dyspnea
    ⋄ respiratory failure
    ⋄ muscle twitching or fasciculation leading to paralysis
    ⋄ decreased blood pressure and pulse
    ⋄ increased salivation
    ⋄ nausea and vomiting
    ⋄ diarrhea

Diagnostic Tests and Findings

+ The Tensilon (edrophonium) test is used to diagnose MG:
    ⋄ Patient is administered the anticholinesterase edrophonium, which inhibits the destruction of acetylcholine and will cause muscle tone to be improved for approximately 5 minutes in MG patients.
    ⋄ Test differentiates between myasthenic crisis and cholinergic crisis.
    ⋄ Patient should be placed on telemetry when being administered edrophonium.
    ⋄ If patient is in a cholinergic crisis, the administration of edrophonium could cause severe bradycardia. For this reason, atropine should be at the bedside when edrophonium is administered.

Treatment and Management

+ For myasthenic crisis:
    ✧ Administer IV fluids.
    ✧ Administer IV immunoglobulin.
    ✧ Administer an anticholinesterase such as edrophonium.
    ✧ The condition can be controlled with medications such as
        • pyridostigmine (Mestinon)
        • steroids
        • muscle relaxants
+ Respiratory failure requires intubation and mechanical ventilation.
+ For cholinergic crisis:
    ✧ Respiratory failure requires intubation and mechanical ventilation.
    ✧ Discontinue anticholinesterase.
    ✧ Administer atropine.

QUICK REVIEW QUESTION

6. A patient suspected of having MG is given a Tensilon (edrophonium) test. What major side effect should the nurse be prepared for?

Guillain-Barré Syndrome

Pathophysiology

Guillain-Barré syndrome is a rare autoimmune disorder in which the immune system attacks healthy cells within the nervous system, rapidly affecting motor function. This disorder is life threatening because of the respiratory depression that can occur when the respiratory muscles are affected. Although there is no cure, treatments are available to improve symptoms and reduce the length of symptoms.

Risk Factors

+ more common in older adults
+ more common in males
+ associated with the campylobacter bacteria acquired by eating undercooked food
+ often developed after a viral illness
    ✧ influenza
    ✧ cytomegalovirus
    ✧ mononucleosis
+ in rare cases, after vaccinations

Signs and Symptoms

+ neuropathy and weakness ascending from lower extremities and advancing symmetrically upward
+ dyspnea because of progression of weakness to respiratory muscles
+ paresthesia in extremities
+ unsteady gait
+ absent or diminished deep tendon reflexes

- autonomic dysfunction:
  - heart block
  - bradycardia
  - hypertension
  - hypotension
  - orthostatic hypotension

Diagnostic Tests and Findings

- electrodiagnostic tests: nerve conduction studies and electromyography
  - slowed nerve conduction velocities in both tests
  - evidence of segmental demyelination in two-thirds of patients undergoing both tests
- CSF analysis
  - increased protein
  - WBC count within normal limits

Treatment and Management

- Treat the symptoms.
- Administer analgesics.
- Administer IV immunoglobulins.
- Patient undergoes plasmapheresis if necessary.
- Patient is intubated if respiratory function is impaired.

QUICK REVIEW QUESTION

7. IV immunoglobulin is the first line of treatment for Guillain-Barré syndrome, but plasmapheresis can also be required. In preparing a patient to begin plasmapheresis, what should the nurse be sure to tell the patient regarding when the plasmapheresis will begin?

Headaches

TEMPORAL ARTERITIS

Pathophysiology

In **temporal arteritis**, the arteries in the temporal area become inflamed or damaged. The inflammation or damage causes the arteries to lose elasticity. The artery walls then become thickened and constrict, causing a narrowing of the lumen in the artery. The result is a reduction in the amount of blood that can flow through the artery.

Risk Factors

- being over 50 years old
- more common in women
- more common in patients of northern European or Scandinavian descent
- excessive use of antibiotics
- history of severe infections

Signs and Symptoms

+ gradual or acute signs and symptoms
+ muscle pain in the jaw or tongue
+ severe, throbbing headache in the temporal or forehead region, combined with scalp pain that is exacerbated with touch
+ systemic symptoms
  ◇ low-grade fever
  ◇ fatigue
  ◇ unexplained weight loss
  ◇ periods of excessive sweating
+ visual disturbances
  ◇ diplopia
  ◇ scotomas
  ◇ ptosis
  ◇ blurred vision
  ◇ loss of vision
    • small period of full or partial blindness in one eye
    • can progress to permanent blindness and may start to affect the other eye

Diagnostic Tests and Findings

+ definitive diagnostic test: biopsy of the temporal artery
  ◇ can be done up to 2 weeks after start of treatment
+ evidence of temporal arteritis in Doppler ultrasound
+ labs
  ◇ elevated ESR
  ◇ elevated C-reactive protein
  ◇ CBC shows anemia

Treatment and Management

+ Administer high-dose corticosteroids such as methylprednisolone.
+ Methotrexate may be given.
+ NSAIDs should be avoided during steroid use to prevent ulcer formation.

QUICK REVIEW QUESTION

8. A patient in the ED is diagnosed with temporal arteritis and is experiencing temporary episodes of blindness in the left eye. What intervention would the nurse anticipate?

MIGRAINE

Pathophysiology

A **migraine** is a neurovascular condition caused by neurological changes that result in vasoconstriction or vasodilation of the intracranial vessels. Chemical changes in the brain stem are believed to trigger migraine attacks.

Risk Factors

+ more common in women
+ family history of migraine
+ changes in sleep patterns
+ sensory stimulation
  ◇ flashing lights
  ◇ strong odors

- stress
- hormonal changes, especially estrogen fluctuations in women
- head trauma
- neck pain
- TMJ pain
- certain foods and drinks (e.g., red wine, aged cheese)

Signs and Symptoms

- intense or debilitating headache lasting from 4 hours to several days
- aura (may occur in the period before the migraine develops)
- typically unilateral symptoms
- nausea and vomiting
- sensitivity to light and sound
- paresthesia

Diagnostic Tests and Findings

- head CT scan with negative findings
- CBC and CMP to check for infection and electrolyte imbalances that could be causing migraine
- urinalysis to check for dehydration

Treatment and Management

- Migraines cannot be cured but can be prevented and managed.
- Administer analgesics.
- Administer antihistamines.
- Administer steroids.
- Administer anti-inflammatories.
- Provide a darkened room for the patient.
- Have the patient apply ice packs to painful area.
- When necessary, start IV fluids for dehydration due to vomiting.
- Administer anti-emetics for nausea and vomiting.
- Discharge teaching:
  - Eliminate triggers such as alcohol, caffeine, and foods with nitrates.

QUICK REVIEW QUESTION

9. A patient presents to the ED with a headache. What signs and symptoms would be indicative of a migraine and would most likely not be present in a patient with a more serious neurological injury?

TENSION HEADACHE

Pathophysiology

Tension headaches are headaches characterized by generalized mild pain without any of the symptoms associated with migraines, such as nausea or photophobia. They can be either episodic or chronic.

Risk Factors

+ sleep disturbances
+ stress
+ TMJ
+ neck pain
+ eyestrain

Signs and Symptoms

+ pain
    ✧ mild to moderate
    ✧ feels like a vise pressing on the head
    ✧ originates in the occipital or frontal area bilaterally
+ episodic
    ✧ occurs fewer than 15 days a month
    ✧ may last 30 minutes to several days
    ✧ typically occurs a few hours after awakening
+ chronic
    ✧ occurs more frequently than 15 days per month
    ✧ constant pain that varies in intensity throughout day

Diagnostic Tests and Findings

+ head CT scan to rule out hemorrhage, lesions, or tumors
+ CBC and CMP to check for infection and electrolyte imbalances that could be causing headache
+ urinalysis to check for dehydration

Treatment and Management

+ Ensure that CT scan is negative before administering NSAIDs.
+ Administer barbiturates or opioids (Fioricet [butalbital, acetaminophen, and caffeine] or morphine) for severe pain.
+ Administer IV fluids to rehydrate.
+ Have patient massage affected area.

QUICK REVIEW QUESTION

10. A patient presents to the ED with a chief complaint of headache that feels like a vise grip. He or she describes being under a great deal of stress lately. What are the priority interventions for this patient?

POST-TRAUMATIC HEADACHE (PTH)

Pathophysiology

Post-traumatic headaches (PTHs) are headaches with an onset within 7 days of a traumatic injury or upon the patient's regaining consciousness after a traumatic injury. They typically resolve within 3 months but can become chronic headaches.

Risk Factors

+ trauma

Signs and Symptoms

+ most commonly resemble migraines
  + pulsating pain
  + nausea and vomiting
  + light and sound sensitivity
  + symptoms worsen with activity

+ occasionally resemble tension headaches
  + nonpulsating pain
  + no nausea or vomiting
  + possible light and sound sensitivity

Diagnostic Tests and Findings

+ CT scan or MRI of head to rule out brain bleed

Treatment and Management

+ No specific medications are indicated for PTHs.
+ Most PTHs are classified and treated as tension headaches or migraines.
+ Administer anti-inflammatories.
+ PTH typically resolves on its own within 3 months.

QUICK REVIEW QUESTION

11. In a patient who does not lose consciousness, how soon after a traumatic head injury would a headache be considered a PTH?

CLUSTER HEADACHE

Pathophysiology

Cluster headaches are characterized by intense unilateral pain in the periorbital or temporal area, with ipsilateral autonomic symptoms. Cluster headaches are usually episodic, lasting from 1 to 3 months, with more than 1 episode of headaches a day. They can go into remission for months to years; for some patients, the cluster headaches never enter a remission period.

Risk Factors

+ primarily affects males
+ age between 20 and 40 years
+ hypothalamic dysfunction

+ alcohol consumption, which can trigger cluster headaches out of remission

Signs and Symptoms

+ headache that happens at the same time each day, often waking the patient at night

+ unilateral pain that always occurs on same side

+ pain that progresses in orbitotemporal distribution
+ intense pain
    ⋄ level can peak within minutes
    ⋄ usually resolves within 30 minutes to 1 hour
+ possible agitation or restlessness
    ⋄ severe restlessness that can lead to bizarre behavior such as banging head on wall
+ autonomic symptoms
    ⋄ nasal congestion
    ⋄ rhinorrhea
    ⋄ lacrimation
    ⋄ facial flushing
    ⋄ Horner syndrome

Diagnostic Tests and Findings

+ no abnormal CT scan or MRI findings

Treatment and Management

+ Give patient 100% oxygen via non-rebreather face mask.
+ Administer analgesic.
+ Anti-inflammatories may be used.
+ Administer IV fluids.

QUICK REVIEW QUESTION

12. A patient in the ED has been diagnosed with an acute cluster headache. The physician orders oxygen therapy. How should the nurse plan to administer the oxygen therapy?

Increased Intracranial Pressure

Pathophysiology

Intracranial pressure (ICP) is the pressure exerted on the skull and brain by the CSF in the subarachnoid space. Normal ICP values vary with age:

+ Adults: 10 – 15 mm Hg
+ Children: 3 – 7 mm Hg
+ Term infants: 1.5 – 6 mm Hg

Increased ICP is an emergent condition that can restrict cerebral blood flow and cause permanent damage to the brain or death. Several underlying conditions can lead to increased ICP. These include an increase in CSF, tumors, trauma, cerebrovascular accidents, hypertension, and infections.

Risk Factors

+ epilepsy
+ seizures
+ hydrocephalus
+ hypertensive brain injury
+ encephalitis
+ lumbar puncture
+ drug use

Signs and Symptoms

+ headache

+ nausea and vomiting

+ increased blood pressure

+ decreased level of consciousness or mental ability

+ diplopia

+ pupils unreactive to light

+ shallow breathing

+ seizures

+ loss of consciousness

+ coma

+ in patients under 12 months old
  ✧ separation of bony plates
  ✧ bulging fontanel

Diagnostic Tests and Findings

+ ICP of 20 mm Hg or higher (for adults)

+ pupils unreactive to light

+ CT scan or MRI
  ✧ may be normal
  ✧ may show abnormality causing the increased pressure (e.g., tumor, infection, or bleed)

Treatment and Management

+ The urgent goal is to reduce the pressure.
  ✧ A shunt is placed through a small hole in the skull (burr hole) or spinal cord.
  ✧ IV mannitol and hypertonic saline are administered.
  ✧ Administer sedatives, if necessary, as anxiety can raise ICP.

+ The following treatments are less common, but are still used:
  ✧ Part of the skull is removed.
  ✧ Patient is placed in a medically induced coma.
  ✧ Hypothermia is induced.

+ The goal is an ICP of less than 20 mm Hg.

+ Cerebral perfusion pressure (CPP) is typically maintained at 70 – 80 mm Hg.
  ✧ CPP is calculated by subtracting the ICP from the mean arterial pressure (MAP): CPP = MAP – ICP.

QUICK REVIEW QUESTION

13. What is the normal ICP, and when is treatment for ICP usually initiated for adults?

Intracranial Hemorrhage

An **intracranial hemorrhage** (or intracranial bleed) is bleeding that occurs within the skull. These hemorrhages are classified according to their location.

EPIDURAL HEMATOMA

Pathophysiology

An **epidural hematoma** occurs when there is bleeding between the skull and the dura mater. Typically, the bleeding occurs from the middle meningeal artery.

Risk Factors

+ trauma

+ skull fractures

Signs and Symptoms

+ characteristic presentation of unconsciousness followed by a coherent "normal" interval and then subsequent rapid deterioration

+ confusion

+ dizziness

+ anisocoria

+ headache

+ nausea and vomiting

+ one-sided oculomotor paralysis

+ contralateral hemiplegia

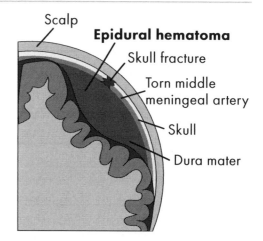

Figure 3.1. Epidural Hematoma

Diagnostic Tests and Findings

+ CT scan may show midline shift or hyperdensities

+ X-rays may show skull fracture

+ MRI showing an area of hematoma

Treatment and Management

+ Maintain patent airway and spinal precautions.

+ Administer IV fluids.

+ Prepare patient for emergent surgery.

+ Monitor for complications:
  ⬥ hydrocephalus
  ⬥ fluid/electrolyte imbalances
  ⬥ seizures

QUICK REVIEW QUESTION

14. A patient is brought in by EMS personnel after sustaining head trauma. They report that the patient was unconscious on scene but is now awake and alert with complaints of a headache and dizziness. The ED nurse should prepare for what priority interventions?

SUBDURAL HEMATOMA

Pathophysiology

A **subdural hematoma** is bleeding that occurs in the subdural space and is usually venous. This type of bleeding may occur immediately after the initial injury or up to weeks afterward.

Risk Factors

+ older age (> 65 years)
+ trauma
+ falls
+ history of bleeding disorders
+ use of anticoagulants
+ alcohol abuse

Signs and Symptoms

+ headache
+ confusion
+ irritability
+ decreased LOC
+ nausea and vomiting

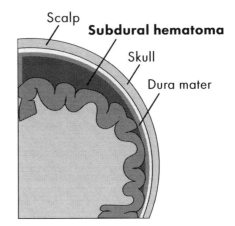

Figure 3.2. Subdural Hematoma

Diagnostic Tests and Findings

+ CT scan may show midline shift or hyperdensities
+ X-rays may show skull fracture
+ MRI showing area of hematoma

Treatment and Management

+ Maintain patent airway and spinal precautions.
+ Administer IV fluids.
+ Smaller or chronic hematomas may require burr holes to drain blood and relieve pressure in brain.
+ Prepare patient for emergent surgery for larger hematomas.

QUICK REVIEW QUESTION

15. A 70-year-old patient presents to the ED with complaints of a headache after falling 2 weeks ago at home. The family says that the patient has been increasingly confused since the fall. In light of the patient's presentation, what type of hemorrhage does the nurse suspect, and what treatment would be anticipated?

SUBARACHNOID HEMORRHAGE

Pathophysiology

A **subarachnoid hemorrhage** is bleeding within the subarachnoid space, which is between the arachnoid membrane and the pia mater. Any patient with a complaint of sudden, severe headache should have a subarachnoid hemorrhage ruled out as the cause.

Risk Factors

+ trauma
+ aneurysms

Signs and Symptoms

+ sudden, intense headache, often described as the worst headache of the patient's life

+ neck pain

+ nausea and vomiting

+ decreased LOC

+ seizures

Diagnostic Tests and Findings

+ CT angiogram showing area of bleeding and arteries within brain

+ MRI showing area of bleeding, surrounding blood vessels, and tissues

+ lumbar puncture may show increased red blood cell counts in all tubes

+ pink or yellow-tinged drainage from lumbar puncture

Treatment and Management

+ Administer pain medications for headaches.

+ Administer anti-emetics for nausea.

+ Administer anticonvulsants for seizures.

+ Prevent increased ICP.

+ Maintain normotensive blood pressure.

+ Prepare patient for emergent surgery to repair bleeding vessels.

QUICK REVIEW QUESTION

16. A patient with a headache presents to the ED. What specific signs and symptoms would lead the nurse to suspect a subarachnoid hemorrhage?

Meningitis

Pathophysiology

Meningitis is an inflammation of the meninges of the brain and spinal cord. The inflammation is caused by infections, usually viral but also bacterial, fungal, or parasitic. Acute meningitis can develop within a few days to a few weeks.

Risk Factors

+ certain age groups more at risk: 0 – 5 years, 15 – 24 years, and > 45 years

+ head injury or brain surgery

+ suppressed immunity (due to medical condition or drug therapy)
  + alcoholism
  + IV drug use
  + previous spleen removal
  + smoking

+ failure to receive the mumps or pneumococcal vaccination

+ living or working with large groups of people
  + college dormitories
  + military housing

+ working with domestic stock animals

+ pregnancy

Signs and Symptoms

+ stiff neck
  - extremely painful to move the neck forward
+ severe headache
+ fever

Diagnostic Tests and Findings

+ CBC showing elevated WBC counts
+ blood culture identifies bacteria
+ MRI or CT scan to note which areas of the brain are inflamed
+ Xpert MTB/RIF test if tuberculous meningitis is suspected
+ CSF analysis (may take a large amount of fluid)
  - aerobic and anaerobic bacterial culture
  - mycobacterial and fungal culture
  - cryptococcal antigen testing
  - antigen or serologic testing
  - special stains
  - cytology

Treatment and Management

+ Ensure standard and droplet isolation precautions until specific cause is determined.
+ Administer corticosteroids.
+ Follow these practices for viral infections:
  - Treat symptoms.
  - Administer IV fluids.
  - Ensure that the patient gets rest.
  - Administer anti-inflammatories.
+ Follow these practices for bacterial infections:
  - Provide prompt treatment with IV antibiotics.
    + Administer penicillin with cephalosporin.
    + For patients resistant to penicillin, administer vancomycin (with or without rifampin), ampicillin, and gentamicin.
  - Practice standard and droplet isolation precautions for at least 24 hours after antibiotic therapy has started for suspected or confirmed meningitis.
+ Follow these practices for fungal infections:
  - Administer amphotericin B and fluconazole (Diflucan).
+ Follow these practices for parasitic infections:
  - Administer benzimidazole derivative or other anthelmintic agent.

QUICK REVIEW QUESTION

17. An 18-year-old college student comes into the ED complaining of a severe headache, a fever, and a stiff neck. On examination, the student is unable to turn his or her head because of stiffness and complains about extreme pain when attempting to move the head forward. What test should the nurse anticipate to prepare the patient for?

Seizure Disorders

TONIC-CLONIC (GRAND MAL) SEIZURES

Pathophysiology

A **seizure** is caused by abnormal electrical discharges in the cortical gray matter of the brain; the discharges interrupt normal brain function. **Tonic-clonic seizures** start with a tonic, or contracted, state in which the patient stiffens and loses consciousness; this phase usually lasts less than 1 minute. The tonic phase is followed by the clonic phase, in which the patient's muscles rapidly contract and relax. The clonic phase can last up to several minutes.

Risk Factors

+ family history of epilepsy

+ brain injury related to head trauma, infection, or stroke

+ sleep deprivation

+ alcohol or drug use or withdrawal

Signs and Symptoms

+ no aura before seizure

+ loss of consciousness

+ falling to ground

+ urinary and fecal incontinence

+ tongue biting and frothing at the mouth

+ initial contraction followed by rapid alternation between contraction and relaxation
    ⬥ usually lasting 1 – 2 minutes

Diagnostic Tests and Findings

+ diagnosis usually based on history of seizure
    ⬥ patients lacking memory of the event (symptoms usually obtained from witnesses)
+ EEG showing abnormal pattern that could help predict probability of another seizure
+ CT scan for those patients with no history of seizure activity to rule out hemorrhage or tumor

Treatment and Management

+ To prevent injury, follow these procedures:
    ⬥ Loosen clothes around the neck.
    ⬥ Place a pillow under patient's head, and remove objects near head.
    ⬥ Roll patient on the left side to avoid aspiration.
    ⬥ Manage patient's airway.
+ Assist with ventilation if it is needed.
    ⬥ Administer oxygen.
    ⬥ Provide mechanical ventilation if it is needed.
+ Administer benzodiazepines, such as diazepam (Valium) or lorazepam (Ativan).
+ Use phenytoin (Dilantin) and carbamazepine (Tegretol) for management.
    ⬥ Blood levels are obtained to ensure levels of these medications are in a therapeutic range.

STATUS EPILEPTICUS

Pathophysiology

Status epilepticus occurs when a seizure lasts longer than 5 minutes or when seizures occur repeatedly without a period of recovered consciousness between them.

Risk Factors

+ history of seizures

+ low levels of antiepileptic drugs in blood

+ low blood sugar

+ brain injury related to trauma, infection, and stroke

Signs and Symptoms

+ seizure activity lasting longer than 5 minutes

+ repeat seizures with no regaining of consciousness between

+ urinary and bowel incontinence

+ clenched teeth

+ irregular breathing

Diagnostic Tests and Findings

+ observation of seizure activity longer than 5 minutes or seizures that repeat without patient's regaining consciousness

Treatment and Management

+ Protect patient from injury.
  ⬦ Do not place objects in or near patient's mouth.

+ Administer benzodiazepines such as diazepam, lorazepam, or midazolam as first-line treatment.

+ Administer levetiracetam (Keppra) or fosphenytoin sodium injection (Cerebyx IV) as second-line treatment.

+ Secure patient's airway.

+ Administer high-flow oxygen.

+ Use sedation and mechanical ventilation as last treatment.

Shunt Dysfunctions

Pathophysiology

Hydrocephalus is treated by placing a shunt inside a brain ventricle to allow for draining of fluid from the brain into another area of the body. A shunt can malfunction when it becomes partly or fully blocked by cells, tissue, or bacterial growth. A shunt can also break down or come apart, or the valve can fail.

Risk Factors

+ more common in pediatric patients
  - 50% of shunts in pediatric patients will experience some degree of dysfunction.
+ bacterial infection in the brain or abdominal area

Signs and Symptoms

+ swelling or redness along shunt tract
+ headache
+ vomiting
+ lethargy
+ irritability
+ confusion
+ gait abnormalities or disturbances
+ seizures
+ urinary urgencies or incontinence
+ special pediatric considerations
  - abnormal head enlargement
  - tense, bulging fontanel

Diagnostic Tests and Findings

+ CT scan or X-ray showing incorrect placement or blockage
+ CBC showing elevated WBC count if there is an infection

Treatment and Management

+ A temporary draining system is put into place until permanent shunt is reinstalled.
+ Surgery is initiated to remove infected or malfunctioning shunt.
+ Measure head circumference to assess for swelling in pediatric patients.

QUICK REVIEW QUESTION

20. How can the nurse assess if a pediatric patient with hydrocephalus and a shunt in place could be experiencing a shunt blockage?

Spinal Cord Injuries

ANTERIOR SPINAL CORD SYNDROME

Pathophysiology

Anterior spinal cord syndrome occurs when the blood flow to the anterior spinal artery is disrupted, resulting in ischemia in the spinal cord. The syndrome typically occurs because of hyperflexion.

Risk Factors

+ trauma
+ spinal cord thrombosis or angioma
+ aneurysms

Signs and Symptoms

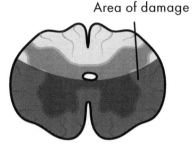

Area of damage

+ complete motor loss below the lesion
+ loss of sensation of pain and temperature below the lesion
+ lower extremities affected more than upper extremities
+ back pain
+ chest pain

Figure 3.3. Anterior Spinal Cord Syndrome

Diagnostic Tests and Findings

+ CT scan and MRI may show spinal cord injury.

Treatment and Management

+ Ensure that patient's spine is immobilized until extent of injury is determined.
+ Maintain patent airway, using jaw-thrust method if necessary to avoid moving neck.
+ Provide supportive treatment.
+ Administer IV fluids.
+ Administer vasopressors if patient is hypotensive.
+ Surgery may be necessary.
+ Steroids may be used in new injuries, but their use is controversial.

QUICK REVIEW QUESTION

21. A patient with a suspected spinal cord injury presents to the ED. What characteristic symptom would lead the nurse to suspect that the patient has an anterior cord injury?

BROWN-SÉQUARD SYNDROME

Pathophysiology

Brown-Séquard syndrome is a type of spinal cord injury caused by complete cord hemitransection. It is typically found at the cervical level.

Risk Factors

+ trauma
+ spinal cord compression
+ disc herniation
+ abscess
+ MS

Signs and Symptoms

+ ipsilateral motor loss below the lesion
+ contralateral loss of sensation of pain and temperature

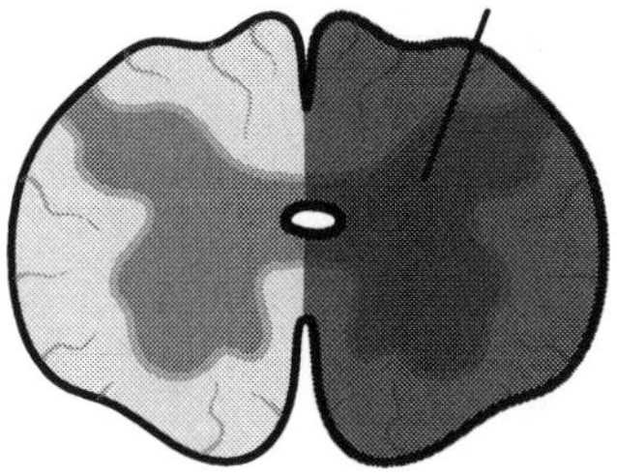

Diagnostic Tests and Findings

+ CT scan and MRI may show spinal cord injury.

Treatment and Management

+ Ensure that patient's spine is immobilized until extent of injury is determined.
+ Maintain patent airway, using jaw-thrust method if necessary to avoid moving neck.
+ Provide supportive treatment.
+ Administer IV fluids.
+ Administer vasopressors if patient is hypotensive.
+ Surgery may be necessary.
+ Steroids may be used in new injuries, but their use is controversial.

Figure 3.4. Brown-Séquard Syndrome

QUICK REVIEW QUESTION

22. A patient with a gunshot wound to the right lower back would exhibit what characteristic sign of Brown-Séquard syndrome?

CAUDA EQUINA SYNDROME
Pathophysiology

Cauda equina syndrome is a type of spinal cord injury typically caused by compression or damage to the cauda equina in the lumbar region. The cauda equina is the nerve bundle that innervates the lower limbs and pelvic organs, most notably the bladder.

Risk Factors

+ herniated discs
+ fractures
+ trauma

Signs and Symptoms

+ sensory loss in the lower extremities
+ bowel and bladder dysfunction
+ severe lower back pain
+ saddle anesthesia (numbness in saddle area)
+ loss of reflexes in upper extremities

Diagnostic Tests and Findings

+ MRI most useful in showing spinal cord injury

Treatment and Management

+ Immediate surgery is necessary.
+ Provide supportive treatment.
+ Administer IV fluids.
+ Administer vasopressors if patient is hypotensive.

QUICK REVIEW QUESTION

23. A patient is being seen in the ED for new onset of leg weakness, back pain, and urinary incontinence. What treatment does the ED nurse anticipate?

CENTRAL CORD SYNDROME

Pathophysiology

Central cord syndrome, the most common type of spinal cord injury, is caused by spinal cord compression and edema, which causes the lateral corticospinal tract white matter to deteriorate.

Risk Factors

+ more common in people > 65 and with degenerative injuries
+ trauma
+ hyperextension injuries

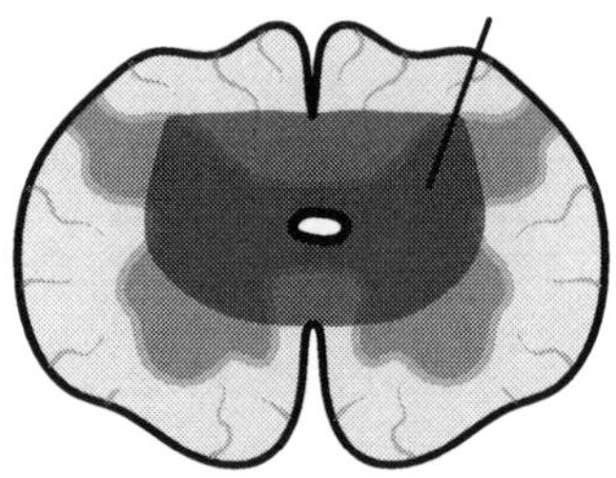

Signs and Symptoms

+ greater motor function loss in the upper extremities than in the lower extremities
+ weakness
+ paresthesia in upper extremities
+ greater deficits in hands

Area of damage

Figure 3.5. Central Cord Syndrome

Diagnostic Tests and Findings

+ CT scan and MRI may show spinal cord injury.

Treatment and Management

+ Ensure that patient's spine is immobilized until extent of injury is determined.
+ Maintain patent airway, using jaw-thrust method if necessary to avoid moving neck.
+ Provide supportive treatment.
+ Administer IV fluids.
+ Administer vasopressors if patient is hypotensive.
+ Surgery may be necessary.
+ Steroids may be used in new injuries, but their use is controversial.

QUICK REVIEW QUESTION

24. What type of motor function loss would be seen in a patient with central cord syndrome?

POSTERIOR CORD SYNDROME

Pathophysiology

Posterior cord syndrome is a rare type of spinal cord injury caused by a lesion on the posterior spinal cord or when the spinal cord artery becomes occluded. It can occur from hyperextension or a disease process.

Risk Factors

+ trauma
+ MS

+ diabetes mellitus
+ neurosyphilis

Signs and Symptoms

+ ipsilateral loss of proprioception, vibration, fine touch, and pressure
+ absent deep tendon reflexes

+ numbness and paresthesia
+ paralysis

Diagnostic Tests and Findings

+ CT scan and MRI may show spinal cord injury.

Treatment and Management

+ Ensure that patient's spine is immobilized until extent of injury is determined.

+ Maintain patent airway, using jaw-thrust method if necessary to avoid moving neck.

+ Provide supportive treatment.

+ Administer IV fluids.

+ Administer vasopressors if patient is hypotensive.

+ Surgery may be necessary.

+ Steroids may be used in new injuries, but their use is controversial.

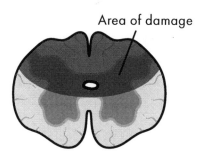

Area of damage

Figure 3.6. Posterior Cord Syndrome

QUICK REVIEW QUESTION

25. A patient with suspected posterior cord syndrome presents to the ED. What priority intervention should the nurse anticipate performing?

NEUROGENIC SHOCK

Pathophysiology

Neurogenic shock is a form of shock caused by an injury or trauma to the spinal cord, typically above the level of T6. Neurogenic shock disrupts the functioning of the automatic nervous system, producing massive vasodilation.

Risk Factors

+ spinal cord injuries at the level of T6 and above

+ epidural anesthesia

+ other anesthesia

+ certain medications
  ⋄ barbiturates
  ⋄ phenothiazine
  ⋄ anti-hypertensives

Signs and Symptoms

+ hemodynamic triad
  ⋄ rapid onset of hypotension
  ⋄ bradycardia
  ⋄ hypothermia

+ wide pulse pressure

+ priapism

+ skin warm, flushed, and dry

Diagnostic Tests and Findings

+ CT scan and MRI may show spinal cord injury.

Treatment and Management

+ Administer IV fluids as first-line treatment.

+ Administer vasopressors and/or inotropes as second-line treatment if hypotension persists.

+ Treat bradycardia with atropine.

+ Ensure that patient's spine is immobilized if spinal cord injury is suspected.

+ Treat underlying cause.

QUICK REVIEW QUESTION

26. What characteristic of neurogenic shock is the opposite of symptoms seen in other types of shock?

AUTONOMIC DYSREFLEXIA

Pathophysiology

Autonomic dysreflexia, an overstimulation of the autonomic nervous system, can follow spinal cord injuries above the T6 level. It occurs when a sympathetic stimulation to the lower portion of the body leads to vasoconstriction below the area of injury, causing cool, clammy skin in that area. This vasoconstriction to lower areas pushes blood to the upper part of the body and causes flushing and sweating in the area above the level of injury.

Risk Factors

+ spinal cord injuries, at the level of T6 and above
+ a full bladder or bowel
+ rapid temperature changes
+ tight, restrictive clothing

Signs and Symptoms

+ flushing and sweating above the level of injury
+ cold, clammy skin below the level of injury
+ bradycardia
+ sudden, severe headache
+ hypertension

Diagnostic Tests and Findings

+ no diagnostic tests available
+ diagnosis based on patient history and physical exam

Treatment and Management

+ Treat underlying cause.
+ Have patient empty the bladder and bowel.
+ Remove tight, restrictive clothing.
+ Administer anti-hypertensives.

QUICK REVIEW QUESTION

27. A patient with a spinal cord injury is experiencing autonomic dysreflexia. They present to the ED with symptoms of hypertension and bradycardia and are sweating above the level of the injury. What should the nurse anticipate as a priority treatment?

Stroke

HEMORRHAGIC STROKE

Pathophysiology

A **hemorrhagic stroke** occurs when a vessel ruptures in the brain or when an aneurysm bursts. The blood that accumulates in the brain leads to increased ICP and edema, which damages brain tissue and causes neurological impairment.

Risk Factors

+ trauma
+ hypertension
+ presence of an AVM
+ taking blood thinners
+ taking oral contraceptives
+ smoking
+ excessive consumption of alcohol
+ cocaine and amphetamine usage

Signs and Symptoms

+ severe, sudden headache
+ sudden onset of weakness
+ difficulty speaking

+ difficulty walking
+ lethargy
+ coma

Diagnostic Tests and Findings

+ CT scan or MRI may show location of bleed.

Treatment and Management

+ Protect patient's airway.
  ⋄ Intubation and mechanical ventilation may be required.
+ Monitor and treat increased ICP.
  ⋄ Keep head of bed at 30-degree angle.
  ⋄ Maintain normotensive blood pressure to reduce cranial pressure.
  ⋄ Administer mannitol IV to reduce increased ICP.
+ Surgery to repair aneurysm may be required.
+ Thrombectomy to remove clots if present may be performed.

QUICK REVIEW QUESTION

28. What is the nursing priority for a patient admitted with a hemorrhagic stroke?

ISCHEMIC STROKE

Pathophysiology

An **ischemic stroke** occurs when blood flow within an artery in the brain is blocked, leading to ischemia and damage to brain tissue. The lack of blood flow can be caused by a thrombosis or an embolus.

Risk Factors

+ history of previous strokes or TIAs
+ atherosclerosis or carotid artery disease
+ history of A-fib
+ hypertension
+ dyslipidemia
+ abdominal obesity

+ diabetes
+ sickle cell disease
+ vasculitis
+ tobacco use
+ cocaine and amphetamine usage

Signs and Symptoms

+ facial drooping, usually on one side
+ numbness, paralysis, or weakness on one side of the body

+ slurred speech
+ inability to speak
+ confusion

- vision changes
- dizziness or loss of balance control
- sudden onset of severe headache
- arm drift may be present

Diagnostic Tests and Findings

- CT scan without contrast to exclude hemorrhage
  - must be done within 25 minutes of arrival at ED
- bedside glucose check to rule out hypoglycemia as cause of symptoms
- CBC and PT/PTT for baseline before administering tPA, if possible
  - immediate administration unless patient has significant history of anticoagulation use
- National Institutes of Health Stroke Scale (NIHSS) to measure patient's neurological deficits
  - predicts severity of stroke
  - scored based on patient's actions during exam
  - 0: lowest score (no deficits)
  - 42: highest score; indicates severe stroke

Treatment and Management

- If CT scan is negative for hemorrhage, tPA should be administered if criteria met:
  - Time is measured from the last time the patient was seen normal.
  - tPA should be administered within 3 – 4.5 hours of this time.
  - tPA dosing is 0.9 mg/kg, with a maximum dose of 90 mg with 10% of dose given as IVP bolus, and the remainder given through infusion.
  - tPA is contraindicated for patients with recent neurosurgery, head trauma, or stroke in previous 3 months.
  - Blood pressure is strictly controlled during tPA administration; it must be kept less than 185 mm Hg systolic and less than 110 diastolic.
  - Monitor patient for signs of bleeding (main side effect of tPA).
- Do frequent neurological checks.
- Monitor blood pressure and heart rhythm.

QUICK REVIEW QUESTION

29. A patient presents to the ED with slurred speech and a left-sided facial droop. What priority interventions should the nurse anticipate?

TRANSIENT ISCHEMIC ATTACK (TIA)

Pathophysiology

A **transient ischemic attack (TIA)**, a sudden, transient neurological deficit resulting from brain ischemia, does not cause permanent damage or infarction. Symptoms will vary depending on the area of the brain affected. Most TIAs last less than 5 minutes and are resolved within 1 hour. A majority are caused by emboli in the carotid or vertebral arteries.

Risk Factors

- older (> 35 years)
- cardiac disorders
  - A-fib
  - history of acute MI
  - infective endocarditis
- diabetes
- obesity
- hypertension
- hypercoagulability
- smoking
- alcoholism

Signs and Symptoms

- usually last less than 1 hour; signs and symptoms similar to stroke
- facial drooping, usually on one side
- numbness, paralysis, or weakness on one side of the body
- inability to speak
- confusion
- loss of vision in one or both eyes
- loss of balance
- dizziness
- sudden, severe headache

Diagnostic Tests and Findings

- most commonly diagnosed retrospectively, according to symptoms
- CT scan to rule out hemorrhage
- diffusion-weighted MRI to rule out infarctions

Treatment and Management

- Focus on identifying the cause and preventing future strokes.
  - Administer antiplatelet medications.
  - Administer statins.
  - Carotid endarterectomy or arterial angioplasty plus stenting may be necessary.
  - Administer anticoagulants.
  - Work with patient to modify risk factors.

QUICK REVIEW QUESTION

30. A patient presents to the ED with complaints of dizziness, headache, and left arm weakness. The patient says these symptoms began about 20 minutes ago and have since improved. The patient has clear speech and answers questions appropriately. What priority interventions should the nurse anticipate?

Traumatic Brain Injury

BASILAR SKULL FRACTURE

Pathophysiology

A **basilar skull fracture** occurs at the base of the skull in either the anterior, the middle, or the posterior fossa. The temporal bone is the most commonly affected. This type of fracture can result in leakage of CSF from the ears or nose.

Risk Factors

+ trauma
+ falls

Signs and Symptoms

+ anterior fossa
  ⋄ anosmia
  ⋄ raccoon eyes
  ⋄ rhinorrhea
  ⋄ epistaxis
  ⋄ leakage of CSF from ears or nose
+ middle fossa
  ⋄ tinnitus
  ⋄ otorrhea
  ⋄ loss of facial sensation
  ⋄ hemotympanum
+ posterior fossa
  ⋄ Battle's sign:
    ⋅ can take up to 24 hours to occur
  ⋄ impaired gag reflex

Diagnostic Tests and Findings

+ Halo test
  ⋄ drop of blood from nose or ear placed onto piece of gauze; if CSF present, a ring or halo will appear around blood
+ X-ray or CT scan of head may show fracture

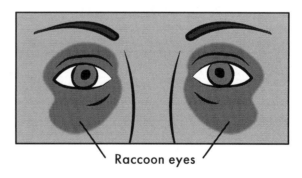

Figure 3.7. Signs of Basilar Skull Fracture

Treatment and Management

+ Fractures typically heal on their own without treatment.

- Patient may be admitted for observation.
- Monitor and prevent increased ICP.
- Patient may require antibiotics.
- Strictly avoid placing anything in patient's nasal cavity. No nasal cannulas, nasogastric tube insertion, or nasal intubation.
- Patient may need surgery if CSF leakage is severe.
- Discharge teaching:
    - Teach patient not to perform activities that increase ICP, such as blowing the nose, sneezing (teach patient how to lessen the force of the sneeze), and bending over to pick things up from the floor.

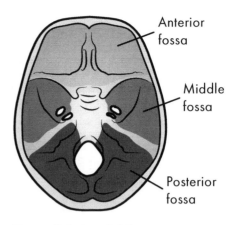

Figure 3.8. Cranial Fossa

QUICK REVIEW QUESTION

31. What characteristic signs would the nurse expect to see in a patient with a basilar skull fracture?

CONCUSSION

Pathophysiology

A **concussion** is a transient and reversible alteration in mental status following trauma to the head. The alteration can last from minutes to anytime less than 6 hours. There are no lesions on the brain, and no neurological residual is noted. Symptoms resulting from short-term injury are temporary and resolve within a few weeks.

Risk Factors

- falls
- motor vehicle accidents
- assault
- participation in sports
    - football, ice hockey, rugby: highest risk rates

Signs and Symptoms

- temporary loss of consciousness: seconds to a few minutes
- confusion
- amnesia
- nausea and vomiting
- headache
- tinnitus
- visual disturbances (e.g., seeing "stars," diplopia, blurry vision)

Diagnostic Tests and Findings

- CT scan rarely abnormal
- GCS mild (14 – 15)

Treatment and Management

+ Usually no treatment is required.

+ Analgesics and anti-emetics may be administered.

+ Discharge teaching:
    ◇ Medication for headaches may be taken.
    ◇ Anti-emetics medication may be taken.
    ◇ Encourage the patient to rest.
    ◇ Advise the patient on restricted activities: no sports, video games, TV, loud music, or intense socialization.
    ◇ Sleep is permitted as needed postconcussion.
    ◇ Patient should be monitored for changes.

QUICK REVIEW QUESTION

32. What findings should the nurse expect for a CT scan of a patient with a concussion?

CONTUSION

Pathophysiology

A **brain contusion** is a bruise of the brain and can be caused by closed or open head trauma. The brain function affected depends on the area of the brain involved and the size of the contusion. Contusions can enlarge hours or days after the initial trauma, leading to neurological deterioration.

Risk Factors

+ falls

+ motor vehicle accidents

+ participation in sports
    ◇ football, ice hockey, rugby: highest risk rates

Signs and Symptoms

+ changes in level of consciousness

+ memory loss

+ behavior changes

+ motor or sensory dysfunction

Diagnostic Tests and Findings

+ CT scan may show hyperdensities from punctate hemorrhages.

Treatment and Management

+ Control bleeding if there is trauma or lacerations.

+ Prevent or reduce swelling in the skull.
    ◇ Monitor blood pressure for hypertension.
    ◇ Monitor sodium levels for hyponatremia.
    ◇ Monitor ABGs for hypercapnia.
    ◇ Surgery may be necessary to reduce ICP.

33. A patient presents to the ED after sustaining head trauma in a motor vehicle accident. What priority diagnostic test should the ED nurse expect to be ordered?

DIFFUSE AXONAL INJURY

Pathophysiology

Diffuse axonal injury (DAI) occurs when there is a widespread damage to axons in the white matter if the soft tissue of the brain rapidly accelerates or decelerates. DAI can also occur secondarily to an initial brain trauma, because of an influx of calcium. The injury can result in edema, which often causes increased ICP. Most patients with severe DAI never regain consciousness.

Risk Factors

+ increased risk for victims of child abuse (shaken-baby syndrome)

+ motor vehicle accidents

+ falls

+ assaults

Signs and Symptoms

+ retinal hemorrhages (seen with shaken-baby syndrome)

+ decreased or complete loss of consciousness

+ decorticate or decerebrate posturing

+ hypertension

+ diaphoresis

+ hyperthermia

+ amnesia

+ confusion

Diagnostic Tests and Findings

+ decreased level of consciousness, typically with a GCS of less than 8
  - ⬦ state may last from hours to months
  - ⬦ patient may never regain consciousness

+ CT scan may show microhemorrhages or small bleeds

+ MRI more useful, but results not always obvious

Treatment and Management

+ Prevent increased ICP.
  - ⬦ Monitor blood pressure for hypertension.
  - ⬦ Monitor electrolytes for imbalances.
  - ⬦ Monitor ABGs for hypercapnia.
  - ⬦ Surgery may be necessary to reduce ICP.

34. With what type of head trauma would the ED nurse expect a DAI to occur in patients?

SECONDARY BRAIN INJURY

Pathophysiology

A **secondary brain injury** occurs after an initial trauma: the initial injury to the brain causes pathological changes of the endogenic neurochemical systems, resulting in secondary injury to the brain. The damage typically occurs anywhere from 12 hours after the initial injury up to approximately 10 days later.

Risk Factors

+ primary brain injuries
    ✧ subdural hemorrhage
    ✧ epidural hemorrhage
    ✧ subarachnoid hemorrhage
    ✧ contusions
    ✧ cerebral lacerations

Signs and Symptoms

+ cerebral edema
+ brain herniation
+ cerebral ischemia
+ hydrocephalus
+ increased ICP
+ hypotension
+ hypercapnia
+ headache
+ nausea and vomiting
+ confusion
+ behavior changes
+ neck pain

Diagnostic Tests and Findings

+ CT scan or MRI may show primary brain injury and/or cerebral edema, herniation, or ischemia.

Treatment and Management

+ Treat underlying cause.
+ Ensure adequate oxygenation and ventilation.
+ Administer IV fluids and vasopressors if patient is hypotensive.
+ ICP monitoring may be done.
    ✧ Administer mannitol IV if ICP is increased.
+ Monitor to prevent neurological damage.
    ✧ Maintain normotensive or slightly elevated blood pressure.
    ✧ Maintain normal glucose levels.
    ✧ Maintain normal body temperature.

QUICK REVIEW QUESTION

35. A patient with a recent contusion from a motor vehicle accident presents to the ED with complaints of headache and dizziness. The patient is found to be hypotensive, with an oxygen saturation of 88% on room air. What priority interventions should the nurse prepare for?

ANSWER KEY

1. A full neurological assessment, including GCS, should be completed. The nurse should expect a CT scan of the head to be ordered to rule out hemorrhage, a urinalysis to rule out a urinary tract infection, a drug panel, an alcohol level, and a CBC and CMP to look for infection and electrolyte imbalances.

2. The nurse should anticipate collecting a urine specimen.

3. A patient with ALS presents with a progressive asymmetrical pattern of weakness that affects both upper and lower extremities.

4. Corticosteroids

5. The nurse should anticipate that the doctor will order noninvasive ventilator support.

6. Administering edrophonium can cause severe bradycardia. The nurse should ensure that the patient is on telemetry monitoring and that atropine is at the bedside.

7. The nurse needs to tell the patient that treatment with plasmapheresis will not start until 2 – 3 days after the last dose of IV immunoglobulin has been given.

8. The nurse should anticipate placing an IV and starting IV methylprednisolone.

9. A patient with a migraine typically will report a history of migraines, have unilateral pain, have photophobia, and experience auras prior to the pain.

10. A neurological assessment should be performed, and the nurse should prepare the patient for a CT scan. An IV line should be placed, labs drawn (CBC, CMP, and urinalysis), and IV fluids administered.

11. The headache would have begun within 7 days after the traumatic injury.

12. The nurse should anticipate administering the oxygen at 100% through a non-rebreather face mask.

13. Normal ICP is between 5 and 15 mm Hg; ICP treatment is usually initiated at 20 mm Hg or above.

14. Because the patient has sustained head trauma, he or she should be placed in spinal precautions and taken for an immediate CT scan of the head/spine. The nurse should closely monitor the patient for subsequent rapid deterioration, which would indicate an epidural hematoma.

15. The increasing change in mental status over the last 2 weeks since the patient fell indicates a subdural hematoma. Priority interventions for this patient include immediate CT scan of the head/neck, protection of the airway, and preparation for surgery.

16. A patient with a subarachnoid hemorrhage typically presents with a sudden, severe headache, often described as the worst headache of his or her life. The patient may also complain of neck pain, nausea, and vomiting. The nurse should prepare the patient for a CT scan of the head/neck and a possible lumbar puncture for diagnosis.

17. The nurse should expect that the physician will order a lumbar puncture to collect CSF.

18. The nurse should be prepared to administer benzodiazepines, such as diazepam or lorazepam.

19. The nurse should anticipate that that patient will be sedated and intubated and that mechanical ventilation will be started.

20. The nurse can measure the head circumference to assess if there is swelling in the cranial area.

21. Patients with anterior cord injuries have a loss of pain and temperature below the lesion. These sensory deficits are usually more pronounced in the lower extremities than they are in the upper extremities.

22. A patient with Brown-Séquard syndrome and a right-sided injury would probably experience right-sided hemiparesis and decreased pain and temperature sensation on the left side.

23. The patient has symptoms indicative of cauda equina syndrome. The ED nurse should expect the patient to have an MRI performed immediately to confirm the diagnosis and then should prepare the patient for immediate surgery.

24. Motor loss is greater in upper extremities than in lower extremities in patients with a central cord injury.

25. Spinal precautions should be maintained until cord injury is ruled out. The nurse should anticipate placing an IV and preparing the patient for an MRI. IV fluids, vasopressors, and steroids may also be administered if necessary.

26. A patient with neurogenic shock typically presents with warm, flushed, and dry skin as compared with other types of shock, which present with pale, cool, and clammy skin.

27. The patient should be checked for bladder or bowel retention and should have any restrictive or tight clothing removed or loosened immediately.

28. The nursing priority is to reduce pressure related to the bleeding and transferring the patient to surgery.

29. The priority intervention for a patient with a suspected ischemic stroke is to get a noncontrast CT scan of the head immediately. After the scan is completed, the ED nurse should conduct a bedside glucose check, place an IV, and draw labs.

30. The nurse should suspect that the patient has had a TIA, in light of symptom presentation. The nurse would anticipate a complete stroke workup, including CT scan of the head, NIHSS, IV placement, lab draw, and admission.

31. The nurse would expect to see raccoon eyes, Battle's sign, hemotympanum, otorrhea, and rhinorrhea in a patient with a basilar skull fracture.

32. The nurse should expect no abnormal findings on the CT exam.

33. Any patient with head trauma should have a CT scan of the head to rule out hemorrhage.

34. A DAI occurs when the head is moved quickly in a back-and-forth motion. Patients with this type of injury have typically experienced trauma or been involved in a motor vehicle accident. Infants may develop DAI after being shaken.

35. A patient with recent head trauma who presents with hypotension and poor oxygenation should be assessed for a secondary brain injury. Oxygenation should be corrected. The nurse should prepare the patient for a CT scan of the head to rule out hemorrhage, herniation, or ischemia. An IV should be placed, and IV fluids and vasopressors administered for hypotension.

FOUR: GASTROINTESTINAL EMERGENCIES

Gastrointestinal Assessment

PHYSICAL ASSESSMENT

+ An initial history of the patient's abdominal pain and symptoms should include:
  - description of the characteristics of the pain
  - length of onset of symptoms
  - family history
  - date of last bowel movement
  - time of last meal eaten
  - medication history, including any recent antibiotic use
  - any history of abdominal surgeries or previous infections

+ A complaint of upper abdominal pain should also have a cardiac origin considered as a possibility.

+ Women, adults over 65, and people with diabetes can present with atypical symptoms when experiencing a cardiac event, one of which is abdominal pain or a complaint of "heartburn" or "indigestion."

+ When a patient presents with a GI complaint, such as abdominal pain, a good rule of thumb is to always consider that the symptom could also be related to the body system *above* (i.e., cardiac) or the body system *below* (i.e., genitourinary).

+ A physical GI assessment should be conducted in the following order:

  1. **Inspection:** Inspection should always be conducted first to visualize the abdomen. Look for distention, bulges, color, hernias, ascites, and/or pulsations.

  2. **Auscultation:** Auscultation should be conducted before percussion or palpation to avoid triggering bowel activity and yielding false bowel sounds. High-pitched gurgling sounds are normal. Auscultate in all 4 quadrants, beginning with the RLQ, and listening for 5 – 35 sounds per minute. Normal bowel sounds can be documented as normal, hypoactive, or hyperactive. Other types of bowel sounds can be heard when auscultating the abdomen:
     + Borborygmi: loud, rumbling sounds caused by shifting of fluids or gas within the intestines; a normal finding
     + High-pitched bowel sounds: often described as tinkling or rushing sounds; may indicate an early bowel obstruction

♦ Absent bowel sounds: an indication of an ileus where no peristalsis is occurring; bowel sounds may be temporarily absent in certain cases (e.g., after surgery), but their absence, combined with abdominal pain, indicates a serious condition.

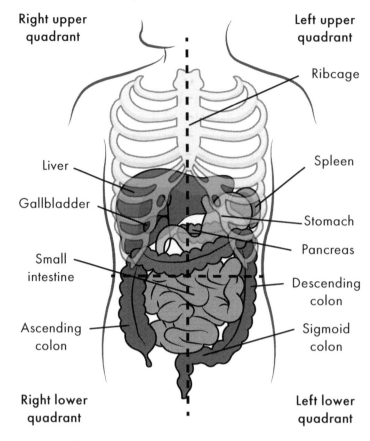

Figure 4.1. Abdominopelvic Quadrants

3. **Percussion:** The nurse percusses the abdomen by tapping on various locations to produce sounds that may give clues toward underlying problems. Tympany (air) sounds are normal, and dull sounds are heard over solid organs (liver and spleen).

4. **Palpitation:** Palpitation should be done last, as it may elicit pain and prevent any further assessment. Check for guarding, rigidity, masses, and/or hernias. Start from an area furthest away from the pain, and move toward the most painful area.

Table 4.1. GI Signs

Name	Description	Indication
Kehr's sign	Left shoulder pain caused when blood below the diaphragm irritates the phrenic nerve	Splenic rupture
Rovsing's sign	Pain in the RLQ with palpation of LLQ (indicates peritoneal irritation)	Appendicitis
Cullen's sign	A bluish discoloration to the umbilical area	Retroperitoneal hemorrhage
Grey-Turner's sign	Ecchymosis in the flank area	Retroperitoneal hemorrhage
Psoas sign	Abdominal pain when right hip is hyperextended	Appendicitis, Crohn's disease
McBurney's point	RLQ pain at point half way between umbilicus and iliac spine	Appendicitis

Name	Description	Indication
Murphy's sign	Cessation of inspiration when RUQ is palpated	Acute cholecystitis
Markle test (heel drop)	Pain caused when patient stands on tiptoes and drops heels down quickly or when patient hops on one leg	Appendicitis, peritonitis

DIAGNOSTIC STUDIES

+ A CT scan produces multiple images of a body part.
  + This exam is quick and painless and is frequently used to diagnose or rule out a cause of abdominal pain.
+ X-rays use a form of radiation to help produce images that can visualize the bowel, bones, and calcifications.
  + Free air, gas, obstructions, foreign bodies, dilatation, fractures, contrast, and surgical clips can all be visualized on X-rays.
+ Ultrasound uses sound waves to visualize blood flow.
  + This tool is frequently used to visualize the gallbladder, liver, pancreas, spleen, and abdominal aorta.
+ Focused assessment sonography for trauma (FAST) exam is a quick bedside exam that uses ultrasound to assess for bleeding after trauma.

Boerhaave's Syndrome

Pathophysiology

Boerhaave's syndrome occurs when the esophageal wall ruptures because of forceful vomiting. This perforation of the esophageal wall may ultimately cause sepsis or other complications.

Risk Factors

+ forceful vomiting
+ excessive eating
+ any activity that causes increased pressure to the esophagus

Signs and Symptoms

+ severe vomiting
+ chest pain
+ tachycardia
+ shock due to blood loss

Diagnostic Tests and Findings

+ free air in mediastinum visible on chest X-ray
+ perforation visible on CT scan

Treatment and Management

+ Immediate endoscopy or surgery to repair esophageal wall may be required.

+ Administer antibiotics.

QUICK REVIEW QUESTION

1. A patient presents to the ED with complaints of chest pain after repeated violent episodes of vomiting after eating at a buffet. The patient is diagnosed with Boerhaave's syndrome, which is confirmed by CT scan. What interventions should the ED nurse prioritize?

Mallory-Weiss Syndrome

Pathophysiology

Mallory-Weiss syndrome is characterized by small tears that occur at the gastroesophageal junction from persistent and forceful vomiting. This condition is usually less severe than Boerhaave's syndrome, and the bleeding typically stops on its own.

Risk Factors

+ vomiting
+ alcohol abuse
+ frequent use of NSAIDs
+ bulimia

+ pregnancy
+ trauma
+ lifting or straining

Signs and Symptoms

+ vomiting
+ hematemesis

+ hematochezia

Diagnostic Tests and Findings

+ endoscopy for diagnosis of bleed

Treatment and Management

+ Maintain airway patency.
  ⋄ The patient is at risk for aspiration because of bleeding.
  ⋄ Suction as needed.
+ Bleeding is usually minor, and treatment is conservative.

+ Administer IV proton pump inhibitor.
+ Administer antiemetics as needed.
+ Cauterization may be needed to stop the bleeding if it is persistent.

QUICK REVIEW QUESTION

2. What would be a priority intervention for a patient who presents to the ED and is diagnosed with Mallory-Weiss syndrome?

Cirrhosis

Pathophysiology

Cirrhosis is a chronic disease in which the liver has permanent scarring and loses cells. The condition impairs the liver's normal functions, which include filtering blood and harmful by-products. Cirrhosis can also decrease blood flow to the liver; the resulting portal hypertension can lead to related conditions, including an enlarged spleen and esophageal varices.

Risk Factors

+ alcohol abuse

+ hepatitis

+ fatty liver disease

+ obesity

Signs and Symptoms

+ bleeding and bruising easily

+ pruritus

+ jaundice

+ ascites

+ nausea

+ spiderlike angiomas

+ confusion and lethargy in presence of hepatic encephalopathy

+ asterixis

+ scratch marks

+ clubbing of nails

+ palmar erythema

Diagnostic Tests and Findings

+ elevated ammonia levels

+ elevated AST, ALT, and/or bilirubin

+ decreased protein, albumin, and fibrinogen

+ decreased WBCs, H/H, and platelets

+ longer PT and PTT, and increased INR

+ CT scan or MRI may show hardening and scarring of liver

Treatment and Management

+ Recommend alcohol cessation.

+ Provide patient with information on weight loss.

+ Have patient begin thiamine and folic acid replacement.

+ Have patient avoid NSAIDs.

+ Avoid giving the patient injections because of risk of bleeding.

+ Administer vitamin K, FFP, and platelets, as needed.

+ Administer lactulose for elevated ammonia levels.

QUICK REVIEW QUESTION

3. A patient presents to the ED with a history of liver failure, alcohol abuse, hypertension, and hyperlipidemia. The patient is confused and appears jaundiced, and the abdomen reveals ascites. What other assessment findings would also be expected in this patient?

Esophageal Varices

Pathophysiology

Esophageal varices occur when the veins in the esophagus dilate and rupture from the pressure caused when liver disease obstructs venous flow and builds up pressure in the veins. Substantial bleeding can occur from varices, making this condition life threatening.

Risk Factors

+   liver disease
+   cirrhosis

+   alcohol abuse
+   portal hypertension

Signs and Symptoms

+   hematemesis
+   melena

+   dizziness
+   hypovolemic shock

Diagnostic Tests and Findings

+   PT and aPTT may be longer
+   decreased H/H
+   decreased platelet counts

+   abdomen ultrasound or CT scan to diagnose varices and visualize areas of bleeding, the liver, and portal veins

Treatment and Management

+   Manage bleeding.
+   Conduct labs:
    ⋄   Monitor H/H every 6 hours for blood loss.
    ⋄   Determine blood type, and crossmatch in preparation for possible blood transfusion.
+   Endoscopy with possible band ligation to tie off bleeding veins may be necessary.

+   Establish an octreotide (Sandostatin) drip to decrease portal pressure.
+   Administer vasopressors if patient is hypotensive.
+   Insert Sengstaken-Blakemore tube to stop or slow bleeding.

QUICK REVIEW QUESTION

4. The physician has ordered an octreotide drip for a patient diagnosed with esophageal varices. The ED nurse knows that this medication is appropriate for this diagnosis because it has what type of action?

Foreign Bodies in the GI System

Pathophysiology

A **foreign body** is any object that enters the GI system either intentionally or accidently. Foreign bodies within the GI system typically present as partial or full obstructions of the esophagus, although objects may also pass to other GI organs. These objects can cause damage, including tears, infection, and obstruction, to the GI system. Objects may pass on their own, be removed with endoscopy, or may require surgery.

Risk Factors

+ children at risk by swallowing objects such as coins or large pieces of food such as grapes
+ obstruction in adults usually caused by meat and bones
+ older adults more susceptible to foreign body aspiration

Signs and Symptoms

+ difficulty swallowing
+ drooling
+ feeling of something "stuck" in throat
+ subcutaneous emphysema present if esophageal perforation

Diagnostic Tests and Findings

+ chest X-ray and neck X-rays

Treatment and Management

+ Priority consideration should always be to maintain the patient's airway.
+ Administer glucagon to promote smooth muscle relaxation.
+ Endoscopy may be required to remove object.

QUICK REVIEW QUESTION

5. A patient presents to triage with complaints of feeling as if something is lodged in her throat after eating dinner. What is the priority intervention for a patient with a foreign body?

Lower GI Bleeding

Pathophysiology

A **lower GI bleed** is any bleeding that occurs below the duodenum. Lower GI bleeds occur less frequently than do upper GI bleeds.

Risk Factors

+ polyps
+ cancer

+ colitis

+ diverticulitis

+ IBS

+ hemorrhoids

+ perirectal abscess

Signs and Symptoms

+ abdominal pain

+ hematochezia

+ fatigue

+ syncope

+ tachycardia

+ hypotension (late sign occurring after significant blood loss)

Diagnostic Tests and Findings

+ positive hemoccult

+ decreased H/H

+ PT and aPTT may be longer

+ colonoscopy for diagnosis

Treatment and Management

+ Conduct labs:
  + Monitor H/H every 6 hours for blood loss.
  + Determine blood type, and crossmatch to prepare for possible blood transfusion.

+ Run CMP to monitor for dehydration and electrolyte imbalances.

+ Administer stool guaiac test.

+ Blood transfusion may be required.

QUICK REVIEW QUESTION

6. A patient presents to the ED with a lower GI bleed. What signs and symptoms would the ED nurse expect to see in this patient?

Upper GI Bleeding

Pathophysiology

An **upper GI bleed** is bleeding that occurs between the esophagus and duodenum.

Risk Factors

+ duodenal and gastric ulcers

+ gastric erosions

+ Mallory-Weiss syndrome

+ esophagitis

+ use of NSAIDs

Signs and Symptoms

+ hematemesis

+ melena

- "coffee-ground" emesis
- weakness
- dizziness
- tachycardia

- syncope
- hypotension
- hypovolemic shock from blood loss

Diagnostic Tests and Findings

- longer PT and aPTT
- decreased H/H
- hemoccult positive

- abdominal X-ray may show free air if ulcer perforation present

Treatment and Management

- Establish 2 large-bore IVs.
- Conduct labs:
    - Monitor H/H every 6 hours for blood loss.
    - Determine blood type, and crossmatch in preparation for possible blood transfusion.
    - Run BUN/creatinine to monitor for dehydration.
- Blood transfusion may be necessary.
- Conduct an abdominal CT scan to detect areas of active bleeding.
- Endoscopy may be necessary.
- Administer a proton pump inhibitor, or establish an octreotide drip.

QUICK REVIEW QUESTION

7. What medications would be a contributing factor to an upper GI bleed?

GI Inflammation

GASTROENTERITIS

Pathophysiology

Gastroenteritis is an inflammation of the stomach and intestines. The cause can be bacterial (e.g., *Salmonella*, *E. coli*, *C. difficile*), viral, or parasitic. Typically, the onset of symptoms is rapid.

Risk Factors

- food poisoning
- viruses

- parasites
- infants, children, and adults > 65

Signs and Symptoms

- nausea and vomiting

- diarrhea

- ✦ diffuse and cramping abdominal pain
- ✦ fever
- ✦ dehydration

Diagnostic Tests and Findings

- ✦ Chemistry panel may show decreased electrolytes from vomiting and/or diarrhea.
- ✦ CBC may show increased WBCs.
- ✦ BUN may be higher if the patient is dehydrated.
- ✦ Bowel sounds are hyperactive.
- ✦ Stool culture may be positive for ova and/or parasites.
- ✦ Urinalysis may show increased osmolality if the patient is dehydrated.

Treatment and Management

- ✦ Electrolyte replacement may be necessary.
- ✦ Administer antiemetics as needed.
- ✦ At discharge, give the patient dietary guidance:
  - ✧ Recommend BRAT diet or other easy-to-digest foods.
- ✦ Administer anticholinergics (to help slow down peristalsis):
  - ✧ dicyclomine (Bentyl)
  - ✧ hyoscyamine (Levsin)
- ✦ Conduct a PO challenge.

QUICK REVIEW QUESTION

8. A patient presents to the ED with nausea, vomiting, and diarrhea for the last 24 hours. The patient is diagnosed with gastroenteritis and is rehydrated with fluids. Upon discharge, the patient should be taught to slowly reintroduce which foods back into his or her diet first?

PERITONITIS

Pathophysiology

Peritonitis is inflammation of the peritoneum (the lining of the abdominal cavity). The inflammation can be caused by a blood-borne organism or from the perforation of an organ. The perforation allows the contents to spill into the peritoneal cavity, causing infection.

Risk Factors

- ✦ trauma
- ✦ organ rupture (e.g., appendix, pancreas, gallbladder)

Signs and Symptoms

- ✦ rigid abdomen
- ✦ fever
- ✦ diffuse pain
  - ✧ usually worsens with movement
  - ✧ relieved by flexing the knees or bending right hip
- ✦ guarding of abdomen, and rebound tenderness

Diagnostic Tests and Findings

+ CT scan or X-ray may show free air or perforation of organ.

+ Markle test is positive.

+ CBC may show increased WBCs because of infection.

Treatment and Management

+ The patient must be kept NPO.

+ Administer broad-spectrum antibiotics (e.g., piperacillin/tazobactam [Zosyn]).

+ Administer antiemetics.

+ Administer analgesics.

+ Prepare the patient for surgery.

QUICK REVIEW QUESTION

9. A patient presents to the ED with severe abdominal pain, guarding, and a fever (temperature, 38.6°C [101.5°F]). The CT scan shows peritonitis from a ruptured appendix. What should be the priority intervention for this patient?

APPENDICITIS

Pathophysiology

Appendicitis is inflammation of the appendix. Obstruction of the appendiceal lumen results in a decrease in blood supply which can lead to necrosis and perforation.

Risk Factors

+ more common in males < 30

+ inflammatory bowel disease (e.g., Crohn's disease or ulcerative colitis)

Signs and Symptoms

+ abdominal pain
    ⬦ dull, steady periumbilical pain
    ⬦ RLQ pain that worsens with movement
    ⬦ pain in RLQ at McBurney's point
+ positive Rovsing's sign

+ positive psoas sign

+ fever

+ anorexia

+ nausea and vomiting

+ rebound tenderness

+ abdominal rigidity

Diagnostic Tests and Findings

+ CT scan is the most precise exam to diagnosis appendicitis.
    ⬦ may show inflammation and/or perforation
+ WBCs may be elevated.

Treatment and Management

+ Keep the patient NPO.

+ Administer analgesics.

+ Administer antiemetics.

+ Administer antibiotics.

+ Prepare the patient for surgery.

QUICK REVIEW QUESTION

10. A patient presents to the ED with RLQ pain, nausea, and vomiting. The patient is diagnosed with appendicitis. What priority interventions should the nurse prepare for?

CHOLECYSTITIS

Pathophysiology

Cholecystitis, acute or chronic inflammation of the gallbladder, usually results from impacted stone in the neck of the gallbladder or in the cystic duct. **Cholelithiasis** is the presence of gallstones in the gallbladder.

Risk Factors

+ the 5 Fs for cholecystitis:
    ◇ Fair (more prevalent in the Caucasian population)
    ◇ Fat (BMI > 30)
    ◇ Female (occurs more often in females than in males)
    ◇ Fertile (one or more children) or pregnant
    ◇ Forty (age > 40)

Signs and Symptoms

+ RUQ pain, which can radiate to back or right shoulder
    ◇ common after eating high-fat meal

+ colicky pain

+ positive Murphy's sign

+ jaundice if obstruction is significant
    ◇ look for jaundice in sclera of eye or inside mouth

+ nausea and vomiting

+ anorexia

+ flatulence

+ atypical symptoms in older patients and patients with type 2 diabetes
    ◇ confusion
    ◇ lack of pain

Diagnostic Tests and Findings

+ increased WBCs, liver enzymes (AST and ALT), and bilirubin

+ elevated amylase and/or lipase may indicate a stone blocking a duct and causing pancreatitis

+ ultrasound: the preferred diagnostic test

Treatment and Management

+ Perform a CT scan of the abdomen to visualize ducts and to monitor for perforation or abscess.

+ Endoscopic retrograde cholangiopancreatography (ERCP) may be performed to remove stones if they are present in the common bile duct.

+ Keep the patient NPO.

+ Administer analgesics.

+ Administer antiemetics.

+ Administer antibiotics.

+ At discharge, teach patient to avoid high-fat foods.

QUICK REVIEW QUESTION

11. Which laboratory test values would the ED nurse expect to see elevated in a patient diagnosed with acute cholecystitis?

DIVERTICULITIS

Pathophysiology

Diverticulitis is inflammation of the diverticula (small outpouchings in the GI tract, usually in the sigmoid colon); the inflammation can cause necrosis and perforation. **Diverticulosis** (also called diverticular disease) is the presence of diverticula without inflammation.

Risk Factors

+ obstruction of diverticula by fecal material or undigested food

Signs and Symptoms

+ LLQ abdominal pain

+ rebound tenderness

+ abdominal distention

+ anorexia

+ nausea and vomiting

+ fever

+ change in bowel habits (diarrhea or constipation)

+ hematochezia

Diagnostic Tests and Findings

+ CBC showing increased WBCs

+ CT scan of abdomen to diagnose or rule out perforation

+ electrolytes monitoring for imbalances

Treatment and Management

+ Administer antibiotics, such as metronidazole (Flagyl) or ciprofloxacin (Cipro).

+ Administer electrolytes as needed.

+ Have patient remain on liquid diet until pain improves.

- Surgery may be necessary if diverticula rupture.
- At discharge, teach patient some practices to prevent a reoccurrence:
    - Recommend stool softeners.
    - Recommend a liquid diet followed by a low-fiber diet until the inflammation is reduced, then a high-fiber diet to prevent straining.

QUICK REVIEW QUESTION

12. A patient diagnosed with diverticulitis has had multiple emergency visits over the past year. What information can the ED nurse implement at discharge to help prevent a reoccurrence?

ESOPHAGITIS

Pathophysiology

Esophagitis is an inflammation of the esophagus. A determination of the cause of esophagitis will guide treatment.

Risk Factors

- reflux
- infections
- medications
- radiation
- ingestion of a caustic substance

Signs and Symptoms

- burning pain within an hour of eating
- sore throat
- pain worsens with increased intra-abdominal pressure (bending, sneezing, lying flat)

Diagnostic Tests and Findings

- diagnosis typically made through a thorough history and physical

Treatment and Management

- Ensure airway patency.
- Elevate the head of the bed to reduce reflux.
- Administer antacid, lidocaine, and anticholinergic (GI "cocktail").
- Administer proton pump inhibitors or H_2 blockers.
- At discharge, teach preventative measures:
    - Stop smoking.
    - Avoid eating or drinking within 1 – 2 hours of bedtime.
    - Avoid foods and beverages that relax the lower esophageal sphincter; these include alcohol, spicy foods, chocolate, and coffee.

QUICK REVIEW QUESTION

13. A patient arrives at the ED with complaints of a sore throat with burning pain. What interventions can the nurse provide to the patient to reduce symptoms while the patient is in the ED?

GASTRITIS

Pathophysiology

Gastritis is the inflammation or irritation of the stomach lining. Without treatment, gastritis can lead to ulcers or GI bleeding.

Risk Factors

+ *Heliobacter pylori* infection

+ stress

+ smoking

+ NSAID use

+ alcohol abuse

Signs and Symptoms

+ epigastric pain

+ nausea and vomiting

+ diarrhea

+ poor appetite

Diagnostic Tests and Findings

+ diagnosis typically made through a history and physical examination

+ endoscopy to visualize inflammation in the stomach

+ positive *H. pylori* infection

Treatment and Management

+ Administer antiemetics.

+ Electrolyte replacement may be needed.

+ Administer H_2 blockers (e.g., ranitidine [Zantac]) to block acid production.

+ Administer antacids (e.g., aluminum hydroxide, magnesium hydroxide [Maalox]) to help neutralize stomach acid.

+ Administer proton-pump inhibitors (e.g., lansoprazole [Prevacid]) to shut down the acid pump in the stomach.

+ At discharge, teach preventative measures:
  ⬦ Avoid NSAIDs, alcohol, and spicy foods.
  ⬦ Eat small meals.
  ⬦ Elevate the head of the bed when sleeping.

PANCREATITIS

Pathophysiology

Pancreatitis is caused by the release of digestive enzymes into the tissues of the pancreas. The condition causes autodigestion, inflammation, tissue destruction, and injury to adjacent structures and organs. It can be acute or chronic, and its onset is usually sudden.

Risk Factors

+ Use the mnemonic **BAD HITS** to recall the causes of pancreatitis:
    ◇ **B**iliary (e.g., gallstones blocking pancreatic duct)
    ◇ **A**lcohol
    ◇ **D**rugs (thiazide diuretics, sulfa drugs, pentamidine, antiretrovirals)
    ◇ **H**ypertriglyceridemia/hypercalcemia
    ◇ **I**diopathic causes
    ◇ **T**rauma
    ◇ **S**corpion sting or surgery (recent ERCP or abdominal surgery)

Signs and Symptoms

+ inability to digest fats, proteins, and/or carbohydrates
+ dull and steady pain, usually in LUQ
+ guarding
+ nausea and vomiting
+ anorexia
+ fever
+ tachycardia

Diagnostic Tests and Findings

+ elevated amylase and lipase
+ elevated glucose
+ CBC and CMP may show increased WBCs, electrolyte imbalances
+ elevated AST and ALT
+ CT scan to diagnose

Treatment and Management

+ Control pain.
    ◇ Avoid morphine because of spasms in the sphincter of Oddi.
+ Keep the patient on NPO.
+ Monitor patient's glucose levels.
+ Monitor for complications:
    ◇ ARDS
    ◇ atelectasis
    ◇ retroperitoneal bleeding

QUICK REVIEW QUESTION

15. A patient presents to the ED with a history of gallstones, and the nurse suspects pancreatitis. What assessment findings would the nurse expect to see in this patient?

GI Trauma

Pathophysiology

GI trauma can be caused by a penetrating injury such as a gunshot or knife wound or can be caused by blunt trauma from a motor vehicle injury or a fall.

Table 4.2. Types of Gastrointestinal Trauma

Organ	Pathophysiology	Signs and Symptoms	Diagnostic Tests and Findings	Treatment and Management
Spleen	Most frequently injured abdominal organ	+ LUQ pain (referred to left shoulder) + LUQ bruising + Distended abdomen	CT scan or FAST exam may show splenic rupture	+ Surgery is indicated. + Administer vasopressors if patient has signs of hypotensive shock.
Liver	+ Largest abdominal organ + Injury most frequently caused by blunt trauma	+ RUQ pain (referred to right shoulder) + RUQ bruising + Rigid abdomen	CT scan may show laceration or hemorrhage	+ Surgery for hemodynamically unstable patients is indicated. + Nonoperative management of stable patients includes establishing IV access, administering IV fluids, and monitoring labs.
Pancreas	Most frequently missed abdominal injury with a high mortality rate	+ Epigastric pain + Rebound tenderness + Elevated pancreatic enzymes	+ CT for diagnosis + Testing for elevated pancreatic enzymes can be delayed in bloodwork up to 6 hours	+ Keep patient NPO. + Control hemorrhage. + For severe injury, surgery is required.
Stomach	Most commonly caused by a penetrating injury	+ Hematemesis + Rigid abdomen + Rebound tenderness	Free air on chest X-ray	Surgery is required.

QUICK REVIEW QUESTION

16. A patient presents to the ED with a penetrating injury to the abdomen. What type of objects could have caused this type of injury?

Hepatitis

Pathophysiology

Hepatitis is a systemic viral disease characterized by inflammation of the liver. There are different types of this disease. Some types resolve without treatment, and others can become chronic illnesses.

Risk Factors

+ Epstein-Barr virus

+ cytomegalovirus

+ specific to type of hepatitis (see table 4.3)

Signs and Symptoms

+ clay-colored stools

+ dark urine (foamy)

+ jaundice

+ steatorrhea

+ flulike symptoms

+ abdominal pain

Diagnostic Tests and Findings

+ elevated liver enzymes (AST and ALT)

+ elevated alkaline phosphatase

+ elevated ammonia

+ low albumin

Treatment and Management

+ Administer lactulose for elevated ammonia levels.

+ At discharge, teach preventative measures:
   ◇ Avoid alcohol.
   ◇ Take small, frequent meals that are low in fat and high in carbohydrates.
   ◇ Avoid steroid medications.
   ◇ Avoid acetaminophen (Tylenol).
   ◇ Always practice proper hand hygiene.
   ◇ Practice safe sex.

Table 4.3. Types of Hepatitis

Hepatitis Type	Route	Comments	Discharge Teaching	Treatment and Management
A	Fecal/oral	+ Vaccine available + Causes epidemic + Short-term illness	+ Wash hands thoroughly after using bathroom. + Avoid handling food eaten by others.	Recommend rest and hydration.
B	Blood/body fluids	+ Vaccine available + Can be acute or chronic	+ Do not donate blood, organs, or other tissue. + Practice protected sex. + Do not share personal items such as toothbrush or razor.	Administer antivirals.

Hepatitis Type	Route	Comments	Discharge Teaching	Treatment and Management
C	Blood/body fluids	+ No vaccine available + Can be acute or chronic + Antivirals available	+ Do not donate blood, organs, or other tissue. + Practice protected sex. + Do not share personal items such as toothbrush or razor.	+ Administer antivirals. + Chronic patients may need liver transplant.
D	Blood/body fluids	+ Occurs simultaneously with hepatitis B + Preventable with hepatitis B vaccine	+ Do not donate blood, organs, or other tissue. + Practice protected sex. + Do not share personal items such as toothbrush or razor.	+ No antivirals are available. + Prevention is key.
E	+ Fecal/oral + Contaminated fish/water	More common in Asia, Mexico	+ Wash hands thoroughly after using bathroom. + Avoid handling food eaten by others.	+ No antivirals are available. + Prevention is key.

Hepatitis A and E are the 2 types transmitted through the fecal/oral route. Remember this mnemonic: the **vowels** hit your **bowels**!

QUICK REVIEW QUESTION

17. A patient presents to the ED with complaints of clay-colored stools; dark, foamy urine; abdominal pain; and flulike symptoms. What factors would contribute to the patient's diagnosis of hepatitis?

Hernia

Pathophysiology

A **hernia** occurs when a portion of the abdominal contents protrudes through the abdominal wall. Common areas for hernias are epigastric, umbilical, inguinal, and femoral. To determine treatment, medical personnel must determine whether the hernia has a good blood supply or is incarcerated (trapped).

Incarcerated inguinal hernias may become strangulated (cut off from blood supply), resulting in ischemia in the trapped tissue. An **incarcerated inguinal hernia** with ischemia is an emergent condition that can lead to bowel necrosis, sepsis, and neurogenic shock.

Risk Factors

+ more common in males
+ heavy lifting
+ straining
+ obesity

Signs and Symptoms

+ pain at hernia site
+ swelling at hernia site, usually a firm, tender mass
+ nausea and vomiting
+ strangulation hernia
  ✧ tachycardia

✧ abdominal distention
✧ fever

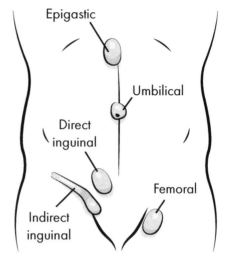

Figure 4.2. Hernias

Diagnostic Tests and Findings

+ physical examination usual method of diagnosis
+ CT scan to rule out incarceration

Treatment and Management

+ If no incarceration is present, the hernia might be manually reduced.
+ If hernia is incarcerated or cannot be reduced, prepare the patient for surgery.

QUICK REVIEW QUESTION

18. A patient arrives at the ED and says he believes he has a hernia. What assessments can the ED nurse perform to confirm?

Inflammatory Bowel Disease

CROHN'S DISEASE

Pathophysiology

Crohn's disease, a type of inflammatory bowel disease, can involve any part of the GI tract. Because the exact cause of Crohn's disease remains unknown, there is no cure; reduction of symptoms is the focus.

Risk Factors

+ smoking
+ family history of inflammatory bowel disease

+ usually diagnosed by age 35
+ NSAID use

Signs and Symptoms

+ loose stools (5 – 6 episodes per day)
+ abdominal pain, typically described as cramping and continuous
+ steatorrhea

+ fever
+ weight loss
+ associated anal fissures or abscesses

Diagnostic Tests and Findings

+ endoscopy for diagnosis

+ abdominal X-rays or CT scan may show perforation, obstruction, or dilation

Treatment and Management

+ Keep the patient NPO.

+ Administer immunosuppressants (e.g., infliximab [Remicade]).

+ Administer corticosteroids.

QUICK REVIEW QUESTION

19. A patient presents to the ED with complaints of cramping abdominal pain, steatorrhea, and several episodes of loose stools throughout the day. What is the probable diagnosis for this patient?

ULCERATIVE COLITIS

Pathophysiology

Ulcerative colitis is a type of inflammatory bowel disease that involves the large colon. The intestines become inflamed, and patients typically have exacerbations and remissions.

Risk Factors

+ family history

Signs and Symptoms

+ hematochezia (10 – 20 episodes per day)

+ weight loss

+ fever

+ tachycardia

+ cramping, abdominal pain, typically in the LLQ

+ dehydration

Diagnostic Tests and Findings

+ abdominal X-rays and/or CT scan may show perforation, obstruction, or dilation

Treatment and Management

+ Administer IV fluids for rehydration.

+ Administer anti-inflammatories.

+ Administer corticosteroids.

QUICK REVIEW QUESTION

20. A patient arrives at the ED with complaints of frequent bloody stools. What further assessment findings would the ED nurse expect to find in a patient diagnosed with ulcerative colitis?

Obstructions, Infarctions, and Perforations

BOWEL OBSTRUCTION

Pathophysiology

A **bowel obstruction** occurs when the bowel stops working or has a physical blockage due to fecal impaction, tumors, or volvulus (a twisted loop of intestine). The majority of bowel obstructions occur in the small bowel as opposed to the large bowel.

Risk Factors

+ diverticulitis
+ previous abdominal surgeries from adhesions
+ carcinomas
+ inflammatory bowel disease

Signs and Symptoms

+ nausea and vomiting
+ diarrhea
+ distended and firm abdomen
+ abdominal pain, typically described as cramping and colicky
+ unable to pass flatus

Diagnostic Tests and Findings

+ increased WBCs
+ elevated BUN and decreased electrolytes from dehydration/vomiting
+ abdominal X-ray may show dilated bowel loops
+ CT scan to diagnose

Treatment and Management

+ Keep the patient on NPO.
+ Insert NG tube for decompression.
+ Run CBC and CMP to monitor for infection/electrolyte imbalances.
+ Administer antiemetics.
+ Administer analgesics.
+ Surgery may be required.

> ### QUICK REVIEW QUESTION
>
> **21.** A patient presents to the ED with abdominal pain, nausea, and vomiting. A bowel obstruction is suspected and then confirmed by CT scan. What interventions should the nurse prioritize for this patient?

INTESTINAL INFARCTION

Pathophysiology

Intestinal infarction, necrosis of part of the intestinal wall, occurs when decreased blood flow in the intestine causes ischemia.

Risk Factors

+ hernias
+ adhesions
+ an embolus

Signs and Symptoms

+ abdominal pain
+ vomiting
+ diarrhea
+ fever
+ hematochezia

Diagnostic Tests and Findings

+ increased WBC
+ CT scan of abdomen to visualize area of ischemia

Treatment and Management

+ Keep the patient NPO.
+ Administer antibiotics.
+ Surgery, either a colostomy or an ileostomy, may be required.

QUICK REVIEW QUESTION

22. A patient presents to the ED with severe abdominal pain, fever, and hematochezia. A bowel infarction is shown on the CT scan. What interventions should the nurse prioritize for this patient?

GASTRIC PERFORATION

Pathophysiology

Gastric perforation is the formation of an opening within the stomach. This hole can lead to peritonitis because of the leakage of stomach contents such as bacteria, acid, food, and/or stool into the peritoneum. Gastric perforation can be due to trauma such as a knife wound or gunshot.

Risk Factors

+ trauma
+ abdominal surgery
+ ulcers
+ cancer
+ long-term steroid use

Signs and Symptoms

+ abrupt onset of severe abdominal pain
+ nausea and vomiting
+ fever
+ tachycardia
+ rigid, board-like abdomen

Diagnostic Tests and Findings

+ abdominal X-ray may show free air
+ abdominal CT scan may show perforation

Treatment and Management

+ Administer antibiotics.
+ Prepare patient for surgery to repair perforation.

INTUSSUSCEPTION

Pathophysiology

Intussusception is a mechanical bowel obstruction caused when a loop of the large intestine *telescopes* within itself. This condition can cut off the blood supply, causing perforation, infection, and bowel ischemia.

Risk Factors

+ usually occurs within first 3 years of life
+ more prevalent in males

Signs and Symptoms

+ red currant-jelly–like stool
+ sausage-shaped abdominal mass
+ colicky pain
+ inconsolable crying
+ absence of stools

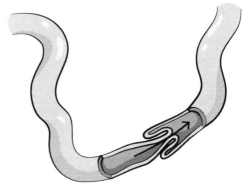

Figure 4.3. Intussusception

Diagnostic Tests and Findings

+ abdominal X-rays to confirm diagnosis
+ CBC to monitor for infection
+ CMP to monitor for electrolyte imbalances
+ urinalysis to monitor for dehydration

Treatment and Management

+ Keep the patient NPO.
+ Give a barium enema; the weight of the barium helps push the telescoped bowel out.

24. A 10-month-old infant patient presents to the ED with persistent crying and red stool with a gelatinous consistency. What condition and treatment does the ED nurse suspect?

PYLORIC STENOSIS

Pathophysiology

Pyloric stenosis is caused by an obstruction of gastric outflow. The pylorus muscle becomes thick and swollen, which prevents food from moving to the small intestine. Children with pyloric stenosis have poor weight gain because of the resulting inability to eat. The condition usually occurs within the first few weeks or months of life.

Risk Factors

+ more common in males
+ family history

Signs and Symptoms

+ projectile vomiting, especially after eating
+ an olive-shaped mass in the RUQ
+ visible peristalsis
+ frequent hunger
+ poor weight gain

Diagnostic Tests and Findings

+ abdominal ultrasound for diagnosis

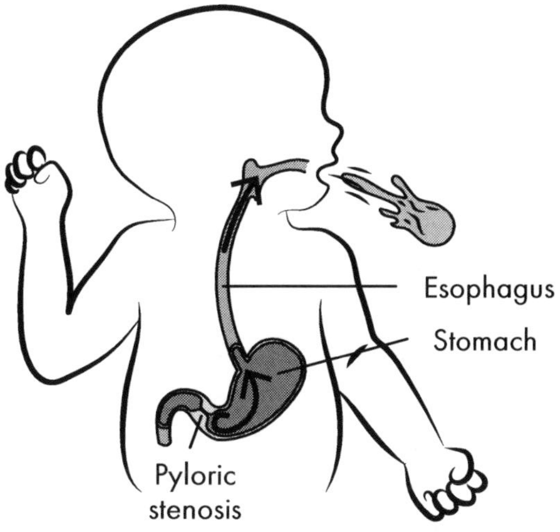

Figure 4.4. Pyloric Stenosis

Treatment and Management

+ Conduct labs to monitor dehydration and electrolyte imbalances.

+ Keep the patient NPO.
+ Surgery is required to fix stenosis.

QUICK REVIEW QUESTION

25. A 2-week-old infant presents to the ED, and the parents state that the child has had poor oral intake and has been projectile vomiting immediately after being fed. What further assessment findings would the ED nurse expect when examining the infant?

Ulcers

Pathophysiology

An **ulcer** is a sore or opening that occurs within the stomach lining (gastric ulcer), duodenum (duodenal ulcer), esophagus, or small intestine. **Peptic ulcers** include both gastric and duodenal ulcers. Duodenal ulcers, which cause the stomach to empty rapidly, are the most common type of ulcer.

Risk Factors

+ frequent use of NSAIDs, or a history of NSAID use

+ stress

+ *H. pylori* infection

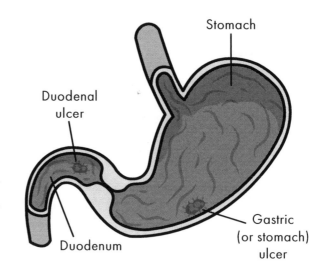

Figure 4.5. Peptic Ulcers

Signs and Symptoms

+ pain described as squeezing or tightness, and may radiate to back

+ burning abdominal and/or throat pain

+ pain may be accompanied by bloating and a feeling of fullness, which may lead to weight loss

+ pain either relieved or worsened by food
    ✧ duodenal ulcer: pain starts before meals; typically relieved by food
    ✧ gastric ulcer: pain chronic; occurs while eating

Diagnostic Tests and Findings

+ testing for *H. pylori* infection

+ endoscopy (esophagogastroduodenoscopy, or EGD)

Treatment and Management

+ Administer antibiotics, if cause is *H. pylori*.

+ Administer H_2 blockers or proton-pump inhibitors.

+ At discharge, teach preventative measures:
    ✧ Avoid NSAIDs.
    ✧ Avoid smoking.
    ✧ Avoid spicy foods.

QUICK REVIEW QUESTION

26. A patient presents to the ED with squeezing and burning abdominal and throat pain. The patient is diagnosed with an ulcer. What information should the ED nurse implement within the discharge teaching for this patient?

ANSWER KEY

1. The patient should be prepared for an emergency endoscopy or surgical intervention to repair the perforation. The patient should have IV access established and IV fluids started. Additionally, the patient's vital signs should be assessed frequently, for any changes in status.

2. Patients with Mallory-Weiss tears may frequently vomit or pass blood through their stools, so controlling bleeding and ensuring airway patency should be the main priorities for these patients.

3. Asterixis, scratch marks, spiderlike angiomas, and palmar erythema are other signs that may be present in the patient who presents with cirrhosis.

4. Octreotide is a vasoconstrictor, which constricts the dilated vessels present in esophageal varices and thereby reduces bleeding.

5. The patient's airway should always be assessed first. It should be assessed for patency, and the nurse should look for signs of airway obstruction, including drooling, the inability to handle secretions, an ineffective cough, and/or stridor.

6. The nurse should watch for early signs of a lower GI bleed, including hematochezia, abdominal pain, and fatigue. A decreased H/H, tachycardia, and hypotension may occur after a significant amount of blood loss and would be seen as late signs of a lower GI bleed.

7. NSAIDs are a class of drug that can cause bleeding and would be a contributing factor to a GI bleed. Types of NSAIDs include aspirin, ibuprofen (Motrin), naproxen (Aleve), ketorolac (Toradol), and indomethacin (Indocin).

8. The patient should begin with bland, easy-to-digest foods, such as those in the BRAT diet. Such foods include bananas, rice, applesauce, and toast.

9. The patient has peritonitis, which can lead to septic shock if the peritonitis is not treated with antibiotics and surgery. Broad-spectrum antibiotics such as a piperacillin/tazobactam infusion should be given, and the patient should be prepared for surgery.

10. Priority interventions for a patient with appendicitis should be keeping the patient NPO, administering antiemetics, analgesics, and antibiotics, and preparing the patient for surgery.

11. A patient with acute cholecystitis can show elevations in WBCs, AST, ALT, and bilirubin. Amylase or lipase may be elevated if the patient has passed gallstones.

12. Patients with acute diverticulitis should start with a liquid diet, with food items such as broth, popsicles, and gelatin, before slowly introducing low-fiber foods. After the acute stage has passed, patients should also be taught to routinely follow a high-fiber diet to help food pass through the colon and to prevent straining. High-fiber foods include fruits, vegetables, and whole grains.

13. The patient has symptoms of esophagitis. The nurse can elevate the head of the patient's bed and administer a GI cocktail and a PPI or an H2 blocker to reduce symptoms.

14. The patient may be dehydrated from vomiting, so administering IV fluids and antiemetics and replacing electrolytes should be priorities. Other medications, such as H2 blockers, proton-pump inhibitors, and antacids may also be given, to reduce symptoms.

15. The nurse would expect the patient to have abdominal pain, nausea, vomiting, and possibly jaundice if the pancreatitis is caused by a gallstone blocking the pancreatic duct. The nurse would also expect to see elevated amylase, lipase, and glucose.

16. Penetrating injuries cause an open wound after an object goes through the skin. These types of injuries would be caused by objects such as a knife, a bullet or shrapnel from a gunshot, or another object that can impale a person (e.g., when a person falls on a protruding object).

17. Contributing factors for hepatitis include the Epstein-Barr virus, cytomegalovirus, unprotected sex, blood transfusions, IV drug use, poor hygiene, alcohol abuse, and excessive acetaminophen use.

18. A full abdominal assessment should be performed to look for a bulge, mass, and/or swelling. The nurse should also gather information about the patient's activities that would cause straining, such as weight lifting. Additionally, a CT scan is necessary to rule out an incarcerated hernia.

19. Cramping abdominal pain, steatorrhea, and 5 – 6 episodes of loose stools are common symptoms of Crohn's disease. Additional symptoms that may be found include fever and weight loss.

20. In addition to hematochezia (up to 20 episodes per day), patients with ulcerative colitis may also have symptoms such as weight loss, fever, tachycardia, and cramping LLQ abdominal pain. Additionally, signs of dehydration may be present because of fluid loss from diarrhea.

21. Patients with bowel obstructions need IV access and IV fluids. They must remain NPO and have an NG tube inserted for decompressing the stomach. Some obstructions may also require surgical intervention.

22. The patient with an intestinal infarction needs to be prepped for surgery, because part of the bowel has limited or no blood supply. To expedite treatment, the nurse should ensure that the patient has IV access, remains NPO, and understands both why surgery is necessary and the associated risks of the surgery.

23. The patient with a gastric perforation has stomach contents spilling out. This condition can quickly lead to sepsis. The nurse should prioritize getting IV access and starting antibiotics while preparations are made for the patient to have surgery to repair the perforation.

24. Red jelly-like stools, along with a sausage-shaped abdominal mass, are hallmarks of intussusception. Intussusception causes the bowel to telescope into itself. A barium enema will help to push the bowel out.

25. In addition to projectile vomiting, an olive-shaped mass is another hallmark of pyloric stenosis. Other findings include visible peristalsis, frequent hunger, and poor weight gain.

26. A patient with an ulcer should be taught to avoid NSAIDs, smoking, and spicy foods, as all of these can lead to stomach irritation.

FIVE: GENITOURINARY & GYNECOLOGICAL EMERGENCIES

Terminology and Assessment

PHYSIOLOGY AND TERMINOLOGY REVIEW

+ **Genitourinary** refers to both the reproductive and urinary organs.

+ The primary functions of the urinary system are to:
    ⬦ regulate fluid and electrolyte balance
    ⬦ excrete waste products
    ⬦ regulate blood pressure
    ⬦ produce erythropoietin to stimulate red blood cell synthesis
    ⬦ metabolize vitamin D

+ **Urine** is formed in the nephrons of the kidneys and flows through the ureters to the bladder.

+ The **urethral sphincter** is a muscle that surrounds the neck of the bladder preventing reflux of urine back into the ureters.

+ Urine is collected in the **bladder** until urination is induced by parasympathetic pathways.

+ The bladder can hold approximately 500 cc of urine but may expand to hold greater amounts if urinary output is restricted or if sympathetic pathways at the level of T12 or higher are disrupted.

+ Urine is passed from the bladder through the **urethra**, exiting the body at the **urinary meatus**.

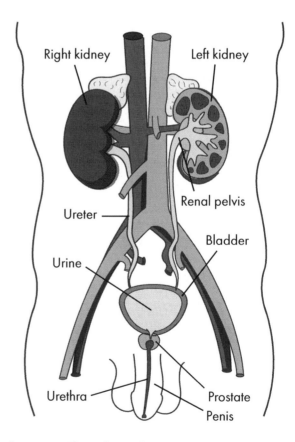

Figure 5.1. The Urinary System

- The primary function of the reproductive system is procreation.
- The urinary and reproductive systems are often assessed concurrently as their structures are in proximity or overlap.
    - The male urethra serves both urinary and reproductive functions, so the term *urogenital* is commonly used in reference to male genitourinary disorders.
- Patients may be reluctant to discuss problems with urinary or sexual function because they are embarrassed.
- Patients may not be able to describe these systems in medical terms, and it is not uncommon for patients to use crude terminology.
- Ensuring patients' privacy and confidentiality is of utmost importance during the assessment.

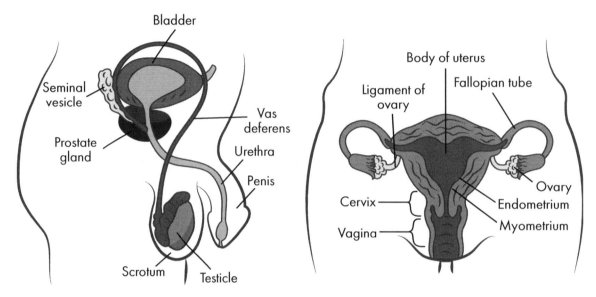

Figure 5.2. Male and Female Reproductive Systems

PHYSICAL ASSESSMENT: URINARY

- Subjective data as reported by the patient should assess for onset of symptoms and history of:
    - polyuria
    - incontinence
    - nocturia
    - enuresis
    - urgency
    - dysuria
    - burning
    - retention
    - decreased force of urine stream
    - visualized hematuria
    - visualized calculi
- Assess objective data.
    - Assess patient's urinary status using the mnemonic **COCA**: **C**olor, **O**dor, **C**larity, **A**mount.
    - Urine output should be measured to assess for diuresis, oliguria, and anuria.
    - Observe clothing to assess for incontinence.
    - Palpate to assess for bladder distension and tenderness in the lower abdomen or lateral flanks.
    - Auscultation of an abdominal bruit may indicate narrowing of the vessels perfusing the kidneys or renal stenosis.
    - Percussion of a distended bladder produces a dull sound.

PHYSICAL ASSESSMENT: MALE

+ Symptoms related to bladder function and urination in males are collectively referred to as **prostatism.**

+ Subjective data as reported by the patient should assess for:

  ⋄ onset of symptoms   ⋄ sexual history
  ⋄ prostatism   ⋄ erectile or sexual dysfunctions

+ Assess objective data.

  ⋄ Assess if the patient is circumcised. If non-circumcised, the nurse may need to retract the foreskin to complete assessment.

  ⋄ Determine if the size and shape of testes are equal and non-edematous.

  ⋄ Look for the presence of a rash, discharge from urinary meatus, or any other abnormalities.

  ⋄ Assess Tanner staging in adolescents.

  ⋄ Palpate inguinal lymph nodes.

  ⋄ Medical provider may perform a digital rectal exam and testicular exam.

PHYSICAL ASSESSMENT: FEMALE

+ Subjective data as reported by the patient should assess for:

  ⋄ onset of symptoms   ⋄ sexual history
  ⋄ urinary patterns and complaints   ⋄ obstetrical history
  ⋄ abdominal tenderness or nausea   ⋄ contraceptive use
  ⋄ date of last menstrual period   ⋄ sexual dysfunctions

+ Assess objective data.

  ⋄ View the external genitalia and note presence of discharge, lesions, rash, skin tears, or other abnormalities of the vulva, labia majora, mons pubis, perineum, and other visible structures.

  ⋄ Assess Tanner staging in adolescents.

  ⋄ Palpate inguinal lymph nodes.

  ⋄ Medical provider may perform a manual pelvic exam and examination of internal structures of the vagina and cervix using a speculum.

+ If vaginal bleeding is present:

  ⋄ Ask patient what their baseline normal menses are compared to the current condition.

  ⋄ Assess for clots, color in relation to frank bleeding versus older blood formation, and amount.

DIAGNOSTIC IMAGING

+ abdominal ultrasound:

  ⋄ used for visualization of the uterus and other internal organs of the female reproductive system

  ⋄ used to confirm viability of pregnancy and assess fetal anatomical structures

  ⋄ can identify presence of free air, fluid, or obstruction in the peritoneal cavity (male or female)

+ bladder scan:

  ⋄ noninvasive bedside test that can be performed by the emergency nurse or delegated to an ED tech or nursing assistant

  ⋄ provides quick assessment of the amount of urine in the bladder

  ⋄ can obtain pre-void and post-void residual data to assess for urinary retention

- pelvic or renal CT scan:
    - produces cross-section images of internal structures of the abdominal cavity including reproductive and urinary organs
    - may be performed with or without contrast
- cystoscopy:
    - visual exam of the bladder performed using a flexible cystoscope
    - most commonly performed in the emergency setting by a medical specialist such as a urologist or gynecologist
- kidney, ureter, bladder (KUB):
    - used to assess size, shape, and position of the anatomical structures
- IV pyelography (IVP):
    - uses contrast to assess images of the kidneys, ureters, and bladder

GYNECOLOGICAL DIAGNOSTIC TESTS

- Pap smear:
    - screening test for cervical cancer or abnormal cells
    - obtained during the pelvic exam with speculum visualization
- vaginal wet mount:
    - sample of vaginal discharge transferred to a microscope slide and examined
    - used to obtain definitive diagnosis of vaginal candidiasis, bacterial vaginosis, and trichomoniasis
- dilation and curettage (D&C):
    - This is most commonly performed in the surgical setting but may be performed with a local anesthetic and light sedation in the emergency setting.
    - The cervical canal is dilated, and a curette is passed through the opening to scrape the endometrial lining for tissue examination, to control abnormal uterine bleeding, or as a therapeutic measure for incomplete abortion (partial miscarriage with retained products of conception).

Abnormal Uterine Bleeding

Pathophysiology

Abnormal uterine bleeding (AUB) is any bleeding from the uterus that is abnormal in volume or timing. This includes menses that occur irregularly, last for an abnormal number of days, or produce excessive blood loss. It occurs most often in adolescents and people approaching menopause.

Risk Factors

- PALM-COEIN:
    - Polyp
    - Adenomyosis
    - Leiomyoma (fibroids)
    - Malignancy
    - Coagulopathy
    - Ovulatory disorder
    - Endometrial
    - Iatrogenic (e.g., IUD insertion)
    - Not otherwise classified

- hormone fluctuations or imbalances:
  - birth control pills
  - pregnancy
  - premenopausal/menopausal
  - hormone replacement therapy
- anovulation
- sudden weight loss
- obesity
- emotional and physical stress

Signs and Symptoms

- metrorrhagia
- menorrhagia:
  - soaking more than 1 pad or tampon per hour
  - greater than 30 cc volume measured via menstrual cup

Diagnostic Tests and Findings

- decreased H/H
- assessment of iron status
- hormone levels (estrogen, progesterone, FSH)
- tests for blood coagulation disorders
- serum qualitative pregnancy test
- ultrasound to rule out polyps or fibroids
- hysteroscopy
- endometrial biopsy to assess pathology and integrity of endometrial lining

Treatment and Management

- For menorrhagia causing hypovolemia:
  - Control bleeding.
  - Administer fluid or blood volume replacement.
- Nonemergent presentations should be referred to a gynecologist/obstetrics specialist.

QUICK REVIEW QUESTION

1. A young female patient accompanied by the mother presents to the ED with a complaint of menorrhagia after experiencing amenorrhea for the past three months. What problem should the nurse anticipate when trying to obtain a truthful and complete history from the patient?

Genitourinary Trauma

Pathophysiology

Genitourinary (GU) trauma can cause injury to the kidneys, bladder, urethra, or external genitalia. GU trauma symptoms can be nonspecific and can be masked by or related to other injuries. Trauma may occur from blunt or penetrating injury.

- Renal: The majority of renal trauma occurs from blunt trauma such as direct impact into the seatbelt or steering wheel in frontal MVCs or from body panel intrusion in side-impact crashes.

- Bladder: The majority of bladder trauma occurs from blunt trauma, usually occurring with a pelvic fracture. Bladder rupture can result from lap belt restraint.

- **Urethral:** Urethral injuries are more common in males and may result from trauma and pelvic fracture or from iatrogenic injuries resulting from catheterization.
- **External genitalia:** These injuries are more common in males due to anatomical presentation and greater participation in physical sports, acts of violence, and war. Up to two-thirds of all genitourinary traumas involve the external genitalia. Injuries to the penis and scrotum may occur from use of penile rings or other sexual pleasure devices, mutilation, or straddle injuries.

Risk Factors

- MVAs
- vehicle-associated pedestrian accidents
- fall from height
- sports injury
- straddle injury
- impairment by alcohol or recreational drug use
- acts of violence and war

Signs and Symptoms

- pain:
  - suprapubic
  - abdominal
  - groin/genital
  - flank
- urinary symptoms:
  - hematuria
  - incontinence
  - dysuria
- bleeding at meatus
- ecchymosis
- distended bladder
- abdominal distention
- foul-smelling vaginal discharge
- edema
- nausea and vomiting
- visible wound, penetration injury, or embedded object

Diagnostic Tests and Findings

- urinalysis for hematuria
- decreased hemoglobin and hematocrit
- monitor for:
  - elevated BUN and creatinine
  - fluid and electrolyte status
- diagnostic imaging:
  - CT scan to assess integrity of renal and urinary organs
  - KUB
  - IVP
  - chest X-ray to assess for concurrent rib fracture
  - renal ultrasound

Treatment and Management

- Administer IV fluids.
- Provide supplemental oxygen as needed.

+ Administer analgesics.

+ Administer antibiotics if injury may lead to infection.

+ Blunt injuries are generally managed nonoperatively; patient given supportive care with bed rest and observation.

+ Penetrating injuries are more likely to require surgical intervention.

+ Consults:

  ✧ trauma surgery

  ✧ urology

  ✧ orthopedic

QUICK REVIEW QUESTION

2. A 16-year-old patient presents to the ED with complaints of nausea and genital pain after sustaining a straddle injury on a skateboard. What further signs and symptoms should the nurse assess to diagnose genitourinary trauma?

Gynecological Trauma

Pathophysiology

Female patients presenting with complaints of genital pain or bleeding should undergo a thorough history and physical examination. External trauma can usually be identified easily; however, internal examination will be required to evaluate for deeper injury. Vulvar injuries may include lacerations and hematomas, while vaginal trauma may present with lacerations. Uterine and cervical injuries are generally associated with pregnancy; however, they can also be caused by vaginal or abdominal trauma. Undiagnosed vaginal trauma may result in secondary issues including dyspareunia, pelvis abscesses, and fistula formations.

Patients may not be forthcoming with the details of the trauma because of fear, embarrassment, or inability to speak (due to age or mental status). The possibility of sexual assault or physical abuse must be considered and should be handled according to the appropriate protocols.

Risk Factors

+ MVA

+ blunt trauma

+ straddle injury

+ consensual sex, particularly first time

+ vaginally inserted foreign object

+ sexual or physical abuse

+ vaginal delivery

Signs and Symptoms

+ pain (vaginal, external, or visceral)

+ vaginal bleeding

+ external laceration, ecchymosis, or mutilation

+ hematuria

+ dysuria

+ foul-smelling vaginal discharge

+ labial edema

+ visible wound, penetration injury, or embedded object

Diagnostic Tests and Findings

+ urinalysis for hematuria

+ decreased H/H

+ CT scan and pelvic/vaginal ultrasound to assess integrity of reproductive organs

Treatment and Management

+ Treatment is based on type and degree of injury.

+ Provide pain management.

+ analgesics

+ cold compresses

+ Administer antibiotics if injury may lead to infection.

+ Sutures may be needed for lacerations.

+ Remove foreign object(s).

+ Teach at discharge:

  ✧ Avoid sexual intercourse and placement of foreign bodies into vaginal cavity until authorized by gynecologist.

QUICK REVIEW QUESTION

3. A 22-year-old female patient seeks treatment in the ED after falling onto a metal hurdle during a track sporting event. In triage, the patient denies vaginal bleeding but complains of throbbing pain "down there." What interventions should the nurse initiate?

Foreign Bodies in the Genitourinary System

Pathophysiology

The most common sources of foreign bodies in the genitourinary system are sexual activity, trauma, or medical intervention. Objects such as pens, pencils, batteries, and wires may be inserted into the urethra; in female patients, larger objects may cause injury to the bladder. Trauma can also result in foreign objects in the bladder, including bullets, shell pieces, and splinters. Medical devices that may be found in the genitourinary system include IUDs, surgical staples, catheter pieces, broken endoscopic parts, and knotted suprapubic catheters. The method used for removal will be based on the patient's age and the object's motility and size.

Risk Factors

+ in young children:
  ✧ curiosity or sexual pleasure
  ✧ abuse

+ penetrating or missile injuries

+ sexual activities while intoxicated

+ drug use

+ mental illness or disability

+ dementia

+ history of self-harm

+ sexual abuse

Signs and Symptoms

+ urinary symptoms:
  ⋄ hematuria
  ⋄ dysuria
  ⋄ frequent urination
  ⋄ acute urinary retention
  ⋄ strangury
+ pain:
  ⋄ lower abdominal
  ⋄ genital

+ dyspareunia
+ acute cystitis
+ urethral discharge
+ signs of infection:
  ⋄ fever
  ⋄ inflammation

Diagnostic Tests and Findings

+ visualization of foreign body during exam
+ X-ray or ultrasound showing presence of foreign body
+ possibly elevated WBC if foreign body is present for several days or more

Treatment and Management

+ Provide analgesics as needed.
+ Remove foreign object endoscopically (first line).
+ cystoscopy
+ suprapubic cystostomy

+ cystolitholapaxy
+ Surgery may be required if object cannot be removed endoscopically.
+ Request psychiatric consult if warranted.

QUICK REVIEW QUESTION

4. A female patient presents to the ED with complaints of acute urinary retention. She reports that her partner was using a pencil to stimulate her the night before while they were both highly intoxicated. A bedside ultrasound reveals that part of the pencil is lodged in her urethra and has entered the bladder. What intervention should the nurse prepare for?

Foreign Bodies in the Gynecological System

Pathophysiology

Foreign objects in the vagina can occur in all age groups. Young children exploring their bodies may insert small objects such as crayons or marker lids; the child may then not be able to remove it and will forget about it. Adolescents beginning menstruation may forget that they have inserted a tampon and leave it in place for days or weeks. Adults may also experience forgotten tampons or have pieces of condoms left behind after sexual activity. Foreign objects may be inserted vaginally for sexual stimulation that cannot subsequently be removed, including sex toys, beads, or marbles. Objects not designed for vaginal use may lead to infection, and objects with batteries may result in chemical burns.

Risk Factors

- in young children:
    - curiosity or sexual pleasure
    - abuse
- sexual activities while intoxicated
- drug use
- mental illness or disability
- dementia
- history of self-harm
- sexual abuse

Signs and Symptoms

- vaginal pain or discomfort
- abdominal or pelvic pain
- vaginal bleeding (usually light)
- vaginal discharge:
    - foul-smelling, yellow, pink, or brown discharge
    - may cause itching or foul odor
- rash in the vaginal area
- swelling of the vagina or vulva
- vulvar discomfort
- dysuria
- dyspareunia
- erythema

Diagnostic Tests and Findings

- visualization of foreign body during exam
- X-ray or ultrasound showing presence of foreign body
- possibly elevated WBC if foreign body is present for several days or more

Treatment and Management

- Provide pain management.
- Object should be removed.
    - Use speculum and forceps to remove object in vagina.
    - Warm water lavage of the vagina may be used for objects that can be easily dislodged.
    - Sedation and/or anesthesia may be required for objects that cannot be removed without causing pain or further injury.
- Administer antibiotics if injury may lead to infection.

QUICK REVIEW QUESTION

5. A 13-year-old female patient presents to the ED with complaints of foul-smelling, yellow-brown vaginal discharge and itching. The girl's mother reports that the girl recently started menstruating. What should the nurse suspect has caused these signs and symptoms?

Infections

CHLAMYDIA

Pathophysiology

Chlamydia is caused by the bacteria *Chlamydia trachomatis*; it is the most commonly reported STI in the United States. The infection can be found in the cervix, urethra, rectum, or pharynx. It is most commonly spread through sexual activity, but it can also spread from the mother's genital tract to the newborn during birth. Chlamydia infections may be asymptomatic for long periods. Left untreated, chlamydia can lead to PID, infertility, and ectopic pregnancy in women.

Risk Factors

+ most common in women ages 15 – 25

+ unprotected vaginal, anal, or oral sex

+ multiple partners

Signs and Symptoms

+ often asymptomatic, especially for men

+ discharge from site of infection (vaginal, penile, or rectal)

+ vaginal bleeding

+ dysuria

+ pruritus

Diagnostic Tests and Findings

+ NAAT performed on urine or swab from urethra, vaginal, pharynx, or rectum

Treatment and Management

+ antibiotics:
    ⋄ azithromycin (Zithromax)
    ⋄ doxycycline

+ supportive treatment for symptoms

+ discharge teaching:
    ⋄ Patients should notify partners and advise them to seek treatment.
    ⋄ Patients should abstain from sexual intercourse for 1 week.

QUICK REVIEW QUESTION

6. A patient asks why they must notify previous partners of their diagnosed chlamydia infection. How should the ED nurse respond?

EPIDIDYMITIS

Pathophysiology

Epididymitis is inflammation of the epididymis, the tube that carries sperm to the testes. It can occur in males of any age and generally occurs in a single testis. Inflammation is usually the result of a bacterial infection secondary to a UTI or sexually transmitted disease. **Chemical epididymitis** is a rare, nonbacterial condition caused by the backflow of urine. Epididymitis occurring frequently or lasting more than 6 weeks is diagnosed as chronic; the symptoms may progress slowly, and the cause may remain unknown.

Risk Factors

+ most common in men ages 18 – 35
+ STIs (most commonly gonorrhea or chlamydia)
+ history of UTIs
+ history of prostate infection or enlargement
+ uncircumcised penis

+ mumps
+ groin injury
+ Foley catheterization
+ GU medical procedures

Signs and Symptoms

+ pain posterior to testes:
  ⋄ gradual onset
  ⋄ can radiate to lower abdomen
+ symptoms of lower UTI:
  ⋄ frequent urination
  ⋄ dysuria
  ⋄ hematuria
  ⋄ fever

+ positive Prehn sign
+ swelling and tenderness in testes
+ tachycardia

Diagnostic Tests and Findings

+ positive STI screening
+ urinalysis to show presence of bacteria

+ elevated WBC count
+ ultrasound showing enlarged epididymis

Treatment and Management

+ Administer antibiotics to treat underlying bacterial infection.
  ⋄ Advise antibiotics for partner(s) if STI is present.
+ Provide pain management.
  ⋄ analgesics
  ⋄ ice packs
  ⋄ scrotal support or elevation
+ Surgery may be required to drain abscess or for severe infection (epididymectomy).

QUICK REVIEW QUESTION

7. What is the primary treatment for a patient newly diagnosed with epididymitis?

GENITAL HERPES

Pathophysiology

Genital herpes is an STI caused by the two strains of the herpes simplex virus (HSV-1 and HSV-2). Both strains cause blisters on the mouth, anus, or genital area. The first outbreak after the initial infection is the most severe; recurrent outbreaks, which vary in frequency and duration, will generally be less severe.

Risk Factors

+ more common in women
+ direct genital or oral contact with an infected person

Signs and Symptoms

+ prodrome of itching, burning, or tingling at infection site
+ vesicles on genitalia, perineum, or buttocks:
  ✧ present for approximately 2 weeks during initial infection
  ✧ present for 6 – 12 days during secondary outbreaks

+ primary infection:
  ✧ fever
  ✧ adenopathy

Diagnostic Tests and Findings

+ PCR on swab of open lesion to confirm infection
+ blood tests when no lesions are present

Treatment and Management

+ There is no cure for HSV.
+ Treatment focuses on alleviating symptoms and reducing recurrence of outbreaks.
+ Prescribe antivirals.
  ✧ acyclovir
  ✧ famciclovir (Famvir)
  ✧ valacyclovir (Valtrex)

QUICK REVIEW QUESTION

8. A patient with a new diagnosis of genital herpes asks how long it will take to cure the condition. How should the nurse respond?

GONORRHEA

Pathophysiology

Gonorrhea is the second highest reported STI in the United States, and law requires notification of a diagnosis to the local CDC. The infection is caused by the gram-negative diplococcus *Neisseria gonorrhoeae*.

Common infection sites include the cervix, vagina, rectum, and pharynx. It is most commonly spread through sexual activity, but it can also spread from the mother's genital tract to the newborn during birth. Left untreated, it can lead to PID, infertility, and ectopic pregnancy.

Risk Factors

+ most common in women ages 15 – 25
+ unprotected vaginal, anal, or oral sex
+ multiple partners

Signs and Symptoms

+ usually asymptomatic
+ discharge from site of infection (vaginal, penile, rectal, or pharynx)
+ dysuria
+ metrorrhagia
+ oropharyngeal erythema
+ in infants:
    ✧ conjunctivitis
    ✧ sepsis

Diagnostic Tests and Findings

+ culture or NAAT of vaginal or urethral swab

Treatment and Management

+ Prescribe antibiotics.
    ✧ ceftriaxone (Rocephin)
    ✧ azithromycin (Zithromax)
+ Fluoroquinolones are not prescribed because some strains of *N. gonorrhoeae* are resistant.
+ Provide supportive treatment for symptoms.
+ Teach at discharge:
    ✧ Patients should notify partners and advise them to seek treatment.

QUICK REVIEW QUESTION

9. A pregnant patient in the ED is diagnosed with gonorrhea and is worried about passing the infection to the newborn when giving birth. How should the nurse respond?

ORCHITIS

Pathophysiology

Orchitis (inflammation of the testes) is usually caused by a bacterial or viral infection. It can occur secondary to epididymitis (epididymo-orchitis). In most cases, only 1 testis is infected.

Risk Factors

+ most common in men ages 18 – 35
+ epididymitis

- STIs (most commonly gonorrhea or chlamydia)
- history of UTIs
- mumps
- urinary tract abnormality
- catheter insertion

Signs and Symptoms

- unilateral, sudden onset of pain in testicle
- swelling and tenderness
- nausea and vomiting
- fever
- tachycardia
- when associated with mumps, will appear 4 – 7 days after signs and symptoms of infection

Diagnostic Tests and Findings

- elevated WBC count
- ultrasound showing increased blood flow to the affected testis

Treatment and Management

- Treatment is based on source of infection.
    - antibiotics for bacterial infection
    - supportive treatment for orchitis secondary to mumps
- Administer anti-inflammatories.
- Give mumps vaccine if warranted.
- Provide pain management.
    - analgesics
    - ice packs
    - scrotal support or elevation

QUICK REVIEW QUESTION

10. A 20-year-old male patient presents to the ED with unilateral testicular pain and tenderness. The patient is currently recovering from the mumps. What treatment should the nurse prepare to provide?

PELVIC INFLAMMATORY DISEASE

Pathophysiology

Pelvic inflammatory disease (PID) is an infection of the upper organs of the female reproductive system, including the uterus, fallopian tubes, and ovaries. The infection, usually an STI, ascends from the cervix or vagina. PID is often asymptomatic; left untreated, it can lead to infertility and increases the risk of cancer.

Risk Factors

- STI (chlamydia or gonorrhea)
- more common in women < 25
- multiple partners

Signs and Symptoms

+ cervical, uterine, or adnexal tenderness
+ vaginal discharge
+ abdominal or low back pain
+ right scapular pain (Fitz-Hugh–Curtis syndrome)
+ postcoital bleeding
+ metrorrhagia
+ dyspareunia
+ pleuritic URQ pain
+ nausea and vomiting
+ temperature > 100.4°F (38°C)
+ chills

Diagnostic Tests and Findings

+ assessment for STI:
    ✧ urinalysis
    ✧ endocervix gram stain
+ elevated ESR
+ elevated C-reactive protein
+ imaging:
    ✧ endometritis
    ✧ transvaginal sonography
    ✧ laparoscopy

Treatment and Management

+ Administer antibiotics.
+ Provide pain management and supportive care for other symptoms.
+ IUD removal will be required for severe infections.
+ Teach at discharge:
    ✧ Patients should notify partners of positive STI and advise them to seek treatment.

QUICK REVIEW QUESTION

11. A patient recently diagnosed with an STI that went untreated for several months complains of vaginal discharge, abdominal pain, fever, and chills. What should the ED nurse consider as a differential diagnosis?

PROSTATITIS

Pathophysiology

Prostatitis (inflammation of the prostate) can be acute or chronic. It is usually caused by bacterial infection (*E. coli*). Left untreated, the infection can lead to sepsis or development of an abscess on the prostate. Prostatitis can also be asymptomatic; this condition is discovered during unrelated assessments and is not usually treated.

Risk Factors

+ benign prostatic hyperplasia
+ recurrent UTIs
+ STI
+ unprotected sex
+ multiple partners

Signs and Symptoms

+ urinary symptoms:
  + frequent urination
  + urgent urination
  + dysuria
  + interrupted stream
  + urinary retention
+ pain:
  + suprapubic or perineal
  + may occur in external genitals
  + low back (chronic prostatitis)

+ general symptoms of infection (acute prostatitis):
  + fever
  + malaise
  + chills
  + nausea and vomiting
+ tachycardia

Diagnostic Tests and Findings

+ elevated WBC count
+ urinalysis to show presence of bacteria

+ bacteria in expressed prostate fluid

Treatment and Management

+ antibiotics

+ NSAIDs

> QUICK REVIEW QUESTION
>
> **12.** A 55-year-old patient in the ED is diagnosed with acute bacterial prostatitis. What signs and symptoms should suggest to the nurse that the patient will require hospitalization?

PYELONEPHRITIS

Pathophysiology

Pyelonephritis, infection of the kidneys, is primarily the result of bacterial infection in the renal parenchyma. Bacteria can reach the kidney via the lower urinary tract or the bloodstream.

Symptoms can be mild to severe and develop over hours or days, with some patients waiting weeks before seeking care. Pyelonephritis can damage organs, be a life-threatening infection, and will lead to renal scarring without prompt diagnosis and treatment.

Risk Factors

+ UTI or history of UTIs
+ urinary tract abnormalities
+ urinary tract procedures

+ recent antibiotic use
+ IV drug abuse

Signs and Symptoms

+ clinical triad:
  - fever
  - nausea and/or vomiting
  - costovertebral pain
+ cloudy or dark urine
+ foul-smelling urine
+ hematuria
+ dysuria

+ suprapubic, cervical, or uterine tenderness
+ chills
+ in patients > 65:
  - fever
  - mental status change
  - dysphasia
  - hallucinations
  - organ failure

Diagnostic Tests and Findings

+ urinalysis to show presence of bacteria
+ urine culture and sensitivity to identify bacteria

+ KUB to show edema
+ electrolytes, creatinine, and BUN to assess renal function

Treatment and Management

+ Provide IV fluid resuscitation (D5W).
+ Administer antibiotics.
+ Administer antipyretics and use cooling measures as needed.

+ Provide supportive care for symptoms.
  - analgesics
  - antiemetics
+ Surgery may be required for complication (e.g., abscess, necrosis).

QUICK REVIEW QUESTION

13. What is the clinical triad associated with pyelonephritis?

SYPHILIS

Pathophysiology

Syphilis is an STI caused by the bacteria *Treponema pallidum*. Syphilis can affect the genitals, mouth, lips, and anus of any gender. It is most commonly spread through sexual activity, but it can also spread from the mother's genital tract to the newborn during birth. The infection progresses through four stages:

+ primary (3 – 90 days after infection)
+ secondary (4 – 10 weeks after infection)

+ latent (3 months – 3 years after infection)
+ tertiary (> 3 years after infection)

Risk Factors

+ more common in men
+ multiple partners

+ unprotected oral, anal, or vaginal sex

Signs and Symptoms

+ primary stage:
    + single or multiple chancres lasting 3 – 6 weeks
    + chancres are firm, round, and painless
+ secondary stage:
    + rough, red rash on torso, hands, soles of feet
    + fever
    + lymphadenopathy
    + fatigue
    + lesions on mucous membranes
    + headache
    + arthritis
+ latent stage:
    + asymptomatic
    + serological tests still positive
+ tertiary stage:
    + gummatous syphilis:
        + lesions that can occur in any body system
    + cardiovascular syphilis:
        + aortitis
        + aneurysms
        + coronary artery stenosis
    + neurosyphilis:
        + most common in tertiary stage but can occur earlier
        + seizures
        + ataxia
        + aphasia
        + personality changes
        + changes in vision or hearing

Diagnostic Tests and Findings

+ positive VDRL test
+ positive RPR test
+ specific treponemal antibody tests
+ LP to test for neurosyphilis

Treatment and Management

+ antibiotics:
    + penicillin
    + doxycycline or tetracycline for those allergic to penicillin
+ supportive care of symptoms (e.g., NSAIDs, cooling measures)

QUICK REVIEW QUESTION

14. A 55-year-old patient is brought to the ED with complaints of ataxia, blurred vision, and behavior impairment. Why should syphilis be included in the differential diagnosis and how would it be diagnosed?

URINARY TRACT INFECTION

Pathophysiology

Urinary tract infections (UTIs) can occur in the lower urinary tract (bladder and urethra) or in the upper urinary tract (kidneys and ureters). UTIs are generally caused by bacteria, and sometimes yeast, entering the urinary tract; *E. coli* is the most common bacteria that causes UTIs.

Risk Factors

- more common in women
- history of UTIs
- urinary tract abnormalities
- sexual intercourse
- STIs
- use of contraceptives in the vagina (diaphragms, spermicide)
- menopause
- kidney stones
- enlarged prostate
- immunosuppression
- diabetes
- urinary catheter use
- GU surgery or procedure

Signs and Symptoms

- burning upon urination
- frequent small amounts of urine
- cloudy urine
- foul-smelling urine
- hematuria
- pelvic, suprapubic, abdominal, or lower back pain or pressure
- urethral discharge
- general symptoms of infection:
  - fever
  - chills
  - malaise
- nausea and vomiting
- in patients > 65:
  - mental status change or confusion
  - increased number of falls
- in children < 2:
  - failure to thrive
  - fever
  - vomiting
  - difficulty feeding

Diagnostic Tests and Findings

- urinalysis to show presence of bacteria
- urine culture and sensitivity to identify bacteria
- KUB to show edema
- electrolytes, creatinine, and BUN to assess renal function

Treatment and Management

- Administer analgesics.
- Administer antibiotics.
- Teach at discharge:
  - Increase fluid intake.
  - Wipe genitals from front to back.
  - Urinate immediately following intercourse.
  - Avoid feminine products such as douches, deodorants, and powders.
  - Consider changing birth control method.

QUICK REVIEW QUESTION

15. A 10-year-old female patient presents to the ED with a diagnosis of a UTI for the third time. The patient asks the nurse to explain why she gets them all the time and her three brothers never do. What can the nurse say to educate this young patient?

VULVOVAGINITIS

Pathophysiology

Vulvovaginitis (inflammation of the vulva and vagina) is usually the result of an infection by bacteria (bacterial vaginosis), yeast (vulvovaginal candidiasis), or trichomoniasis, a protozoan parasite.

Risk Factors

+ bacterial vaginosis:
    ⬥ multiple partners
    ⬥ unprotected sex
    ⬥ douching
    ⬥ frequent use of spermicide
    ⬥ IUD
+ vulvovaginal candidiasis:
    ⬥ diabetes mellitus
    ⬥ use of antibiotics
    ⬥ diet high in sugar

+ trichomoniasis:
    ⬥ multiple partners
    ⬥ unprotected sex

Signs and Symptoms

+ bacterial vaginosis:
    ⬥ malodorous white-grey vaginal discharge
+ vulvovaginal candidiasis:
    ⬥ thick, white vaginal discharge with no odor (often described as "cottage cheese" like)
    ⬥ dyspareunia
    ⬥ dysuria
    ⬥ vulvovaginal pruritis
    ⬥ vaginal inflammation
    ⬥ vaginal edema

+ trichomoniasis:
    ⬥ frothy, green-yellow vaginal discharge
    ⬥ dyspareunia
    ⬥ dysuria
    ⬥ vaginal inflammation ("strawberry cervix")

Diagnostic Tests and Findings

+ bacterial vaginosis:
    ⬥ vaginal pH > 4.5

    ⬥ wet mount

- vulvovaginal candidiasis:
  - normal vaginal pH
  - microscopic exam
  - vaginal culture
- trichomoniasis:
  - vaginal pH > 5.4
  - presence of parasites in wet mount

Treatment and Management

- bacterial vaginosis:
  - antibiotics:
    - metronidazole (Flagyl) or clindamycin
- vulvovaginal candidiasis:
  - antifungals:
    - fluconazole (Diflucan) or nystatin
- trichomoniasis:
  - nitroimidazoles

QUICK REVIEW QUESTION

16. A 22-year-old female patient presents to the ED with white, foul-smelling vaginal discharge but no itching or urinary symptoms. What medication will the patient most likely require?

Ovarian Cyst

Pathophysiology

Ovarian cysts form in the ovaries, usually a result of an unreleased egg (follicular cyst) or failure of the corpus luteum to break down (corpus luteum cyst). Ovarian cysts are usually asymptomatic and are often found during assessments related to other conditions. However, the cysts can burst, causing intense pain; they can also increase the risk of ovarian torsion.

Risk Factors

- endometriosis
- infertility treatment
- hormonal imbalances
- hypothyroidism
- tubal ligation
- pelvic infection or inflammation
- smoking

Signs and Symptoms

- often asymptomatic
- pelvic pain, feeling of fullness, or discomfort
- dyspareunia
- irregular menstrual cycle
- rupture:
  - sudden, severe, unilateral pelvic pain
  - nausea and vomiting
  - fever
  - tachypnea
  - tachycardia

Diagnostic Tests and Findings

+ pelvic ultrasound

+ might be seen during laparoscopic procedures

+ hCG test to rule out pregnancy

Treatment and Management

+ treat pain with NSAIDs or opioids

+ for complications:
  ⬦ blood products in case of severe hemorrhage

+ surgical intervention in rare cases of continued bleeding or large cyst

QUICK REVIEW QUESTION

17. A patient arrives at the ED with vaginal bleeding and pain on the right side of the abdomen. The pregnancy test is negative, and the nurse suspects an ovarian cyst. What method definitively diagnoses an ovarian cyst?

Priapism

Pathophysiology

Priapism is an unintentional, prolonged erection that is unrelated to sexual stimulation and is unrelieved by ejaculation. **Ischemic (low-flow) priapism** occurs when blood becomes trapped in the erect penis. **Non-ischemic (high-flow) priapism** is the unregulated circulation of blood through the penis resulting from a ruptured artery in the penis or perineum. Ischemic priapism is considered a medical emergency requiring immediate intervention to preserve function of the penis.

Risk Factors

+ trauma:
  ⬦ straddle injury
  ⬦ acute spinal cord injury

+ medications:
  ⬦ antidepressants
  ⬦ anticoagulants
  ⬦ prostaglandin E1
  ⬦ testosterone

+ common underlying conditions:
  ⬦ sickle cell disease
  ⬦ leukemia
  ⬦ malaria

+ recent urologic surgery

+ cocaine use

Signs and Symptoms

+ ischemic priapism:
  ⬦ rigid, painful erection unrelated to sexual activity lasting > 4 hours

+ nonischemic priapism:
  ◇ recurrent episodes of persistent erections (may be partial)
  ◇ difficulty maintaining full erection
  ◇ no pain
  ◇ trauma (usually straddle injury)
  ◇ delay between injury and priapism

Diagnostic Tests and Findings

+ ultrasound showing obstructed or decreased blood flow
+ venous blood gas dark or black

Treatment and Management

+ For patients with ischemic priapism, blood should be drained from the penis within 4 – 6 hours to prevent permanent damage.
  ◇ First-line treatment is aspiration with intracavernosal phenylephrine injection.
  ◇ Second-line treatment is a shunt (T-shunt, Al-Ghorab's shunt, or Ebbehoj's shunt).
  ◇ Penile prostheses can be inserted for priapism lasting > 36 hours.
+ Treatment for nonischemic priapism should be conservative, as the condition will often spontaneously resolve.
  ◇ Monitor condition.
  ◇ First-line treatment, if needed, is elective arterial embolization.

QUICK REVIEW QUESTION

18. A 22-year-old patient in the ED is diagnosed with nonischemic priapism resulting from a straddle injury and is currently under observation. The patient is becoming increasingly anxious and tells the nurse he wants to be treated so he won't lose function in his penis. How should the nurse explain to the patient why he is not receiving medical intervention?

Penile Fracture

Pathophysiology

Penile fractures occur when there is a rupture of the corpus cavernosum and the tunica albuginea, usually as a result of abrupt bending of the erect penis. The injury may also include the urethra and vasculature within the penis. Penile fractures are medical emergencies that require immediate treatment.

Risk Factors

+ abrupt blunt trauma:
  ◇ sexual intercourse
  ◇ industrial accidents
  ◇ forceful masturbation
  ◇ turning in bed with an erection
+ kneading of penis to achieve detumescence (common in Middle East)

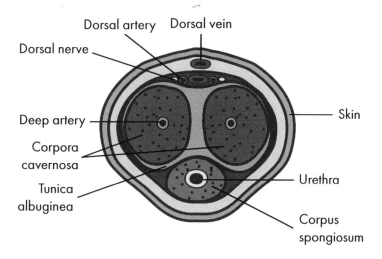

Figure 5.3. Anatomy of the Penis

Signs and Symptoms

+ popping, snapping, or cracking noise
+ sudden detumescence
+ may present with pain
+ penile deformity ("eggplant" or "aubergine sign")
+ ecchymosis
+ swelling
+ urethral damage:
    ✧ blood at meatus
    ✧ gross hematuria
    ✧ difficulty voiding bladder

Diagnostic Tests and Findings

+ based on signs and symptoms
+ MRI to identify site and extent of injury
+ urethrography if damage to urethra is suspected

Treatment and Management

+ Administer IV fluids.
+ Administer analgesics.
+ Prepare patient for surgery.
+ During surgical delays, provide:
    ✧ cold compresses
    ✧ pressure dressings

QUICK REVIEW QUESTION

19. A 19-year-old male patient arrives at the ED with symptoms of a penile fracture. What intervention should the nurse prepare for?

Renal Calculi

Pathophysiology

Renal calculi (kidney stones) are hardened mineral deposits (most often calcareous) that form in the kidneys. Renal calculi are usually asymptomatic but will cause debilitating pain and urinary symptoms once they pass into the urinary tract, where they are referred to as urinary calculi.

Risk Factors

+ dehydration
+ excess protein, sodium, or oxalate in diet
+ obesity
+ inflammatory bowel disease
+ renal tubular acidosis
+ hyperparathyroidism
+ gout
+ medications:
  ✧ topiramate (Topamax)
  ✧ ciprofloxacin
  ✧ sulfa antibiotics
  ✧ diuretics
  ✧ decongestants
+ UTIs

Signs and Symptoms

+ flank pain:
  ✧ severe
  ✧ sudden and sharp
  ✧ intermittent
  ✧ can radiate to abdomen or groin
+ nausea and vomiting
+ dysuria
+ hematuria
+ urine frequency
+ urinary urgency
+ fever
+ chills
+ tachycardia

Diagnostic Tests and Findings

+ urinalysis for hematuria, pyuria, acidic urine
+ 24-hour urinalysis to monitor elevated calcium, oxalate, and sodium; decreased volume
+ imaging to diagnose calculi:
  ✧ CT scan
  ✧ abdominal X-ray
  ✧ ultrasound
  ✧ intravenous urography (with dye)

Treatment and Management

+ Treatment is based on cause and size of stone(s).
+ For small stones (< 5 mm) with minimal symptoms:
  ✧ Small stones will pass spontaneously.
  ✧ Administer analgesics.
  ✧ Alpha blockers can help the stone pass.
  ✧ Patients should drink 2 to 3 quarts of water a day.

- Large stones (> 5 mm) with symptoms require surgical intervention.
  - ESWL
  - uteroscopic stone removal
  - percutaneous nephrolithotomy

QUICK REVIEW QUESTION

20. A patient presents to the ED with complaints of bloody urine and severe side and back pain. What imagining study should the nurse anticipate will be ordered?

Testicular Torsion

Pathophysiology

Testicular torsion occurs when the spermatic cord, which supplies blood to the testicles, becomes twisted, leading to an ischemic testicle. The condition is considered a medical emergency that requires immediate treatment to preserve the function of the testicle. Most testicular torsion cases are caused by **bell-clapper deformity**, in which the testicle is not correctly attached to the tunica vaginalis.

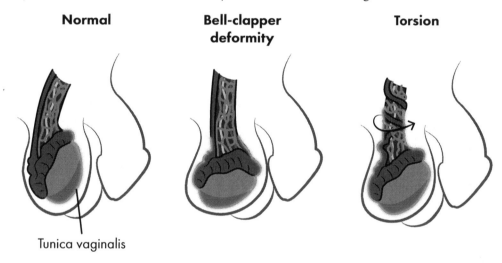

Normal **Bell-clapper deformity** **Torsion**

Tunica vaginalis

Figure 5.4. Testicular Torsion

Risk Factors

- male ages 10 – 25
- bell-clapper deformity
- trauma
- cold weather (especially sudden shift from warm to cold)

Signs and Symptoms

- sudden, severe unilateral scrotal pain
- high-riding testicle
- absent cremasteric reflex
- nausea and vomiting
- signs of inflammation in scrotal skin:
  - edematous
  - warm
  - indurated

Diagnostic Tests and Findings

+ Due to risk of ischemia in testicle, diagnosis is made based on signs and symptoms.

+ Ultrasound will show reduced or absent blood flow to affected testicle.

Treatment and Management

+ Administer analgesics.

+ Prepare patient for immediate exploratory surgery.

QUICK REVIEW QUESTION

21. What is the primary risk factor for testicular torsion?

Urinary Retention

Pathophysiology

Urinary retention is the inability to void the bladder. The condition can be acute or chronic and is most often caused by either an obstruction (e.g., prostatic hyperplasia, organ prolapse) or an infection (e.g., prostatitis, vulvovaginitis). Acute urinary retention is a medical emergency that can result in bladder injuries, kidney infections, and sepsis if left untreated.

Risk Factors

+ obstruction:
  ⋄ prostatic hyperplasia (BPH) or cancer
  ⋄ organ prolapse
  ⋄ urinary calculi
+ infection:
  ⋄ prostatitis
  ⋄ vulvovaginitis
  ⋄ urethritis
+ neurological:
  ⋄ herpes zoster
  ⋄ Guillain-Barré syndrome
  ⋄ spinal cord injury or disease (neurogenic bladder)

+ medications:
  ⋄ tricyclic antidepressants
  ⋄ anticholinergics
  ⋄ antihistamines
  ⋄ hormones
  ⋄ muscle relaxants
  ⋄ trauma

Signs and Symptoms

+ inability to urinate
+ urinary frequency or urgency

+ pelvic pressure or pain

- depending on underlying cause of retention, may include:
  - dysuria
  - hematuria
  - vaginal discharge
  - urethral discharge
  - enlarged prostate

Diagnostic Tests and Findings

- urinalysis to assess for infection
- prostate-specific antigen to assess for cancer or BPH
- BUN, creatinine, electrolytes to assess for renal failure
- ultrasound to measure post-void residual
- imaging to identify cause of retention:
  - renal/bladder ultrasound
  - CT scan

Treatment and Management

- Priority intervention is immediate voiding of bladder via catheter.
- After bladder is voided, provide treatment for underlying cause of retention.

QUICK REVIEW QUESTION

22. A patient in the ED states that he has not voided for 16 hours, and a bladder scan shows 600 ml of urine in the bladder. What is the nurse's priority?

Sexual Assault and Battery

Sexual assault is any unwanted sexual or physical contact or behavior that occurs without the explicit consent of the recipient. Victims of sexual assault can be male or female, adult or pediatric. It is a significantly underreported crime, and many victims know the assailant. Any patient presenting with a report of sexual assault should be treated with respect and dignity.

Treatment and Management

- Assess for serious or emergent conditions that may require immediate treatment.
- For female patients, take a complete OB/GYN history.
- The physician or a certified sexual assault nurse examiner (SANE) may perform a sexual assault medical forensic exam (also called a sexual assault forensic exam or "rape kit") to document injuries and collect evidence.
- Follow hospital protocols for STI screening (some hospitals require it while others do not).
- All patients reporting sexual assault should be offered postexposure prophylaxis.
  - emergency contraception (after negative hCG test)
  - antibiotics and antiprotozoals (ceftriaxone, metronidazole, azithromycin and/or doxycycline)
  - HIV postexposure prophylaxis (PEP)
  - HPV vaccine

+ Provide emotional support to patient.

+ Provide patient with access to available resources for survivors of sexual assault, including hospital counselors and community sexual assault centers.

Legal Considerations

+ Nurses should keep in mind that patients' medical records are legal documents that may be used in criminal or civil court proceedings.

+ All interactions with patients should be carefully documented.

+ Nurses who are asked to testify in court should confer with the hospital's legal team.

QUICK REVIEW QUESTION

23. A patient arrives at the ED stating they have been beaten and sexually assaulted. What is the nurse's priority?

ANSWER KEY

1. A young female patient may not disclose a history of sexual activity or potential pregnancy in the presence of a parent. The nurse should create an opportunity to ask these questions in a private setting such as a bathroom or exam room.

2. Common symptoms of straddle injuries, in addition to nausea and genital pain, include suprapubic or abdominal pain and dysuria.

3. The patient likely sustained a straddle injury and is experiencing soft tissue swelling of the labia and external genitalia. A urine sample should be obtained and the patient prepped for a manual pelvic exam. Cold compresses can be provided to decrease swelling and provide localized pain relief.

4. The nurse should prepare the patient for endoscopic removal of the object.

5. The start of menses can be challenging for young women. The patient may have accidently left a tampon in her vagina, which after a few weeks would cause the reported signs and symptoms.

6. The nurse should tell the patient that the risk of the infection spreading and causing permanent harm to future and past partners is high.

7. Antibiotics should be prescribed based on the presentation and history provided by the patient. Pain control should be provided through the use of medications and non-pharmacological methods such as scrotal support, ice, and rest.

8. The nurse should explain to the patient that the outbreaks are treatable and mostly preventable; however, the disease has no cure. Education should be provided to the patient to prevent the spread of the virus.

9. Gonorrhea can be transferred to the newborn via vaginal birth and cause complications, including eye infections. However, gonorrhea is treatable, and with regularly scheduled checkups and no reoccurrences before delivery, the newborn should be unaffected.

10. The nurse should provide supportive treatment for orchitis secondary to mumps. This includes analgesics, ice packs, and scrotal elevation.

11. The nurse should consider PID, with the main contributing factor being the fact that the STI went untreated. The symptoms suggest an exacerbation of pelvic inflammatory disease.

12. While most cases of prostatitis can be treated in the ED with antibiotics, patients who have obstructive anuria or show signs and symptoms of sepsis will require hospitalization.

13. The clinical triad consists of fever, nausea and/or vomiting, and costovertebral pain.

14. Tertiary stage syphilis presents with a wide range of symptoms that can manifest in almost any body system. For a patient with neurological symptoms, an analysis of CSF can confirm or rule out a diagnosis of syphilis.

15. The nurse should explain that *E. coli* found in feces is the most common cause for UTIs and explain the importance of wiping from front to back. In addition, girls have a much shorter urethra than boys, making it easier for feces to enter a girl's bladder.

16. A white, foul-smelling vaginal discharge with no other signs or symptoms is characteristic of bacterial vaginosis. The patient will likely be treated with a course of antibiotics such as metronidazole or clindamycin.

17. Ultrasound of the ovaries, usually transvaginal, is used to determine if there is an ovarian cyst and the status of the cyst (e.g., intact, ruptured, etc.).

18. The nurse should explain that during episodes of nonischemic priapism, blood continues to move through the penis and the chance of permanent damage is very low. The nurse should further explain that this type of priapism usually resolves on its own but that treatment options are available if it does not.

19. The patient should be prepared for surgery. Historically, penile fracture was treated conservatively using cold compresses and anti-inflammatories, but current protocol is for immediate surgical repair.

20. The patient has symptoms of urinary calculi. A CT scan is the preferred imaging study to visualize the location, size, and composition of the calculi.

21. Bell-clapper deformity, a genetic condition in which the testicles are not attached to the scrotum, is found in 90 percent of testicular torsion cases.

22. The nurse should assist the patient with voiding by placing a straight catheter or a Foley catheter.

23. The nurse's priority is to assess the patient for serious or life-threatening injuries. Further interventions, including forensic exams and prophylaxis, will be provided based on the patient's wishes.

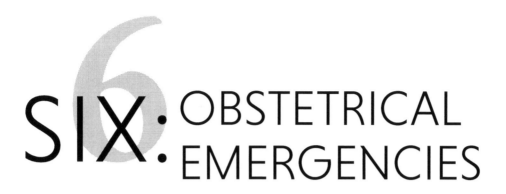

SIX: OBSTETRICAL EMERGENCIES

Eclampsia and Related Emergencies

PREECLAMPSIA

Pathophysiology

Preeclampsia is a syndrome caused by abnormalities in the placental vasculature. The syndrome is characterized by hypertension in the mother paired with either proteinuria or end-organ dysfunction. Symptoms can appear after the twentieth week of pregnancy and most commonly appear after 34 weeks. In most cases, preeclampsia will resolve after delivery, but symptoms can develop up to 4 weeks postpartum. Because preeclampsia is usually diagnosed during routine prenatal care, postpartum preeclampsia most commonly presents in the ED.

Preeclampsia is classified as being either with or without severe features. Preeclampsia with severe features can lead to life-threatening complications, including eclampsia, pulmonary edema, and abruptio placentae.

Risk Factors

+ age > 35
+ personal or family history of preeclampsia
+ obesity
+ pregestational diabetes

+ nulliparity
+ multifetal pregnancy
+ pregestational hypertension
+ chronic kidney disease

Signs and Symptoms

+ hypertension:
  ✧ systolic BP > 140 mmHg or diastolic BP > 90 mmHg
  ✧ two measurements 4 hours apart

+ facial edema
+ rapid weight gain (> 5 pounds a week)

- severe preeclampsia:
  - severe headache
  - visual abnormalities
  - epigastric pain
  - pitting edema
- signs and symptoms of pulmonary edema:
  - chest pain
  - dyspnea
  - oxygen sat < 94%

Diagnostic Tests and Findings

- proteinuria diagnosed through urine sample:
  - 24-hour urine protein: ≥ 0.3 g
  - urine dipstick protein: $\geq 1+$ (mild preeclampsia) to $\geq 3+$ (severe preeclampsia)
- serum creatinine: > 1.2 mg/dL indicates severe preeclampsia

Treatment and Management

- Administer antihypertensives (labetalol, hydralazine, or short-acting nifedipine).
- Prophylactic magnesium prevents progression to eclampsia.
- Patient should be admitted to OB for monitoring and possible delivery.
- Postpartum preeclampsia patients should be admitted for observation and magnesium infusion.

QUICK REVIEW QUESTION

1. A patient who is 37 weeks pregnant presents to the ED. Assessment finds BP 162/112, P 88, R 24, reflexes +3/+4, and her urine tests positive for ketones. What intervention should the nurse be prepared for?

ECLAMPSIA

Pathophysiology

Eclampsia is the onset of tonic-clonic seizures in women with preeclampsia. Eclampsia can occur ante-, intra-, or postpartum. It is an emergent condition that requires immediate medical intervention.

Risk Factors

- preeclampsia

Signs and Symptoms

- signs and symptoms of preeclampsia
- tonic-clonic seizure(s)

Diagnostic Tests and Findings

- urine protein consistent with preeclampsia diagnosis

Treatment and Management

+ Maintain airway during and after seizures.
  - Roll patient onto left side.
  - Use raised and/or padded bed rails when appropriate.
  - Administer oxygen via non-rebreather face mask after seizure.
+ Administer magnesium sulfate to prevent further seizures.
+ Administer antihypertensives.
+ Patient should be admitted to OB for management and emergent delivery.

QUICK REVIEW QUESTION

2. A pregnant patient experiences a seizure in the ED waiting room. What actions should the nurse take?

HELLP SYNDROME

Pathophysiology

HELLP syndrome is currently believed to be a form of preeclampsia, although the relationship between the two disorders is controversial and not well understood. Around 85% of women diagnosed with HELLP will also present with symptoms of preeclampsia (hypertension and proteinuria). HELLP is characterized by:

+ hemolysis (H)
+ elevated liver enzymes (EL)
+ low platelet count (LP)

As with preeclampsia and eclampsia, symptoms of HELLP may develop ante-, intra-, or postpartum.

Risk Factors

+ preeclampsia or history of preeclampsia
+ history of HELLP
+ Caucasian
+ prior births

Signs and Symptoms

+ hypertension:
  - systolic > 140 mmHg or diastolic > 90 mmHg
+ abdominal pain:
  - epigastric
  - RUQ
+ nausea and vomiting
+ severe headache
+ visual disturbances

Diagnostic Tests and Findings

+ urine protein consistent with preeclampsia diagnosis
+ schistocytes on blood smear
+ platelets: ≤ 100,000 cells/μL
+ total bilirubin: ≥ 1.2 mg/dL
+ AST: > 70 units/L

Treatment and Management

+ Administer antihypertensives (labetalol, hydralazine, or short-acting nifedipine).
+ Administer magnesium sulfate.
+ Patient should be admitted to OB for management and emergent delivery.

Ectopic Pregnancy

Pathophysiology

In an **ectopic pregnancy**, the blastocyst implants in a location other than the uterus. In > 95% of cases, implantation occurs in the fallopian tubes (tubal pregnancy), but implantation can also occur in the ovaries, cervix, or abdominal cavity. Ectopic pregnancies are most often caused by tubal irregularities that are congenital or the result of infection or surgery. A tubal pregnancy may rupture the fallopian tube, causing a life-threatening hemorrhage.

Risk Factors

+ age > 35
+ history of ectopic pregnancy
+ PID
+ STIs (chlamydia and gonorrhea)
+ infertility
+ fertility treatments
+ tubal surgery
+ smoking

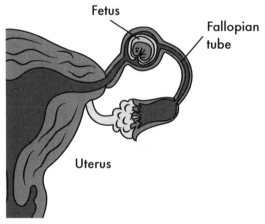

Figure 6.1. Ectopic Pregnancy (Tubal Pregnancy)

Signs and Symptoms

+ may be asymptomatic
+ vaginal bleeding
+ abdominal pain
+ signs and symptoms of pregnancy:
  + amenorrhea
  + nausea and vomiting
  + breast tenderness
  + fatigue
+ signs and symptoms of hemorrhage:
  + hypotension
  + dysrhythmias
  + dyspnea
  + syncope

Diagnostic Tests and Findings

+ pregnancy confirmation with urine or serum hCG

+ pelvic exam to confirm source of bleeding

+ transvaginal ultrasound to locate pregnancy

+ FAST ultrasound to assess for hemorrhage if suspected

Treatment and Management

+ Administer RhoGAM if mother is Rh negative.

+ For hemodynamically unstable patients:
    ⬧ Stabilize patient.
    ⬧ Prepare for emergency surgery.

+ For hemodynamically stable patients:
    ⬧ OB referral for surgery or treatment with methotrexate.

QUICK REVIEW QUESTION

4. A sexually active 19-year-old presents to the ED with vaginal bleeding and intermittent LLQ abdominal pain. Vital signs are stable, abdomen is tender, and the patient's uterus is soft and slightly enlarged. An ultrasound assessment confirms an ectopic pregnancy. What will be the most likely intervention for this patient?

Hyperemesis Gravidarum

Pathophysiology

Hyperemesis gravidarum is severe nausea and vomiting that occurs during pregnancy. While there is no definitive diagnostic line between hyperemesis and common "morning sickness," hyperemesis is generally defined as frequent vomiting that results in weight loss and ketonuria. Severe vomiting can lead to dehydration, hypovolemia, and electrolyte imbalances. Hyperemesis usually presents around 6 weeks gestation and resolves around 16 to 20 weeks. However, for some women it may persist until delivery.

Risk Factors

+ personal or family history of hyperemesis

+ previous nausea and vomiting related to:
    ⬧ estrogen-based medications
    ⬧ motion sickness

+ multifetal pregnancy

+ young age

+ hydatidiform mole

Signs and Symptoms

+ persistent vomiting (> 3 times per day)

+ weight loss of > 5 pounds or > 5% of body weight

+ signs and symptoms of hypovolemia:
    ⬧ thirst
    ⬧ decreased urine volume
    ⬧ tachycardia
    ⬧ tachypnea
    ⬧ hypotension
    ⬧ delayed CRT

Diagnostic Tests and Findings

- elevated BUN
- elevated urine specific gravity
- serum electrolytes showing hypokalemia or other imbalances
- urinalysis positive for ketones
- elevated AST and ALT

Treatment and Management

- Administer IV fluids.
    - initial infusion of lactated Ringer's followed by dextrose
    - urine output 100 ml/hour
- Replace lost vitamins and minerals.
    - IV thiamine
    - IV multivitamin
    - IV magnesium, calcium, or phosphorus as indicated by labs
- Administer antiemetics.
    - doxylamine-pyridoxine (Diclegis)
    - ondansetron
    - antihistamines (dimenhydrinate or diphenhydramine)
    - promethazine
- Admit to hospital if electrolyte imbalances or vomiting continue.
- Educate patient:
    - BRAT diet
    - diet high in protein
    - triggers to avoid (e.g., brushing teeth, tight clothing)

> ### QUICK REVIEW QUESTION
> **5.** How is hyperemesis gravidarum differentiated from morning sickness?

Labor and Delivery

Pathophysiology

Labor and delivery occurs in 3 stages.

- Stage 1: onset of labor to full cervical dilation (12 – 16 hours)
    - latent phase: gradual cervical dilation
    - active phase: rapid cervical dilation
- Stage 2: cervical dilation to expulsion of fetus (2 – 3 hours)
    - passive phase: before active maternal pushing
    - active phase: during active maternal pushing
- Stage 3: delivery of placenta (10 – 12 minutes)

Delivery is **imminent** if the fetus is visible and/or the mother reports the urge to push with contractions. Alternatively, delivery can be considered imminent if the cervix is fully dilated (10 cm) and contractions are < 2 minutes apart.

Contractions and cervical dilation before the thirty-seventh week of gestation is **preterm labor**. If preterm labor begins between 34 and 37 weeks with no other complications, the patient should be transferred to the labor and delivery setting if delivery is not imminent. When preterm labor begins at < 34 weeks, the mother should be transferred to OB for treatment to delay delivery.

Risk Factors

+ emergent delivery:
    ✧ unrecognized pregnancy
    ✧ unrecognized signs of labor
    ✧ lack of prenatal care
    ✧ trauma
+ preterm labor:
    ✧ history of preterm labor
    ✧ short cervical length
    ✧ infections (e.g., bacterial vaginosis, UTI, STIs)
    ✧ multifetal pregnancy
    ✧ underweight mother
    ✧ obese mother
    ✧ diabetes

Signs and Symptoms

+ ruptured amniotic membrane ("water broke")
+ dilation of cervix
+ contractions
+ urge to push

Diagnostic Tests and Findings

+ pelvic exam:
    ✧ Assess cervical dilation.
    ✧ Identify presentation and location of fetus.
+ fetal Doppler to assess fetal heart rate
+ transabdominal ultrasound:
    ✧ Identify presentation and number of fetus(es).
    ✧ Assess placenta and cord for possible complications.

Treatment and Management

+ Assess patient to determine stage of labor and gestational age.
    ✧ OB consult is required stat for complications (e.g., preeclampsia, cord prolapse, breech presentation).
    ✧ Patients in preterm labor should be transferred stat to OB for treatment and possible delivery.

- If delivery is not imminent, patient should be transferred to OB for delivery.
- If delivery is imminent and no complications have been identified, delivery will take place in the ED.
+ Monitor maternal blood pressure, heart rate, and contractions.
+ Monitor fetal heart rate.
+ Position mother is lithotomy position for delivery.
+ Clean perineum with antiseptic.
+ Care of newborn postdelivery:
  - Wipe nose and mouth; suction airway if obstructed.
  - Dry and stimulate newborn.
  - Assign Apgar score; 0 to 2 points for:
    + neonatal heart rate
    + respiratory effort
    + muscle tone
    + reflex irritability
    + color
+ Care of mother postdelivery:
  - Deliver placenta.
  - Administer oxytocin IM or perform fundal massage.
  - Monitor for signs of hemorrhage.

QUICK REVIEW QUESTION

6. A 25-year-old full-term patient presents to the ED stating her water broke and that she is in labor. A quick assessment reveals the cervix is fully dilated and the head is crowning. What is the nurse's priority?

Neonatal Resuscitation

Pathophysiology

The transition to extrauterine life requires a complex series of changes in the cardiopulmonary system of a neonate. The alveoli in the neonate's lungs expand, usually beginning with the first breath, and the lungs are cleared of fluid. In addition, the clamping of the umbilical cord combined with the expansion of the lungs raises the neonate's blood pressure and pushes blood into the vasculature of the lungs.

A small number of neonates (around 10%) will require intervention to establish ventilation. Poor respiratory performance can have a number of causes:

+ blocked airway
+ lack of respiratory effort (usually the result of musculature or neurological deficits)
+ persistent pulmonary hypertension in the newborn
+ heart or lung defects
+ preterm labor (lungs are not mature enough to clear and expand)

Risk Factors

+ age > 35
+ maternal diabetes
+ maternal hypertension
+ premature or postmature delivery

+ fetal heart or lung defects
+ narcotic use immediately before birth
+ alcohol use
+ cocaine use

Signs and Symptoms

+ absence of spontaneous breath
+ absence of vigorous cry
+ airway obstruction (nares and/or trachea)

+ cyanosis
+ poor muscle tone

Resuscitation Procedures

+ Stimulate the neonate by rubbing back, feet, and/or chest vigorously.
+ Prevent heat loss by placing child in warmer.
+ Clear airway of obstructions using bulb suction or wall suction (low suction).
+ If stimulation and warming do not work, activate neonatal resuscitation code.
+ Neonatal resuscitation is a specialized skill and requires supplemental education and certification.
+ The ED nurse should be prepared to provide basic resuscitation of a neonate until the appropriate caregivers can arrive.
  ⟡ Apply oxygen with positive pressure ventilation.
  ⟡ If the neonate is apneic and the heart rate is < 60, initiate CPR.

> ### QUICK REVIEW QUESTION
> **7.** A neonate delivered in the ED is receiving resuscitation measures. What assessment criteria would indicate that resuscitation measures have been successful?

Obstetrical Trauma

Pathophysiology

Trauma is the leading nonobstetric cause of death for pregnant people. Common causes of trauma include MVAs, falls, and intimate partner violence. Trauma is categorized as major if it involves the abdomen, includes high force, or results in vaginal bleeding or decreased fetal movement. Minor trauma does not involve the abdomen and may include no obvious signs and symptoms. However, minor trauma can still be fatal for mother or fetus, so a thorough assessment should be done on any trauma patient who may be pregnant.

In the ED, the patient should be assessed and stabilized before the fetus is assessed. Pregnant patients presenting to the ED should be evaluated for any non–pregnancy-related issues and then referred to OB if necessary.

Physiological changes to the mother during pregnancy that may affect assessment include:

+ 50% increase in blood volume
+ 50% increase in respiratory rate
+ delayed gastric emptying
+ elevated diaphragm

Risk Factors

+ MVAs
+ falls
+ intimate partner violence
+ GSW
+ epilepsy
+ self-harm
+ iatrogenic injury

Signs and Symptoms

+ visible signs and symptoms of injury, including ecchymosis and lacerations
+ vaginal bleeding
+ tense abdomen
+ decreased uterine tone
+ presence of amniotic fluid due to membrane rupture

Diagnostic Tests and Findings

+ pregnancy confirmation with urine or serum hCG (if needed)
+ transvaginal ultrasound to assess fetus, locate placenta, and assess for abruption
+ FAST ultrasound to assess for hemorrhage if suspected
+ no speculum or digital exam of cervix until location of placenta is confirmed via ultrasound
+ routine trauma labs (CBS, coagulation, etc.)

Treatment and Management

+ Treatment and management are determined by severity of injury to mother and fetus.
+ Assess mother's ABCs.
    ⋄ oxygen and respiratory intervention as needed (keep oxygen sat > 95%)
    ⋄ cardiac resuscitation as needed
    ⋄ cesarean delivery to be performed after maternal cardiac arrest if fetus is > 23 weeks
+ Administer IV fluids or blood products as needed.
+ Monitor fetus and uterine contractions for at least 24 hours.
+ Administer RhoGAM if mother is Rh negative.
+ Administer Tdap vaccine if not already given during pregnancy.
+ Administer betamethasone for imminent delivery of fetus < 34 weeks.
+ OB consult for all obstetric trauma patients.
+ Patients with contractions, bleeding, membrane rupture, or an abnormal fetal heart rate should be admitted to OB for management.

+ Perimortem cesarean delivery can be performed in cases of maternal death if there is a reasonable possibility of preserving the life of the fetus.

QUICK REVIEW QUESTION

8. A patient in the third trimester is admitted to the ED after a fall. The assessment shows no vaginal bleeding, but the patient's H/H is low. What should the nurse suspect?

Placental Disorders

ABRUPTIO PLACENTAE

Pathophysiology

Abruptio placentae (placental abruption) occurs when the placenta separates from the uterus after the twentieth week of gestation but before delivery. Abruption can lead to life-threatening conditions, including hemorrhage and DIC. Blood loss due to abruption can be difficult to quantify as blood may accumulate behind the placenta (**concealed abruption**) rather than exiting through the vagina.

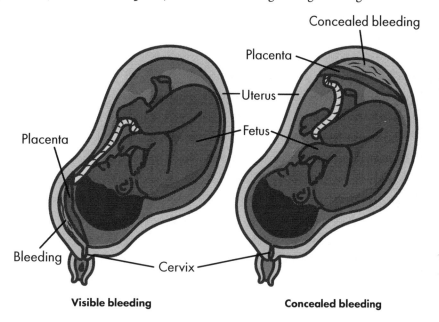

Figure 6.2. Abruptio Placentae

Risk Factors

+ personal or family history of abruption

+ hypertension

+ preeclampsia

+ fetal abnormalities

+ blunt trauma

+ smoking

+ cocaine use

Signs and Symptoms

+ vaginal bleeding (light to heavy)

+ firm uterus

+ contraction

+ abdominal or back pain (depending on location of placenta)

+ signs and symptoms of hemorrhage:
    ⬦ hypotension
    ⬦ tachycardia
    ⬦ abnormal fetal heart rate

Diagnostic Tests and Findings

+ transabdominal ultrasound to confirm abruption

+ decreased fibrinogen suggestive of DIC

Treatment and Management

+ Begin fetal heart rate monitoring.

+ Monitor mother for signs of hemodynamic instability.

+ Administer RhoGAM if mother is Rh negative.

+ Monitor vaginal bleeding.

+ Administer IV fluids.

+ Patient should be admitted stat to OB for management.

QUICK REVIEW QUESTION

9. What signs or symptoms indicate a significant separation of the placenta from the uterus?

PLACENTA PREVIA

Pathophysiology

Placenta previa occurs when the placenta partially or completely covers the internal orifice of the cervix. A low lying placenta is located ≤ 2 cm from the cervix but does not cover it. Placenta previa is usually asymptomatic and is found on routine prenatal ultrasounds. The presence of previa makes the placenta susceptible to rupture or hemorrhage and necessitates a cesarean delivery.

Placenta previa is correlated with **placenta accreta**, particularly in women who have had multiple previous cesarean deliveries. In placenta accreta, the placenta attaches abnormally deeply into the myometrium. Because the placenta cannot detach from the uterus after delivery, placenta accreta can lead to hemorrhage and requires a hysterectomy.

Risk Factors

+ age > 35

+ history of placenta previa

+ multifetal pregnancy

+ previous cesarean delivery

+ infertility treatment

+ smoking

+ cocaine use

Signs and Symptoms

+ vaginal bleeding

Table 6.1. Differentiating Abruptio Placentae and Placenta Previa

	Abruptio Placentae	Placenta Previa
Onset of Symptoms	sudden and intense bleeding with pain	asymptomatic or painless bleeding
Bleeding	bleeding may be vaginal or concealed	vaginal bleeding
Uterine Tone	firm	soft and relaxed

Diagnostic Tests and Findings

+ transabdominal or transvaginal ultrasound to confirm location of placenta over cervix

+ no rectal or cervical exam until placenta placement is known

Treatment and Management

+ Begin fetal heart rate monitoring.

+ Monitor mother for signs of hemodynamic instability.

+ Administer RhoGAM if mother is Rh negative.

+ Administer IV fluids and blood products if patient shows signs of hypovolemia.

+ If patient presents with vaginal bleeding, admit to OB for management and possible emergent delivery.

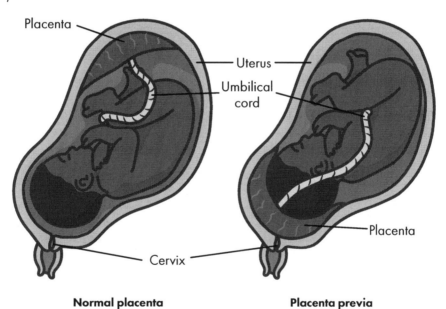

Normal placenta   **Placenta previa**

Figure 6.3. Placenta Previa

QUICK REVIEW QUESTION

10. A patient presents to the ED at 32 weeks gestation with heavy vaginal bleeding. What signs or symptoms would guide the nurse to suspect placenta previa over placental abruption?

Postpartum Emergencies

POSTPARTUM HEMORRHAGE

Pathophysiology

Postpartum hemorrhage is bleeding that occurs any time after delivery up to 12 weeks postpartum and exceeds 1000 ml or that causes symptoms of hypovolemia. Primary hemorrhage occurs during the first 24 hours after delivery; secondary hemorrhage occurs between 24 hours and 12 weeks postpartum. The etiology of both primary and secondary hemorrhage varies.

Causes of primary hemorrhage:

+ trauma: lacerations to uterus or vagina
+ uterine atony: failure of the uterus to contract after delivery, often because of placental disorders
+ retained tissue
+ coagulation disorders

Causes of secondary hemorrhage:

+ subinvolution of the placental site: persistence of dilated arteries in placenta or uterus postpartum
+ retained tissue
+ infection
+ coagulation disorders

Risk Factors

+ placental disorders (accreta or previa)
+ preeclampsia, eclampsia, or HELLP
+ failure to progress in labor
+ retained products of conception

Signs and Symptoms

+ vaginal bleeding
+ signs and symptoms of hypovolemia:
    ⋄ hypotension
    ⋄ tachycardia
    ⋄ tachypnea
    ⋄ syncope
    ⋄ delayed CRT

Diagnostic Tests and Findings

+ decreased fibrinogen
+ decreased RBC count
+ elevated WBC, indicating infection
+ decreased platelet count
+ decreased H/H

Treatment and Management

+ Monitor for signs of hemodynamic instability.
+ Administer IV fluids.

- Administer blood products for patients with coagulopathies.

- Administer tranexamic acid.

- Prepare patient for surgery to diagnosis and treat underlying cause of bleeding.

QUICK REVIEW QUESTION

11. A patient presents to the ED with heavy vaginal bleeding after a home birth. Her blood pressure is 110/65 mm Hg, her HR is 118, and her RR is 24. What interventions should the nurse prepare for?

POSTPARTUM INFECTION

Pathophysiology

Postpartum patients are frequently discharged soon after delivery and may develop **postpartum infections** at home that require further treatment. Possible sites of infection include the endometrium (**endometritis**), surgical incisions, breasts (**mastitis**), and urinary tract. The infection may spread and lead to septicemia, peritonitis, or sepsis. Endometritis is the most common postpartum infection.

Risk Factors

- cesarean delivery

- vaginal infections

- manual rupture of membranes

Signs and Symptoms

- fever of ≥ 100.4°F (38°C):
    - on more than 2 of the first 10 days postpartum
    - maintained over 24 hours after the end of the first day postpartum
- endometritis:
    - tachycardia
    - uterine tenderness
    - midline lower abdominal pain

- surgical incision infection:
    - erythema and inflammation at incision
    - purulent exudate
- mastitis:
    - erythema and tenderness in breast
- UTI:
    - signs and symptoms consistent with UTI

Diagnostic Tests and Findings

- Increased WBC count indicates infection.

- Elevations in ESR will be present in endometritis.

- Cultures taken from cervical discharge, urine, or wound will identify bacteria causing infection.

- Ultrasound of breast tissue may show abscess related to infection.

Treatment and Management

- endometritis and UTI:
    - Administer broad-spectrum antibiotics.
    - Treat for fever and pain as needed.

- surgical incision:
  - Drain, irrigate, and debride wound.
  - Antibiotics are not usually needed.
- mastitis:
  - Treat for fever and pain as needed.
  - Empty breast of milk.
  - Administer broad-spectrum antibiotics if infection persists.

12. A postpartum patient returns to the ED 4 days following discharge from an uncomplicated vaginal delivery. She has a temperature of 101 °F (38.3 °C) and assessment shows erythema and discharge with an odor at her episiotomy site. What interventions should the nurse anticipate?

Spontaneous Abortion

Pathophysiology

Spontaneous abortion (miscarriage) is the loss of a pregnancy before the twentieth week of gestation. (Death of the fetus after the twentieth week is commonly referred to as a **stillbirth**.) Spontaneous abortions are a common complication of early pregnancy. They can occur because of chromosomal or congenital abnormalities, material infection or disorders, or trauma.

Spontaneous abortions are classified by the location of the embryo/fetus and cervical dilation.

- **missed abortion**: occurs when the embryo/fetus is nonviable but has not been passed from the uterus and the cervix is closed
- **threatened abortion**: occurs when the patient has vaginal bleeding before 20 weeks and the cervix is closed; may progress to incomplete or complete abortion
- **inevitable abortion**: occurs when the patient has vaginal bleeding and the cervix is dilated but the embryo/fetus remains in the uterus; often accompanied by abdominal pain or cramps
- **incomplete abortion**: occurs when the patient has vaginal bleeding, the cervix is dilated, and the embryo/fetus is found in the cervical canal
- **complete abortion**: occurs when the embryo/fetus has been completely expelled from the uterus and cervix and the cervix is closed
- **septic abortion**: occurs when the abortion is accompanied by uterine infection; it is a life-threatening condition that requires immediate medical intervention

Risk Factors

- age > 35
- history of spontaneous abortion
- underweight mother
- obese mother
- pregestational hypertension
- infection, particularly with fever
- endocrine disorders
- smoking
- cocaine use
- alcohol use

Signs and Symptoms

+ vaginal bleeding
+ passage of fetal tissue
+ radiating pelvic pain
+ signs and symptoms of cessation of pregnancy (e.g., nausea, breast tenderness)

+ signs and symptoms of infection with septic abortion:
  ✧ fever
  ✧ chills
  ✧ tachycardia
  ✧ tachypnea

Diagnostic Tests and Findings

+ pelvic exam to assess cervical dilation
+ fetal Doppler to assess for fetal cardiac activity
+ transvaginal ultrasound to confirm pregnancy loss

Treatment and Management

+ Administer RhoGAM if mother is Rh negative.
+ Manage pain.
+ Monitor patient for hemodynamic instability if bleeding is heavy.
+ Refer to OB for management.

+ For septic abortion:
  ✧ Take blood and endometrial cultures.
  ✧ Administer broad-spectrum antibiotics.
  ✧ Prepare patient for immediate surgery to evacuate uterus.

QUICK REVIEW QUESTION

13. A patient in the first trimester is admitted to the ED with complaints of abdominal cramping and spotting over the last 18 hours. During the assessment the nurse is palpating the breast for tenderness and the patient states that the tenderness is gone. Why is the lack of tenderness to the breast a concern for the nurse?

Umbilical Cord Prolapse

Pathophysiology

Umbilical cord prolapse occurs when the cord presents alongside (occult) or ahead of (overt) the presenting fetus during delivery. Exposure of the cord makes it vulnerable to compression or rupture, which disrupts blood flow to the fetus.

Risk Factors

+ premature delivery
+ small fetus
+ breech, transverse, or oblique presentation
+ low-lying placenta

+ obstetric interventions:
  ✧ rupture of amniotic sac
  ✧ forceps or vacuum
  ✧ intrauterine pressure catheter
  ✧ balloon catheter

Signs and Symptoms

+ cord may protrude from vagina or be palpated during vaginal exam

+ fetal bradycardia (< 120 bpm)

+ sudden increase then decrease in fetal activity

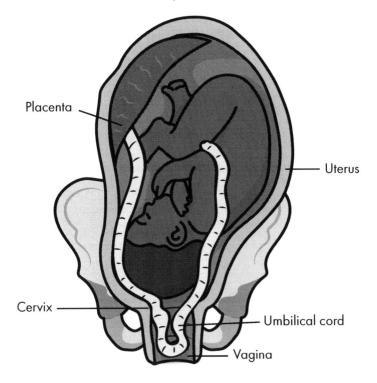

Figure 6.4. Umbilical Cord Prolapse

Treatment and Management

+ Prepare patient for emergent delivery.
    ⬦ Delivery should be cesarean unless vaginal delivery is judged to be quicker.

+ Monitor fetal heart rate.

+ Apply saline-soaked sterile gauze to exposed umbilical cord.

+ Administer intrauterine resuscitation measures until patient is ready for delivery.
    ⬦ Elevate presenting part of fetus manually or through positioning.
    ⬦ Place patient in Trendelenburg or knee-chest position.
    ⬦ Retrofill bladder.

QUICK REVIEW QUESTION

14. During an emergent delivery in the ED, the umbilical cord exits the vaginal canal ahead of the fetus. What interventions should the nurse be prepared for?

ANSWER KEY

1. The patient is presenting with signs and symptoms of preeclampsia. The nurse should be prepared to administer antihypertensives and magnesium and to begin maternal and fetal monitoring.

2. The nurse's priority is to protect the patient's airway and prevent trauma to the patient. The nurse should roll the patient onto the left side and clear objects and people away from the patient. After the seizure, the nurse should prepare for the patient to be admitted to the ED, assessed for eclampsia, and treated with magnesium sulfate to prevent further seizures.

3. Hemolysis (H), elevated liver enzymes (EL), and a low platelet count (LP).

4. Because the patient is stable, refer to OB for assessment. The pregnancy will most likely be terminated using methotrexate or surgically.

5. Morning sickness is the common term for mild nausea and vomiting during early pregnancy. It does not usually affect fluid levels and can be managed with lifestyle changes. Hyperemesis gravidarum is defined as persistent nausea and vomiting in early pregnancy that leads to weight loss (> 5 pounds), dehydration, and possible hypovolemia and electrolyte imbalances.

6. The nurse should prepare for the patient for delivery. Obtain maternal vital signs and fetal heart rate. Place the mother in the lithotomy position and raise the head of the bed. Clean the perineum with antiseptic. Continue to check fetal heart rate and be prepared to aid with delivery of newborn.

7. The goal of resuscitation is for the neonate to have spontaneous respiration and a heart rate ≥ 100 bpm. The neonate's oxygen saturation should also be monitored and should reach 85% to 95% by 10 minutes postdelivery.

8. The nurse should suspect occult bleeding. The patient will require an ultrasound to assess for an abruption or other sources of bleeding, and may need blood products. This patient will likely be admitted to OB.

9. Significant separation of the placenta results in hemorrhage and rapid blood loss. Patients will show signs of hypovolemia, including heavy vaginal bleeding (unless abruption is concealed), hypotension, tachycardia, tachypnea, reduced urine output, and abnormal fetal heart rate.

10. The nurse should suspect placenta previa if the patient presents with no complaints of abdominal or pelvic pain and if the uterus is soft. The diagnosis will be confirmed via ultrasound.

11. The patient is showing early signs of hypovolemia (tachycardia and tachypnea accompanied by heavy blood loss). The nurse should monitor the patient for signs of hemodynamic instability and be prepared to deliver fluids or blood products as necessary. Once stable, the patient should be prepared for surgery.

12. The patient most likely has a postpartum infection at the episiotomy site. The nurse should be prepared to drain and clean the wound and provide treatment for pain (ice packs or NSAIDs). The nurse may also be asked to order a culture and sensitivity of the discharge and administer broad-spectrum antibiotics.

13. A loss or lack of tenderness indicates hormone levels have decreased and a spontaneous abortion is in progress or is imminent.

14. The patient will likely be prepared for an emergency cesarean delivery. While the patient is prepped, the nurse should expect to alleviate pressure on the cord by repositioning the patient and possibly retrofilling the bladder with saline. The nurse may also need to manually alleviate pressure on the cord by donning sterile gloves and gently pushing the presenting part of the fetus back into the vaginal canal.

SEVEN: PSYCHOSOCIAL EMERGENCIES

Psychosocial Assessment

+ Psychosocial emergencies can present as the patient's primary complaint or they can present with comorbid issues.

+ A psychosocial assessment is performed on every emergency patient regardless of chief complaint.

+ Key nursing considerations for such an assessment include:
  + relevant past medical history of mental illness
  + screening for weapons or contraband on the patient's person
  + lifestyle questions:
    + alcohol, tobacco, and recreational drugs
    + sexual activity (number of partners, condom use, and contraceptive use)
  + self/other harm assessment:
    + suicidal ideation
    + homicidal ideation
  + psychological assessment:
    + cognitive examination (mental status of the patient, including reasoning and language and executive functions)
    + behavioral assessment (affect, disposition, and speech abnormalities)
    + visual assessment (overall appearance of the patient and abnormal behaviors)
    + clinical impairment (Does the patient appear to be under the influence of alcohol or drugs?)

+ Depending on the patient's presentation and other factors, a medical assessment should be performed in conjunction with the psychosocial assessment.

+ Voluntary commitment for mental health concerns occurs when a patient and a physician determine that the patient would benefit from inpatient mental health care, and the patient consents to such an admission.

+ Involuntary commitment for mental health concerns occurs when a physician determines that a patient is at an acute risk of harming themselves or others and that the patient cannot be left to make a decision to voluntarily seek inpatient mental health care. Involuntary commitment laws are governed at the state level. Generally, an ED physician performs an evaluation and initiates the involuntary commitment paperwork that is then sent to the local official, after which the local law enforcement agency serves the patient with the legal document stating that they have been involuntarily committed.

Abuse and Neglect

Characteristics

Patients presenting in the ED with concern for **abuse** and **neglect** generally fall into one of three categories: domestic abuse, child abuse/neglect, and geriatric abuse/neglect. Nursing assessment for each of these concerns begins at triage, and every patient presenting to the ED should be screened for signs or indications of neglect. Abuse can include both physical and emotional abuse; neglect may be on the part of caregivers or self.

Signs and Symptoms

+ physical manifestations of abuse and neglect:
    ⋄ unexplained injuries
    ⋄ fractures or bruising at different stages of healing
    ⋄ poor hygiene
    ⋄ weight loss or gain
    ⋄ alopecia from hair pulling or lack of repositioning

+ emotional manifestations of abuse and neglect:
    ⋄ severe mood swings or changes
    ⋄ agitation
    ⋄ depression
    ⋄ withdrawal
    ⋄ sleep disturbance
    ⋄ suicidal ideation

Treatment and Management

+ Protected populations (including pediatric and geriatric patients) require obligatory reporting of suspected abuse and neglect.

+ The priority treatment of the abused or neglected patient should focus on physical injuries. Consideration should also be made for emotional needs that result from abuse and neglect, such as providing same-gender caregivers or a same-gender chaperone for exams, using organizational resources to provide support for the patient, asking permission to touch the patient or narrating the physical exam and warning the patient when and where they will be touched during the exam, and contacting local authorities or agencies where appropriate (in cases of child or elder abuse).

QUICK REVIEW QUESTION

1. A male pediatric patient arrives at the ED with a chief complaint of abdominal pain. Upon assessment, the nurse discovers bruising to the abdomen, back, and arms that appears to be in different stages of healing. The mother of the patient is at the bedside. What is the nurse's next action?

Aggressive or Violent Behavior

Characteristics

Aggressive or violent behavior in patients may occur for many reasons. These include:

+ crisis or psychosis

+ altered mental status

+ influence of drugs or alcohol

+ underlying organic processes:
  ⋄ traumatic brain injuries
  ⋄ urosepsis, especially in patients > 65
  ⋄ acute dementia or Alzheimer's disease

Treatment and Management

+ Management ranges from verbal de-escalation to mechanical restraint of the violent patient.
+ De-escalation strategies:
  ⋄ verbal redirection
  ⋄ allowing the patient to express needs
  ⋄ allowing the patient to exercise
  ⋄ decreased environmental stimulation (quiet room time)
  ⋄ PRN medication administration (as requested by patient)
+ Restraints may be used.
  ⋄ should be used conservatively
  ⋄ only for patients whose behavior cannot be controlled through less restrictive measures
  ⋄ require frequent assessment:
    + every 5 – 15 minutes depending on organizational policy
    + check vitals, assess pain, assess circulation and skin integrity of all restrained extremities, and address restroom needs
  ⋄ should be removed as soon as they are deemed unnecessary for patient and staff safety
+ In patients with acute agitation, medications can be administered.
  ⋄ olanzapine (Zyprexa)
  ⋄ haloperidol (Haldol)
  ⋄ risperidone (Risperdal)

QUICK REVIEW QUESTION

2. A patient was placed in mechanical restraints after demonstrating violent and aggressive behavior toward nursing staff. It has been 15 minutes since the restraints were applied, and the nurse is preparing to assess the patient. What will the nurse include in her assessment?

Anxiety and Panic

Characteristics

Anxiety is feelings of fear, apprehension, and worry that can be characterized as mild, moderate, or severe (panic). Anxiety will impact other functions such as the respiratory, cardiac, and gastrointestinal systems.

A key nursing consideration is to assess for organic causes for reported symptoms, as other life-threatening illnesses may present with similar symptoms.

Signs and Symptoms

+ physical manifestations:
  ⬩ palpitations or chest pain
  ⬩ dizziness
  ⬩ shortness of breath
  ⬩ diaphoresis
  ⬩ nausea

+ sudden onset of fear, worry, concern
+ extreme vigilance

Treatment and Management

+ Treatment of anxiety should be targeted at the level of anxiety the patient presents with (mild to panic).
+ Both non-pharmacological and pharmacological management should be considered.
+ Non-pharmacological interventions include:
  ⬩ Place patient in calm environment.
  ⬩ Encourage rhythmic breathing.
  ⬩ Offer social support if possible.
+ Pharmacological interventions (fast-acting anxiolytics) include:
  ⬩ benzodiazepines (diazepam [Valium], lorazepam [Ativan])
  ⬩ antihistamines (hydroxyzine)
+ Allow the patient time to overcome the episode.
+ In the case of chronic anxiety, consider long-term treatment.

QUICK REVIEW QUESTION

3. A patient presents to the ED stating he was in a movie theater and suddenly began to feel fearful, apprehensive, and on edge. He is feeling mild chest pain and shortness of breath. What should the nurse ask in the assessment of this patient?

Bipolar Disorder

Characteristics

Bipolar disorder (also known as manic-depressive illness) is characterized by shifts in mood accompanied by changes in activity and energy. These shifts are categorized as manic behaviors or depressive behaviors. Severe episodes of either mania or depression can also result in psychosis, characterized by hallucinations or delusions.

There are four classifications of bipolar disorder that are differentiated by the pattern of change in mood and behavior:

- Bipolar I disorder is characterized by manic episodes lasting a minimum of 7 days and depressive episodes lasting 2 weeks or longer. Symptoms of mania in bipolar I often lead to hospitalization.

- Bipolar II disorder is characterized by patterns of depression and hypomania (less severe manic episodes). These patterns can be predictable and symmetrical.

- Cyclothymic disorder does not meet the criteria for bipolar disorder, but patients have many episodes of depressive and hypomanic symptoms over at least a 2-year period.

- Other unspecified bipolar and related disorders characterize patients with bipolar-like symptoms that do not meet diagnostic criteria for the above diagnoses.

Signs and Symptoms

- manic behavior:
  - feelings of elation
  - high levels of energy and increased activity
  - difficulty sleeping; may not sleep for several days
  - increased rate of speech
  - engaging in high-risk activities (excessive spending, risky sexual activity)

- depressive behavior:
  - deep or intense feelings of sadness
  - decreased energy levels with associated decreased activity
  - sleep disturbances; either too much or too little sleep
  - appetite disturbance
  - suicidal ideation or focus on death
  - feelings of anxiety or worry

Treatment and Management

- Treatment is driven by patient presentation.

- Treatment in ED addresses the exacerbations of the disorder (i.e., patients "in crisis").

- Extreme or long-term mania requires immediate hospitalization and medical attention.

- Medications used to treat symptoms of exacerbations include:
  - mood stabilizers:
    - lithium
    - lamotrigine (Lamictal)
    - valproic acid
  - atypical antipsychotics:
    - risperidone
    - aripiprazole (Abilify)
    - ziprasidone (Geodon)
  - antipsychotics and antidepressants (usually used long-term):
    - olanzapine
    - quetiapine (Seroquel)
    - paroxetine (Paxil)

QUICK REVIEW QUESTION

4. A patient who is in a manic state in the emergency department refuses medical care. What is the next action that should be considered by the health care team?

Depression and Dysthymic Disorder

Characteristics

Depression is a mood disorder that has both emotional and physical symptoms. Patients who are depressed report feelings of sadness and hopelessness that last longer than two weeks, and they often will report feelings of suicidality along with feelings of hopelessness and sadness. Depression can manifest as an exacerbation of bipolar disorder or as its own disease process.

Signs and Symptoms

+ feelings of sadness or tearfulness
+ irritability, increased anger, outbursts
+ decreased interest in things that were once interesting
+ sleep changes (too much or too little sleep)
+ trouble concentrating
+ increased anxiety

Treatment and Management

+ Every patient presenting to the ED should be screened for depression or feelings of depression.
+ Nurses should also screen these patients for suicidal ideation.
+ Management of depression is long-term treatment with antidepressants and therapy.
+ Symptoms associated with depression can result from an underlying illness (e.g., metabolic disorders).
  + Such disorders should be ruled out prior to diagnosis and treatment for depression.

QUICK REVIEW QUESTION

5. A nurse is performing an assessment of a patient with a chief complaint of fatigue. The patient tells the nurse that he has felt hopeless recently and has not slept well for the last 2 or 3 weeks. What follow-up questions should the nurse ask this patient?

Homicidal Ideation

Characteristics

Homicidal ideation is characterized by feelings of intent to harm other people, either groups or individuals.

Treatment and Management

+ Assess for level of intent.
+ If the patient identifies an individual or group, the nurse and physician should determine if they are obligated to report the threat to law enforcement or to the individual or group.

QUICK REVIEW QUESTION

6. During triage, a patient expresses to the triage nurse that he wants to kill his boss. What should the nurse do next?

Mania

Characteristics

Mania is a state of high energy, increased activity, and feelings of elation and immortality. Mania is a manifestation of bipolar disorder in some patients.

Signs and Symptoms

+ reported feelings of increased productivity and focus
+ not sleeping for days or extended periods of time
+ poor financial decisions
+ unsafe decisions about sexual activity or safety

Treatment and Management

+ Patient may require hydration or other interventions if self-care has been neglected.
+ Treat acute cases of mania with medication.
    ⬦ antipsychotics and atypical antipsychotics:
        ‣ aripiprazole
        ‣ cariprazine
        ‣ clozapine
        ‣ olanzapine
    ⬦ mood stabilizers:
        ‣ lithium
        ‣ gabapentin
        ‣ lamotrigine
        ‣ oxcarbazepine
        ‣ valproic acid
    ⬦ may require a combination of these medicines
+ Screen the patient for unsafe behaviors.
    ⬦ recreational drug use
    ⬦ risky sexual encounters

> QUICK REVIEW QUESTION:
>
> 7. What are some key considerations in the assessment of a patient on the third day of a manic episode?

Psychosis

Characteristics

A patient experiencing an episode of **psychosis** will have delusions, hallucinations, paranoia, suicidal or homicidal ideation, and disturbances in thinking and perceptions. Psychosis can be the result of organic illnesses or an exacerbation of an existing or new-onset mental illness such as schizophrenia or bipolar disorder.

Treatment and Management

+ pharmacological intervention if patient is a threat to self or others
+ psychiatric consult

- assessment and treatment of underlying causes of psychosis
- involuntary commitment to inpatient mental health unit

QUICK REVIEW QUESTION

8. What are key nursing interventions for a patient in the ED presenting with acute psychosis?

Schizophrenia

Characteristics

Schizophrenia is a chronic psychotic condition that is characterized by bouts of psychosis, hallucinations, and disorganized speech. Positive symptoms of schizophrenia are those not normally seen in healthy persons, and negative symptoms are disruptions of normal behaviors.

Signs and Symptoms

- positive
  - delusions and hallucinations
  - disorganized speech
  - odd or confusing behavior
- negative
  - social withdrawal
  - paranoia
  - flattened affect
  - poverty of speech

Treatment and Management

- Treatment largely depends on how the patient presents to the ED.
- Organic causes for odd behavior should be ruled out.
  - DKA
  - hypoglycemia
  - stroke
  - sepsis
  - electrolyte imbalance
- Patients with known history of schizophrenia should be tested to rule out lithium toxicity.
- Perform further testing for alcohol and recreational drugs.
- Administer benzodiazepines for acute crisis.
- Crisis intervention response should be considered after medical evaluation is performed.

QUICK REVIEW QUESTION

9. A known schizophrenic patient presents to the ED after neighbors called the police concerned for her behavior. The patient appears unkempt, unclean, and not appropriately dressed for the weather. What key elements should the nurse assess this patient for?

Situational Crisis

Characteristics

A **situational crisis** is an acute change or event in a patient's life that may lead to feelings of anxiety, fear, depression, or other mental or emotional illness concerns. Examples of a situational crisis can include:

+ divorce
+ rape or sexual assault
+ domestic violence or abuse
+ loss of a job/retirement from a job
+ loss of a family member
+ any event that creates crisis from a patient's perspective

Nurses should understand that the crisis is as problematic as the patient perceives it to be. The key distinction is not the nature of the event, but the patient's response to the event. Patients may self-refer for situational crises, or the ED nurse may discover that the patient is experiencing a situational crisis during the course of the ED visit.

Signs and Symptoms

+ self-harm
+ aggression
+ hysteria
+ suicidal ideation
+ depression
+ psychosis

Treatment and Management

+ Management is determined by the patient's presentation.
+ Assess for patient safety and suicidal ideation.
+ Provide a safe environment for the patient.
+ Administer anxiolytic medications as necessary.
+ Refer to the appropriate crisis resources.

> ### QUICK REVIEW QUESTION
>
> **10.** A nurse is caring for a patient in the ED who has presented with a situational crisis. The patient has made a recent attempt at self-harm. What is the nurse's priority intervention for this patient?

Suicidal Ideation and Behavior

Characteristics

Suicidal ideation is characterized by feelings or thoughts of attempting or considering suicide. Patients exhibiting suicidal ideation may have vague thoughts without a distinct plan, or they may have a specific plan and the means to carry it out.

Risk Factors

+ populations at increased risk for suicide:
  ⬥ male < 20 or > 65
  ⬥ access to firearms
  ⬥ family history of suicide

+ situational factors:
  ✧ recent loss
  ✧ financial difficulty
  ✧ family difficulties such as divorce or strain
  ✧ physical or emotional abuse

+ chronic depression or mental illness such as bipolar disorder
+ substance abuse

Signs and Symptoms

+ Screen for suicidal ideation in all patients.
  ✧ Ask directly if the patient is considering suicide or has recently or in the past attempted suicide.
  ✧ If so, does the patient have a concrete plan to carry it out?
  ✧ Determine the presence of risk factors such as history of substance abuse or recent loss of a family member.
+ Assess the presence of social supports for the patient.

Treatment and Management

+ Secure all weapons in the patient's possession.
+ Secure a contract of safety with the patient. (Patient will sign a contract that states they will remain safe while in the hospital and in the future.)
+ Create an environment of safety for the patient.
+ Establish 1:1 watch or line-of-sight supervision for the patient.
+ Assess for admission based on the severity of suicidal ideation or behavior.
+ Before discharge, patient will be evaluated by psychiatrist, or ED provider will consult psychiatry.

QUICK REVIEW QUESTION:

11. How can the nurse address patient and staff safety when a patient reports thoughts of self-harm?

ANSWER KEY

1. The nurse should complete the physical assessment and discuss these findings with the ED physician. She should then complete the screening for child abuse and follow local policy on mandatory reporting of suspected child abuse.

2. The nurse should assess the status of the patient, including orientation, vital signs, neurovascular status of the extremities restrained, and skin integrity at the restraint points.

3. The nurse should obtain prior medical history to include cardiac and respiratory concerns and find out if the patient has a history of anxiety reactions in the past. The nurse should be prepared to address all life-threatening illnesses before addressing anxiety.

4. The ED physician should determine if the patient meets criteria for involuntary commitment because of concerns for the patient's safety.

5. The nurse should use the statements from the patient to consider organic causes for the fatigue and difficulty sleeping but should also ask further questions regarding the patient's emotional and psychological state, including those about suicidal ideation and feelings of safety.

6. The nurse should determine if the patient is in possession of any weapons and follow organizational policy regarding notifying security and the emergency physician of the patient's intent.

7. The nurse should do a physical assessment to include vital signs and sleep and eating habits to determine if the patient is adequately hydrated and fed. The nurse should determine if the patient has participated in any high-risk activities that may have either long-term or acute consequences to their health.

8. Address underlying causes of psychosis as well as resultant symptoms or injuries; request psychiatric consultation; prepare for involuntary commitment; provide a safe environment for the patient until the crisis can be addressed.

9. The nurse should perform a head-to-toe physical assessment to determine if any physical harm has come to the patient. The nurse should assess electrolyte balance, and determine if the patient is using recreational drugs or alcohol.

10. Providing for the patient's safety while in the ED is the nurse's priority.

11. The nurse should get a detailed accounting of the patient's plan for self-harm as well as determine if the patient is in possession of any objects or weapons that could cause harm to the patient or to the staff.

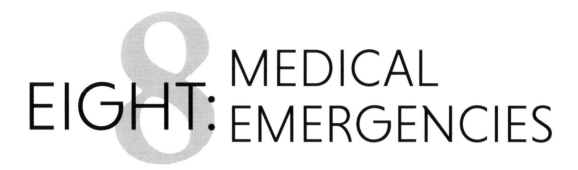

EIGHT: MEDICAL EMERGENCIES

Electrolyte Imbalances

Electrolytes are positively or negatively charged ions located in both the intracellular fluid (ICF) and the extracellular fluid (ECF). These ions are necessary for the maintenance of homeostasis, cellular excitability, and the transmission of neural impulses. Important electrolytes include sodium, potassium, magnesium, calcium, and phosphate. Electrolyte concentrations are influenced by fluid intake and output, dietary intake, medications, underlying disease, and trauma.

HYPONATREMIA (LOW SODIUM)
Normal values: 135 – 145 mEq/L

Clinical Manifestation

+ tachycardia
+ hypotension
+ weakness
+ dizziness
+ presyncope (lightheadedness and weakness)

+ headache
+ cerebral edema
+ increased ICP
+ seizures

Treatment and Management

+ Initiate sodium replacement: do not exceed 12 mEq/L in a 24-hour period. Rapid rise in sodium levels can cause demyelination and consequently impair neurological responses.

+ Administer PO sodium replacement as tolerated.

+ Administer isotonic IV solutions (lactated Ringer's or 0.9% normal saline).

+ Hypertonic fluid may be used to decrease cerebral edema in advanced cases.

+ Restrict patient's fluid intake, and monitor fluid intake and output.

HYPERNATREMIA (HIGH SODIUM)
Normal values: 135 – 145 mEq/L

Clinical Manifestation

- hypertension
- tachycardia
- pulmonary edema
- elevated body temperature

- hyperreflexia, including twitching
- polydipsia
- lethargy or decreased LOC
- seizures

Treatment and Management

- Restrict the patient's dietary sodium.
- Increase the patient's PO fluid or free-water intake.
- Administer diuretics.

- Administer D5W or other hypotonic IV solutions.
- Employ seizure precautions.

HYPOKALEMIA (LOW POTASSIUM)
Normal values: 3.5 – 5 mEq/L

Clinical Manifestation

- dysrhythmias:
  - flat or inverted T waves
  - prominent U waves
  - ST depression
  - prolonged PR interval

- hypotension
- altered mental status
- leg cramps or muscle cramps
- hypoactive reflexes
- flaccid muscles

Treatment and Management

- Replace potassium PO or IV:
  - For IV administration, do not exceed 20 mEq/h.
  - Do not exceed 40 – 80 mEq in a 24-hour period.
  - Never give IVP.
- Assess for phlebitis: potassium chloride irritates the vein, causing a burning sensation.
- Stop the infusion if the urine output is less than 30 cc/h.
- Cardiac monitoring is appropriate.

HYPERKALEMIA (HIGH POTASSIUM)
Normal values 3.5 – 5 mEq/L

Clinical Manifestation

+ dysrhythmias or cardiac arrest:
    + tall, peaked T waves
    + prolonged PR interval
    + wide QRS complex
    + absent P waves
    + ST depression
+ abdominal cramping and diarrhea
+ anxiety

Treatment and Management

+ Administer the following based on severity of symptoms:
    + calcium gluconate
    + IV insulin and D50
    + loop diuretics (furosemide)
    + sodium polystyrene sulfonate (Kayexalate)
    + sodium bicarbonate
    + beta 2 agonists (albuterol)
    + hypertonic IV solution (3% normal saline)
+ Perform ECG and continue cardiac monitoring.
+ Restrict PO intake of potassium-containing foods.
+ Patient may require dialysis.

HYPOMAGNESEMIA (LOW MAGNESIUM)
Normal values: 1.3 – 2.1 mEq/L

Clinical Manifestation

+ dysrhythmias:
    + torsades de pointes
    + flat or inverted T waves
    + ST depression
    + prolonged PR interval
    + widened QRS complex
+ hypertension
+ tetany
    + Chvostek sign
    + Trousseau sign
+ seizures
+ hyperreflexia

Treatment and Management

+ Replace magnesium PO or IV:
    + Administer magnesium sulfate IV, 1 – 2 g over 60 minutes.
    + Magnesium sulfate acts as a vasodilator and causes flushing and hypotension.
+ Employ seizure precautions.
+ Monitor swallowing.
+ Monitor for magnesium toxicity, and treat with calcium gluconate.
+ Cardiac monitoring is appropriate.

HYPERMAGNESEMIA (HIGH MAGNESIUM)
Normal values: 1.3 – 2.1 mEq/L

Clinical Manifestation

+ dysrhythmias or cardiac arrest:
    ✧ prolonged PR interval
    ✧ wide QRS complex
    ✧ peaked T waves

+ bradycardia (more common) or tachycardia
+ bradypnea
+ respiratory paralysis
+ altered mental status, lethargy, or coma

Treatment and Management

+ Administer calcium gluconate.
+ Administer loop diuretics.
+ Administer isotonic IV solutions (lactated Ringer's or 0.9% normal saline).

+ Mechanical ventilation may be needed.
+ Dialysis may be appropriate.

HYPOCALCEMIA (LOW CALCIUM)
Normal values: 4.5 – 5.5 mEq/L

Signs and Symptoms

+ dysrhythmias or cardiac arrest:
    ✧ prolonged QT interval
    ✧ flattened ST segment
+ hypotension
+ third space fluid shift
+ decreased clotting time

+ laryngeal spasm or bronchospasm
+ seizures
+ Chvostek sign
+ Trousseau sign
+ hyperactive deep tendon reflexes

Treatment and Management

+ Administer PO or IV calcium replacement:
    ✧ Administer calcium gluconate, 10 – 20 mL, over 5 – 10 minutes.
    ✧ Dilute IV solution with D5W only, never with normal saline.

+ Give vitamin D supplements (to enhance absorption).
+ Employ seizure precautions.

HYPOPHOSPHATEMIA (LOW PHOSPHATE)
Normal values:

+ adults: 1.8 – 2.3 mEq/L

+ children: 2.3 – 3.8 mEq/L

Signs and Symptoms

+ respiratory distress or failure

+ tissue hypoxia

- chest pain
- cardiomyopathy
- seizures

- decreased LOC
- increased susceptibility to infection
- nystagmus

Treatment and Management

- Administer PO or IV phosphate replacement.
  - Replace slowly if patient is on TPN.

- Protect for infection.
- Employ seizure precautions.

HYPERPHOSPHATEMIA (HIGH PHOSPHATE)
Normal values:

- adults: 1.8 – 2.3 mEq/L

- children: 2.3 – 3.8 mEq/L

Signs and Symptoms

- tachycardia
- tetany
  - Chvostek sign
  - Trousseau sign

- hyperreflexia
- soft-tissue calcifications

Treatment and Management

- Correct hyperphosphatemia:
  - Dialysis may be appropriate.
  - Limit dietary intake of phosphates.
  - Administer diuretics.
  - Administer aluminum hydroxide.

- Correct hypocalcemia:
  - Administer PO or IV calcium replacement.
  - Give vitamin D supplements.
- Administer isotonic IV solution (0.9% normal saline).

QUICK REVIEW QUESTION

1. A patient arrives at the ED in cardiac arrest, with a torsades de pointes waveform showing on the ECG monitor. What electrolyte should the nurse anticipate hanging?

Fever

Pathophysiology

Fever is an elevation in core body temperature. Normal core temperature is 98.6°F (37°C) and varies within 1°C in healthy people. Fever is classified as any one time temperature of 101°F (38.3°C) or any temperature > 100.4°F (38°C) for > 1 hour.

Core body temperature is mediated by the thermostatic set point in the thermoregulatory center of the hypothalamus. Fever occurs when the thermostatic set point resets to a higher value in response to circulating pyrogens and cytokines. The hypothalamus will not raise the body temperature above 105.8°F (41°C).

Fevers higher than this indicate damage to the thermoregulatory center and may result from seizure activity, hyperthermic states, and cerebral injuries. All fevers increase the metabolic rate and oxygen consumption.

Risk Factors

+ newborns < 6 weeks old
+ children from 6 months – 5 years old: at risk for febrile seizures
+ infection
+ inflammation
+ malignancies (neutropenic fever)
+ dehydration, heat stroke, heat exhaustion, and environmental exposure

+ head injury or unconsciousness
+ spinal cord injury (T6 and above)
+ anaphylaxis and allergic reactions
+ seizures and postictal states
+ meningitis

Signs and Symptoms

+ one time temperature of 101°F (38.3°C)
+ temperature of > 100.4°F (38°C) for > 1 hour
+ hot, flushed skin
+ piloerection, shivering, or chills
+ diaphoresis

+ weakness
+ fatigue
+ loss of appetite
+ headache
+ dehydration

Diagnostic Tests and Findings

+ fevers of unknown origin:
    ◇ CBC with differential to identify source
    ◇ blood cultures and serum lactate before the administration of antibiotics and to rule out bacteremia
    ◇ chest X-ray to rule out pneumonia
    ◇ urinalysis and urine culture, if indicated, to rule out UTI
+ additional workup if source of infection still unidentified after above tests:
    ◇ CT scan of abdomen to rule out peritonitis, appendicitis, or abscess
    ◇ CT scan of head to rule out malignancies
+ wound culture
+ lumbar puncture
    ◇ if source of infection still unidentified
    ◇ standard for fever in infants < 90 days old

Treatment and Management

+ Administer antipyretic medications.
    ◇ Do not administer aspirin for pediatric patients (≤ 18 years).

- ✦ Use cooling techniques:
    - ◇ Use a hypothermia blanket.
    - ◇ Adjust the environmental temperature.
    - ◇ Minimize patient's clothing and bedding.
    - ◇ Apply ice packs to armpits, groin, and forehead and behind neck.
- ✦ Administer IV fluids for volume replacement.

QUICK REVIEW QUESTION

2. A 4-week-old infant arrives at the ED with lethargy and fever (temperature of 104.5°F [40.3°C]). What diagnostics should the nurse anticipate?

Hypersensitivity Reactions

ALLERGIC REACTIONS

Pathophysiology

An **allergic reaction** occurs when an irritant or allergen protein enters the body by inhalation, ingestion, or topical exposure. The allergen initiates a response from the immune system, which triggers acute inflammation and vasodilation. Allergic reactions can be topical, localized or systemic, and the onset of symptoms can occur immediately or later. Common mild allergens include plant and tree pollens, animal dander, detergents, soaps, and perfumes.

Risk Factors

- ✦ age ≤ 18 years (for new onset)
- ✦ family history of allergies or asthma
- ✦ previous allergy
- ✦ food sensitivities
- ✦ immunocompromised conditions
- ✦ asthma

Signs and Symptoms

- ✦ topical dermatitis
- ✦ urticaria (hives)
- ✦ rhinorrhea
- ✦ sneezing
- ✦ itchy skin, nose, or mouth
- ✦ watering, itchy eyes
- ✦ circumoral tingling or pallor
- ✦ mild nausea or abdominal discomfort

Diagnostic Tests and Findings

- ✦ diagnosis based on history and signs and symptoms

Treatment and Management

- ✦ Treat with a combination of medications, depending on signs and symptoms and medical provider's preferences.
    - ◇ Administer PO or IV H1 antihistamines (diphenhydramine [Benadryl]).

- Administer PO or IV H2 antihistamines (famotidine, ranitidine, cimetidine).
- Administer PO or IV glucocorticoid (methylprednisolone, prednisone).
- Have patient use a bronchodilator such as albuterol inhalation.
- Administer PO nonsedating antihistamines (cetirizine [Zyrtec], fexofenadine [Allegra], levocetirizine [Xyzal], loratadine [Claritin]).
- Apply topical antihistamines and steroid-containing creams, gels, or lotions.

QUICK REVIEW QUESTION

3. A patient arrives at the ED with diffuse poison ivy to the lower extremities, upper extremities, chest, and neck. The patient describes having taken 50 mg of loratadine (Claritin) by mouth prior to arrival. What other medications should the nurse anticipate administering?

ANAPHYLACTIC SHOCK

Pathophysiology

Anaphylactic shock (or anaphylaxis) is a life-threatening, severe allergic reaction that causes symptomatic vasodilation and bronchoconstriction. The most common causes of anaphylactic shock are food allergens, medications, and insect venom.

Risk Factors

+ age ≤ 18 years (for new onset)
+ family history of allergies or asthma
+ previous allergic reaction
+ immunocompromised conditions
+ asthma

Signs and Symptoms

+ respiratory distress (can be severe):
    - dyspnea
    - wheezing
    - cough > 5 per minute
+ throat tightness
    - hoarseness
    - dysphagia
+ edema in face, lips, or tongue
+ skin pallor or flushing
+ hypotension
+ weakness
+ weak thread pulse
+ syncope or presyncope
+ vomiting or diarrhea
+ altered mental status
    - sense of doom
    - anxiety
    - confusion
+ uterine contractions in pregnant females

Diagnostic Tests and Findings

+ CBC elevated total WBC count
    - differential elevation of basophils and eosinophils

Treatment and Management

+ First-line treatment for all anaphylactic reaction is epinephrine:
    ⬥ Epinephrine may be delivered as a standard dose via an EpiPen auto-injector (as prescribed for home use) or as a weight-based dose obtained from a multidose vial (per facility policy or medical provider order).
    ⬥ Epinephrine in all forms used for the management of anaphylaxis is only to be given via IM injection.
+ Administer EpiPen:
    ⬥ EpiPen Jr, 0.15 mg IM (for patients < 65 pounds [< 30 kg]).
    ⬥ EpiPen, 0.3 mg IM (for patients ≥ 65 pounds [≥ 30 kg]).
+ IM injections are to be given in the lateral thigh and may be given through clothing if the patient is dressed.
+ May repeat IM dose after 5 minutes.
+ Patients who have self-administered an EpiPen should be monitored for at least 4 hours.
+ Administer epinephrine: 1:1,000 IM 0.01 mg/kg, for a maximum dose of 0.5 mg.
+ Initiate a second-line treatment after administering epinephrine:
    ⬥ Administer medications for allergic reactions.
    ⬥ Provide supplemental oxygen.
    ⬥ Administer IV glucagon.
    ⬥ Initiate fluid resuscitation with 0.9% normal saline bolus.

QUICK REVIEW QUESTION

4. A patient from an MVC is sent to radiology for a CT scan with contrast. Upon returning, the patient complains of dyspnea and dizziness and has hoarseness. What medication should the nurse anticipate giving?

Immunocompromised Conditions
ACQUIRED IMMUNODEFICIENCY SYNDROME (AIDS)
Pathophysiology

Acquired immunodeficiency syndrome (AIDS) is the end-stage progression of an infectious disease caused by the **human immunodeficiency virus (HIV)**. Patients with AIDS have a depletion of T lymphocytes and are susceptible to opportunistic and sometimes life-threatening infections and conditions, including candidiasis, aphthous ulcers, encephalopathy, Kaposi's sarcoma, Burkitt's lymphoma, tuberculosis, and pneumonia.

Treatment and Management

+ Employ immunosuppression and neutropenic precautions.
+ Treat underlying infections if present.
+ Support nutrition and hydration.
+ Administer supplemental oxygen.
+ Provide mechanical ventilation as needed.
+ Offer supportive care for the patient and family.

CHEMOTHERAPY

Chemotherapy is conducted with a class of cytotoxic medications that destroy cancer cells by disrupting cell mitosis and DNA replication. The treatment can cause bone marrow depression, nausea, anorexia, dehydration, fluid and electrolyte imbalances, alopecia, elevated uric acid levels, and aphthous ulcers. The presence of cancerous tumors puts the patient at risk for metastasis, spinal cord compression, superior vena cava syndrome, and tumor lysis syndrome.

Treatment and Management

+ Employ immunosuppression and neutropenic precautions.

+ Follow bleeding precautions for thrombocytopenia.

+ Provide supplemental oxygen.

+ Provide nutritional support for anemia.

+ Give fluids for volume replacement.

+ Provide pain management.

+ Changes in neurological status may indicate metastasis to the brain, side effects from chemotherapy medications, or alterations in fluid volume status.

LEUKEMIA

Pathophysiology

Leukemia, cancer of the WBCs, occurs in the bone marrow, disrupting the production and function of WBCs. In the absence of functioning WBCs, the patient becomes immunocompromised.

The types of leukemia are differentiated by which WBCs are affected (lymphocytes or myeloid cells). Leukemia is further categorized as either acute or chronic. There are 4 main types of leukemia:

+ **Acute lymphocytic leukemia (ALL):** Most common in children; can also occur in adults.

+ **Acute myelogenous leukemia (AML):** Occurs in children and adults.

+ **Chronic lymphocytic leukemia (CLL):** Most common chronic adult leukemia. The patient may feel well for years without needing treatment.

+ **Chronic myelogenous leukemia (CML):** Affects mainly adults. The patient may be asymptomatic for months or years before entering a phase in which the leukemia cells grow more quickly.

Risk Factors

+ previous cancer treatment with chemotherapy and/or radiation

+ genetic disorders such as Down syndrome or Fanconi anemia

+ smoking

+ exposure to chemicals such as benzene or Agent Orange

+ family history of leukemia

Signs and Symptoms

+ fever

+ persistent fatigue or weakness

+ frequent or severe infections

+ weight loss

+ adenopathy

+ enlarged liver or spleen

+ night sweats

+ bone pain or tenderness

+ easy bleeding or bruising:
  ✧ recurrent epistaxis
  ✧ petechiae
  ✧ ecchymosis (> 1 cm spots of subcutaneous bleeding not attributable to trauma)
  ✧ gingival bleeding

Diagnostic Tests and Findings

+ CBC:
  ✧ WBC count with >20% immature blast cells
  ✧ PLT showing thrombocytopenia
  ✧ RBC showing decrease of total erythrocytes

+ increased uric acid levels

+ bone marrow biopsy or aspiration

Treatment and Management

+ Treat presenting patient's complaints and symptoms, usually fever and infection.

+ Treatments for leukemia include the following:
  ✧ chemotherapy
  ✧ radiation
  ✧ stem cell transplant
  ✧ bone marrow transplant

QUICK REVIEW QUESTION

7. An 8-year-old child arrives at the ED with fever, weakness, and a recent weight loss as reported by the parents. What additional clinical findings would lead the nurse to suspect acute lymphocytic leukemia?

Metabolic Emergencies

ACUTE ADRENAL CRISIS (ADDISONIAN CRISIS)

Pathophysiology

Acute adrenal insufficiency (Addisonian crisis) occurs when the adrenal cortex cannot produce enough corticosteroids to meet the body's needs. It is usually an acute escalation of preexisting adrenal insufficiency but can also be caused by trauma to the adrenal glands. Acute adrenal crisis is rapid onset, causes shock, and requires immediate treatment.

Risk Factors

+ causes of adrenal insufficiency:
    ⬦ Addison's disease
    ⬦ adrenal adenoma
    ⬦ pituitary adenoma
    ⬦ infections (e.g., tuberculosis)
    ⬦ autoimmune conditions
    ⬦ HIV infection

+ precipitating events for adrenal crisis:
    ⬦ infection or sepsis
    ⬦ steroid withdrawal
    ⬦ physiological stress after surgery (e.g., MI, fluid volume loss)
    ⬦ trauma to adrenal or pituitary glands

Signs and Symptoms

+ dehydration
+ hypotension
+ hyperpigmentation
+ nausea and vomiting
+ abdominal pain
+ weakness or fatigue
+ dizziness

+ tachycardia
+ respiratory distress
+ history of
    ⬦ weight loss
    ⬦ anorexia
    ⬦ craving for salt

Diagnostic Tests and Findings

+ electrolyte imbalances:
    ⬦ hyperkalemia
    ⬦ hyponatremia
    ⬦ hypercalcemia
+ decreased serum glucose (blood glucose)
+ increased serum BUN
+ increased serum creatinine

+ decreased serum cortisol
+ ACTH
+ ECG (for cardiac dysrhythmias associated with electrolyte imbalances)
+ X-ray, CT scan to determine cause (e.g., tumor or adrenal atrophy)

Treatment and Management

+ Treatment is based on clinical appearance and is not delayed pending diagnostic test results.

+ Provide IV fluid replacement.
+ Administer IV corticosteroids.

+ Provide supplemental oxygen.

+ Provide mechanical ventilation if needed.

QUICK REVIEW QUESTION

8. A 19-year-old patient who has recently stopped a course of prednisone for asthma exacerbation arrives at the ED with a blood pressure of 78/40 mm Hg, a HR of 135 bpm, fatigue, and extreme thirst. What classification of medication does the nurse anticipate giving this patient?

DIABETES INSIPIDUS

Pathophysiology

Diabetes insipidus occurs when there is a deficiency of antidiuretic hormone (ADH) (also called vasopressin) produced by the posterior lobe of the pituitary gland. ADH deficiency affects the renal tubules' ability to concentrate urine, causing large amounts of undiluted urine to be excreted from the body. The result is acute dehydration.

Risk Factors

+ tumor

+ head injury or trauma

+ CNS infection

+ use of some medications (e.g., lithium carbonate and demeclocycline)

Signs and Symptoms

+ polydipsia

+ polyuria

+ dehydration

+ weakness

Diagnostic Tests and Findings

+ decreased urine specific gravity

+ decreased urine osmolality

+ increased serum osmolality

+ decreased sodium

+ decreased potassium

+ water deprivation test

+ CT scan or MRI of head

Treatment and Management

+ Provide fluids for volume replacement.

+ Monitor fluid intake and output.

+ Treat electrolyte imbalances.

+ Administer vasopressin.

QUICK REVIEW QUESTION

9. The nurse is performing a bedside urinalysis on a patient with diabetes insipidus. What finding is consistent with this diagnosis?

DIABETES MELLITUS

Pathophysiology

Diabetes mellitus is a metabolic disorder affecting insulin production and insulin resistance. It requires long-term management with insulin or oral hypoglycemics. Diabetes mellitus is classified as type 1 or type 2.

+ **Type 1**: an acute-onset autoimmune disease most prominent in children, teens, and adults < 30. Beta cells in the pancreas are destroyed and are unable to produce sufficient amounts of insulin, causing blood sugar to rise.

+ **Type 2**: a gradual-onset disease most prominent in adults > 30, but it can develop in individuals of all ages. Type 2 diabetes is not an autoimmune disease. Instead, the person develops insulin resistance, which prevents the cellular uptake of glucose and causes blood sugar to rise.

Risk Factors

+ type 1:
    ✧ family history
    ✧ autoimmune disease and environmental factors (mechanisms not well understood)
+ type 2:
    ✧ family history
    ✧ obesity
    ✧ more prevalent in African American, Hispanic, and Native American populations
    ✧ sedentary lifestyle
    ✧ history of gestational diabetes

Signs and Symptoms

+ polyuria
+ polyphagia
+ polydipsia
+ fatigue
+ weakness
+ altered mental status
+ abdominal pain
+ nausea and vomiting
+ recurrent infections
+ slow-healing wounds

Diagnostic Tests and Findings

+ elevated blood sugar
+ elevated glucose tolerance test
+ elevated Hbg A1C

Treatment and Management

+ Treat symptoms of hypo- or hyperglycemia as indicated.
+ Peripheral neuropathy can cause loss of sensation in feet:
    ✧ Assess feet carefully for signs of diabetic ulcers.
    ✧ Never trim toenails or start IV access in the foot of a patient with diabetes.

- Diabetic retinopathy can cause visual deficits and lead to further complications, including diabetic macular edema and cataracts:
    - Treat emergent conditions as warranted.
    - Initiate an ophthalmology referral and consult.
- For patients with diabetes but presenting with unrelated complaints:
    - Dosing of insulin or oral hypoglycemics may change in light of presenting complaint.
    - Patients will need to eat regularly and may be on a restricted diet.
    - Administer IV fluids with dextrose for NPO patients.
    - Use of metformin is contraindicated with IV contrast. Patients should be instructed to discontinue metformin for at least 48 hours after receiving contrast.

QUICK REVIEW QUESTION

10. A patient with a history of type 1 diabetes arrives at the ED after sustaining a shoulder dislocation and is put on NPO status in anticipation of surgical intervention. The nurse should anticipate an IV infusion of what fluid to maintain a therapeutic blood glucose level?

HYPERGLYCEMIA

Pathophysiology

Hyperglycemia occurs when serum glucose concentrations are elevated in response to a decrease in available insulin or to insulin resistance. The condition is most often associated with diabetes mellitus but can also be caused by medications (such as corticosteroids and amphetamines), infection, sepsis, and endocrine disorders.

Diabetic ketoacidosis (DKA) is a hyperglycemic state characterized by an insulin deficiency that stimulates the breakdown of adipose tissues. This process results in the production of ketones and leads to metabolic acidosis. DKA develops quickly (< 24 hours) and is most common in people with type 1 diabetes.

Hyperosmolar hyperglycemic state (HHS) is a severe hyperglycemic state characterized by profound hyperosmolarity and the absence of acidosis. HHS develops gradually over days to weeks. Volume depletion occurs as the result of osmotic diuresis caused by prolonged hyperglycemia. HHS is more common in persons with type 2 diabetes and has a much higher mortality rate than does DKA.

HHS was previously referred to as hyperglycemic hyperosmolar nonketotic coma (HHNC). The name of the condition changed to reflect that coma is not always present in HHS, although mental status changes and seizures are common.

Risk Factors

- hyperglycemia:
    - diabetes mellitus
    - use of medications that affect glucose use (e.g., glucocorticoids or dobutamine)
    - trauma
    - infection or sepsis

- DKA:
    - type 1 diabetes, particularly new onset
    - type 2 diabetes (less common)
    - precipitating events: acute illness, poor insulin compliance, or use of medications that affect glucose use

- HHS:
    - type 2 diabetes
    - persons >50 years old
    - precipitating events: acute illness, poor insulin compliance, or use of medications that affect glucose use

Signs and Symptoms

- common to hyperglycemia, DKA, and HHS:
    - polyphagia
    - polydipsia
    - polyuria
    - dehydration
    - weight loss
    - tachycardia
    - hypotension
- DKA:
    - Kussmaul respirations
    - fruity odor on breath
    - abdominal pain
    - nausea and vomiting
- HHS:
    - lethargy
    - delirium
    - seizures
    - coma

Diagnostic Tests and Findings

- elevated serum glucose concentration:
    - hyperglycemia: > 200 mg/dL
    - DKA: usually 350 – 800 mg/dL
    - HHS: usually > 800 mg/dL
- elevated BUN and creatinine
- DKA:
    - presence of ketones in urine, and elevated serum ketones
    - elevated serum lactate
    - reduced serum bicarbonate
    - decreased serum pH
- HHS: elevated plasma osmolality

Treatment and Management

- Administer IV fluids for volume replacement.
- Administer IV potassium for patients with potassium deficiency.
- Administer insulin: subcutaneous fast-acting or IV regular, depending on patient need.
- Administer sodium bicarbonate for DKA patients with severe acidosis.

HYPOGLYCEMIA

Pathophysiology

Hypoglycemia occurs when blood sugar (glucose) concentrations fall below normal. Patients will typically show symptoms when serum glucose is < 70 mg/dL, but the onset of symptoms will depend on the patient's tolerance.

Risk Factors

+ diabetes mellitus (type 1 or 2)
+ too much insulin
+ skipping meals

+ low carbohydrate intake
+ increased physical activity

Signs and Symptoms

+ shakes/tremors
+ tachycardia
+ changes in mental status:
    ⋄ anxiety or nervousness
    ⋄ irritability
    ⋄ confusion
    ⋄ altered LOC
+ cold, clammy skin

+ presyncope or dizziness
+ hunger
+ blurred vision
+ circumoral tingling
+ fatigue or sleepiness
+ lack of coordination, or impaired gait
+ seizures

Diagnostic Tests and Findings

+ Blood sugar < 70 mg/dL

Treatment and Management

+ Give 15 – 30 grams of carbohydrates PO to the patient who is conscious and alert.
+ If patient is unconscious or unable to ingest PO carbohydrates:
    ⋄ Administer IM glucagon.
    ⋄ Administer D50 IV.
+ Continue to monitor capillary blood glucose levels until stable, continue to monitor.

THYROTOXIC CRISIS

Pathophysiology

Thyrotoxic crisis, also known as a **thyroid storm**, is a rapid increase in circulating thyroid hormones. The surge in hormones speeds up metabolism in all body systems and increases oxygen demand. Thyrotoxic crisis is the result of untreated or undertreated hyperthyroidism and is a lift-threatening emergency that requires immediate medical intervention.

Risk Factors

+ hyperthyroidism:
  ⋄ Graves' disease
  ⋄ exogenous hyperthyroidism
  ⋄ toxic goiter
  ⋄ thyroid nodules
  ⋄ thyroid adenoma

+ precipitating events:
  ⋄ trauma
  ⋄ pregnancy
  ⋄ stress (physiological or emotional)
  ⋄ discontinuation of thyroid medications

Signs and Symptoms

+ hyperpyrexia
+ tachycardia
+ respiratory distress
+ altered mental status:
  ⋄ agitation
  ⋄ delirium
  ⋄ manic state

+ abdominal pain
+ nausea and vomiting
+ diarrhea
+ ophthalmopathy
+ stupor or coma

Diagnostic Tests and Findings

+ decreased TSH
+ elevated free T4, total T4 and T3
+ elevated thyroid-stimulating immuno-globulins

+ elevated thyrotropin receptor antibodies

Treatment and Management

+ Treatment is based on clinical appearance and is not delayed pending thyroid study results.
+ Use cooling measures, including antipyretics, to reduce core body temperature.
+ Provide supplemental oxygen:
  ⋄ Administer mechanical ventilation if needed.
+ Administer IV fluids for volume replacement.
+ Administer medications:
  ⋄ thyroid-hormone-inhibiting medications (PTU or MMI)
  ⋄ corticosteroids
  ⋄ iodine
  ⋄ beta blockers
  ⋄ digoxin

13. A patient arrives at the ED in a thyrotoxic crisis. What therapeutic interventions can the nurse initiate to reduce core body temperature while waiting for antipyretics to take effect?

Platelet Disorders

THROMBOCYTOPENIA

Pathophysiology

Thrombocytopenia is an abnormally low platelet level that can lead to severe bleeding or thrombosis. The condition has a diverse etiology:

+ **Heparin-induced thrombocytopenia (HIT):** an acute-onset condition in patients receiving heparin therapy.

+ **Idiopathic thrombocytopenic purpura (ITP):** an autoimmune disorder that reduces the lifespan of platelets; also called immune thrombocytopenia.

+ **Gestational thrombocytopenia:** occurs during pregnancy and presents with little risk of bleeding.

+ Thrombocytopenia can occur secondary to cancer or chemotherapy, bone marrow disorders, infections, chronic liver disease, and autoimmune diseases.

Risk Factors

+ heparin use > 1 week
+ history of autoimmune disease
+ cancers
+ bone marrow suppression
+ chemotherapy
+ infection by HIV, hepatitis C, or *Helicobacter pylori*
+ trauma
+ surgery

Signs and Symptoms

+ petechiae, purpura, or ecchymosis
+ gingival bleeding
+ epistaxis
+ heavy menstrual cycle
+ occult or frank blood in stools, urine, or emesis
+ acute hemorrhage

Diagnostic Tests and Findings

+ low platelets:
  + mild: 100,000 – 150,000/µL
  + moderate: 50,000 – 100,000/µL
  + severe: < 50,000/µL

Treatment and Management

+ Mild thrombocytopenia with no bleeding usually does not require treatment in the ED; the patient can be referred to a hematologist.

+ For patients with thrombocytopenia and severe bleeding:
    ⋄ Use bleeding precautions.
    ⋄ Give immediate platelet transfusion.
    ⋄ Administer IVIG.
    ⋄ Administer corticosteroids.

+ Treat underlying cause if known.

> ### QUICK REVIEW QUESTION
> **14.** A 28-year-old patient with a history of idiopathic thrombocytopenic purpura is diagnosed with acute appendicitis. What type of precautions should the nurse implement?

DISSEMINATED INTRAVASCULAR COAGULOPATHY (DIC)
Pathophysiology

Disseminated intravascular coagulopathy (DIC) is a coagulation disorder with simultaneous intervals of clotting and bleeding. Micro clots cascade throughout the vascular system, causing hypoxia and ischemia to multiple organs. In response to these clots, fibrinogens release profuse amounts of anti-clotting factors, triggering both internal and external hemorrhages. DIC may present as acute or chronic:

+ **Acute (or decompensated) DIC**: characterized by severe bleeding.

+ **Chronic (or compensated) DIC**: more likely to lead to thrombosis than to bleeding; can be asymptomatic.

Risk Factors

+ sepsis
+ cancers (especially leukemia)
+ obstetrical complications:
    ⋄ preeclampsia
    ⋄ placental abruption
    ⋄ retained products of conception
+ trauma to CNS
+ cardiac arrest

Signs and Symptoms

+ spontaneous hemorrhage
+ petechiae or ecchymosis
+ abnormal bleeding (oozing to profuse hemorrhage) from orifices and injection sites
+ tachycardia
+ hypotension
+ diaphoresis
+ respiratory distress
+ progresses to MODS; symptoms vary with organ affected

Diagnostic Tests and Findings

+ decreased platelets
+ decreased hemoglobin
+ decreased fibrinogen levels
+ prolonged PT, aPTT, and thrombin time
+ elevated D-dimer

Treatment and Management

+ Treatment is focused on the underlying cause.
+ Administer IV fluids for volume replacement.
+ Provide supplemental oxygen.
+ Correct electrolyte imbalances as needed.
+ Administer vasopressors.
+ Give transfusions of one of these blood products:
  ✧ cryoprecipitate
  ✧ FFP
  ✧ packed RBCs
+ Administer heparin for chronic DIC.

QUICK REVIEW QUESTION

15. A trauma patient arrives at the ED with active hemorrhaging from multiple lacerations. Lab values reveal a markedly decreased hemoglobin, hematocrit, and platelet count. What other lab studies should the nurse expect to see if this patient is experiencing DIC?

Red Blood Cell Disorders

HEMOPHILIA

Pathophysiology

Hemophilia is a recessive, X-chromosome-linked bleeding disorder characterized by the lack of coagulation factor VIII (hemophilia A), factor IX (hemophilia B), or factor XI (hemophilia C). Hemophilia A is the most common form of the condition. Hemophilia C is mild and very rare; it occurs mainly in Ashkenazi Jewish populations. In general, the condition is seen in males. Females usually only act as carriers, but female carriers can develop symptoms.

The deficiency in coagulation factors causes abnormal bleeding after an injury or medical procedures, and spontaneous bleeding can occur in patients with severe hemophilia. Hemophilia is usually diagnosed in infancy or childhood, but mild forms may not be diagnosed until the patient experiences injury or surgery later in life. **Hemarthrosis**, bleeding into the joints, is one of the most common presentations of hemophilia.

Risk Factors

+ family history of hemophilia

Signs and Symptoms

+ excessive bleeding
+ easy bruising
+ hemorrhage after minor trauma

+ hemarthrosis:
    ⬦ painful joints
    ⬦ swelling in joints
                                        ⬦ muscle pain

Diagnostic Tests and Findings

+ prolonged aPTT

+ normal platelet count

+ normal PT

+ decreased activity level for factors VIII, IX, or XI

Treatment and Management

+ Treatment of severe bleeding for patients with hemophilia should be initiated within 30 minutes of injury and should not be delayed for assessment.

+ Administer factor VIII for hemophilia A and factor IX for hemophilia B.

+ Manage symptoms of hemarthrosis:
    ⬦ Administer NSAIDs.
    ⬦ Apply ice packs to affected joint(s).

+ Use bleeding precautions.

QUICK REVIEW QUESTION

16. An 8-year-old boy with a known history of hemophilia A arrives at the ED after sustaining a closed radial ulna fracture when he fell off a swing at school. What intervention should the nurse anticipate performing first?

SICKLE CELL DISEASE

Pathophysiology

Sickle cell disease is an inherited form of hemolytic anemia that causes deformities in the shape of the RBCs. When oxygen levels in the venous circulation are low, the RBCs dehydrate and form a sickle shape. This process can be exacerbated by exposure to cold temperatures or high altitudes. Sickle cell disease is a chronic disease that can lead to complications that require emergency care:

+ **Sickle cell crisis** (also called vaso-occlusive pain): sickle-shaped cells clump together and restrict blood flow, causing localized ischemia, inflammation, and severe pain.

+ **Acute chest syndrome (ACS)**: vaso-occlusion in the lungs (often after an infection) that exacerbates the sickle formation of RBCs.

+ **Aplastic crisis**: anemia that occurs after an infection, usually by human parvovirus; rapid decline of hemoglobin caused by the inability of the bone marrow to produce new cells.

+ **Splenic sequestration**: pooling of RBCs in the spleen; can lead to anemia and hypovolemia.

+ **Infection**: the leading cause of death for children with sickle cell disease; common infections include bacteremia, pneumonia, and osteomyelitis.

+ **Acute infarctions**: blood clots caused by clumped sickle-shaped cells; can lead to hypoxia and infarction (MI, stroke, PE, DVT, etc.).

+ **Priapism**: a common complication for men with sickle cell disease.

Risk Factors

+ family history of sickle cell anemia or sickle cell trait
+ most common among:
    ⋄ people of African, Middle Eastern or Mediterranean descent
    ⋄ Hispanic people from Central or South America

Signs and Symptoms

+ sickle cell crisis:
    ⋄ intense, localized pain in absence of injury
    ⋄ inflammation
+ ACS:
    ⋄ fever
    ⋄ chest pain
    ⋄ respiratory distress
+ aplastic anemia:
    ⋄ fatigue
    ⋄ dyspnea
    ⋄ tachycardia
    ⋄ jaundice
+ splenic sequestration:
    ⋄ enlarged spleen
    ⋄ pallor
    ⋄ tachycardia
    ⋄ tachypnea
+ signs and symptoms specific to other complications (e.g., DVT, priapism, infection)

Diagnostic Tests and Findings

+ reticulocyte count elevated
+ indirect bilirubin increased
+ low H/H (anemia)
+ hemoglobin electrophoresis, HgB S increased (80 – 100%)

Treatment and Management

+ Treatment depends on the patient's signs and symptoms and diagnosis.
+ Many complications of sickle cell disease (including ACS, splenic sequestration, and symptomatic anemia) require transfusion of packed RBCs.
+ For ACS:
    ⋄ Administer IV fluids.
    ⋄ Provide pain management.
    ⋄ Provide supplemental oxygen.
    ⋄ Administer low-molecular-weight heparin.
    ⋄ Administer hydroxyurea.
+ For sickle cell crisis, administer analgesics (usually IV opioids).
+ Follow standard treatment protocols for other complications (e.g., DVT, priapism, infection).

QUICK REVIEW QUESTION

17. A 26-year-old male with a history of sickle cell disease arrives at the ED with fever, jaundice, and priapism. What symptom is most urgent to address?

Renal Failure

Pathophysiology

Acute renal failure (ARF), also called acute kidney injury, is an acute decrease in the kidneys' ability to filter the blood. ARF causes an accumulation of waste in the bloodstream. Often the effects of ARF are reversible with prompt treatment. ARF has a diverse etiology:

+ **Prerenal**: decreased renal perfusion
  + hypovolemia
  + systemic vasodilation (e.g., shock)
+ **Intrinsic renal**: disease within the kidneys
  + infection
  + acute tubular necrosis

+ **Postrenal**: blocked drainage of urine
  + prostatic hypertrophy
  + renal calculi

Chronic kidney disease, the progressive and irreversible loss of kidney function, occurs over months or years. The most common causes of chronic kidney disease are diabetes mellitus and hypertension. Chronic kidney disease is classified as stage 1 through 5. Stage 1 signifies minimal kidney damage, and stage 5 signifies complete kidney failure and end-stage disease that may require dialysis or transplant.

The remainder of this section discusses the symptoms and treatment of ARF that require emergency medical intervention.

Risk Factors

+ any condition causing a decrease in renal perfusion:
  + sepsis
  + shock
+ trauma

+ chronic use/abuse of NSAIDs
+ liver failure
+ exposure to nephrotoxins

Signs and Symptoms

+ oliguria or anuria
+ hypertension
+ edema
+ lethargy

+ confusion
+ vomiting
+ diarrhea
+ may be asymptomatic

Diagnostic Tests and Findings

+ elevated serum creatinine:
  + stage 1: 1.5 – 1.9 times normal
  + stage 2: 2.0 – 2.9 times normal

  + stage 3: > 3 times normal

+ elevated BUN

+ decreased GFR

+ low H/H (anemia)

+ X-ray KUB to assess for renal calculi, obstruction, hydronephrosis, and size of kidneys

Treatment and Management

+ Treat underlying cause.

+ Administer IV fluids for patients with hypovolemia.

+ Discontinue medications causing ARF.

+ Correct electrolyte imbalances, and monitor for related complications:

    ⋄ Provide a sodium-, phosphate-, magnesium-, and potassium-restricted diet.

    ⋄ Conduct cardiac monitoring.

+ Administer bicarbonate for patients with metabolic acidosis.

+ Initiate a nephrology consult and transfer for dialysis and management.

QUICK REVIEW QUESTION

18. The nurse is assessing a patient with acute renal failure. What is the most effective way to monitor for a decrease in renal perfusion?

Sepsis

Pathophysiology

Sepsis, a massive inflammatory response to systemic infection, can lead to multi-organ failure and death. The most common sites of initial infection are blood (bacteremia), the lungs (pneumonia), the urinary tract or kidneys, and the abdominal area (e.g., peritonitis or ruptured appendix). Sepsis progresses through 4 stages:

1. systemic inflammatory response syndrome (SIRS)

2. sepsis

3. severe sepsis

4. septic shock

Multiple organ dysfunction syndrome (MODS) refers to the dysfunction of one or more organs and requires supportive therapy in an acute illness. MODS is sometimes placed on the most severe end of the sepsis spectrum.

Risk Factors

+ adults ≥ 65 years

+ children < 12 months

+ existing infection

+ immunocompromised conditions

+ long-term in-dwelling catheters

+ malnourished or homeless population

+ comorbidities:

    ⋄ diabetes

    ⋄ cancers

    ⋄ lung disease

    ⋄ renal disease

    ⋄ valve replacement

Table 8.1. Signs and Symptoms and Diagnostic Tests and Findings for Sepsis Conditions

SIRS	Sepsis	Severe Sepsis	Septic Shock
+ temperature > 101°F (38.3°C) or < 96.9°F (36°C) + HR > 90 bpm + RR > 20 per minute + PaCO$_2$ < 32 mm Hg + WBC > 12,000/mm^3 or < 4,000/mm^3 or > 10% bands	+ 2 or more signs or symptoms of SIRS, plus suspected or confirmed infection + serum lactate > 2 mmol/L	+ sepsis, plus new or acute onset of organ dysfunction + urine output <30 cc/h + altered mental status + respiratory distress + tachycardia + abdominal pain + systolic BP < 90 mm Hg + MAP < 60 mm Hg + serum lactate >4 mmol/L + thrombocytopenia + elevated liver enzymes	+ severe sepsis, plus persistent hypotension and hypoperfusion that does not respond to fluid volume replacement

Treatment and Management

+ Provide supplemental oxygen for all patients and mechanical ventilation as needed.

+ Administer IV fluids.

+ Administer broad-spectrum antibiotics.

+ Administer vasopressor for patients with persistent hypotension.

QUICK REVIEW QUESTION

19. A patient with septic shock has a blood pressure of 84/38 mg Hg after receiving a 1 L normal saline bolus. What medication should the nurse anticipate administering?

ANSWER KEY

1. Administer 1 – 2 g of magnesium sulfate, and follow ACLS protocol for the length of the code.

2. Workup for fever of unknown origin in an infant includes blood cultures, chest X-ray, urinalysis, and lumbar puncture.

3. Loratadine is an H1 blocker. H2 blockers, steroids, bronchodilators, and topical antihistamines will also help reduce the allergic response to poison ivy.

4. The nurse should expect to administer epinephrine 1:1,000 IM 0.01 mg/kg. Epinephrine 1:1,000 is the correct dosage for IM injections and is the first-line treatment for anaphylactic symptoms. Doses of 1:10,000 – 1:100,000 are used IV for cardiac arrest.

5. The patient is exhibiting signs of progression to the AIDS stage of the HIV infection and may be immunocompromised. In addition, the patient is at risk for rapid decline and will require swift assessment and interventions.

6. The nurse should suspect septic pneumonia. Chemotherapy immunocompromises patients, making them more susceptible to infection.

7. The nurse should look for diffuse petechiae, generalized ecchymosis, or gingival bleeding; these all present with thrombocytopenia.

8. The patient will likely receive IV corticosteroids to treat Addisonian crisis related to the abrupt discontinuation of the prednisone.

9. The nurse should expect to find low specific gravity because the urine is quite diluted in diabetes insipidus.

10. The nurse will administer D5W or other dextrose-containing IV fluids.

11. DKA presents with hyperglycemia, Kussmaul respirations, abdominal pain, and vomiting. HHS presents with hyperglycemia and neurological changes, including delirium or coma.

12. Establish IV access, and push 1 ampule of D50. The patient is unconscious and cannot be given PO therapy, because of the risk of aspiration. The patient needs glucose immediately.

13. The nurse can use a hypothermia blanket, can apply ice packs to the armpits and groin and behind the neck, and can reduce the room temperature.

14. The patient is at great risk for surgical hemorrhage. The nurse should initiate bleeding precautions.

15. The nurse should expect to see elevated D-dimer and prolonged aPTT and PT in a patient with DIC.

16. Factor VIII transfusion should be initiated immediately if not previously started by the parent or school nurse.

17. Priapism can lead to permanent impotence, sexual dysfunction, and tissue necrosis. This symptom requires immediate treatment to restore blood flow.

18. The nurse should insert a Foley catheter with an attached urometer. Output of less than 30 cc/h indicates inadequate renal perfusion.

19. Vasopressors such as dobutamine hydrochloride, norepinephrine (Levophed), and phenylephrine hydrochloride (Neo-Synephrine) are used for supportive therapy of organ perfusion related to hypotension.

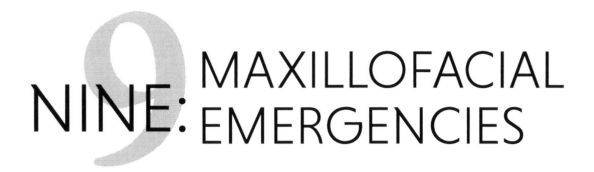

NINE: MAXILLOFACIAL EMERGENCIES

Cranial Nerves

+ The 12 **cranial nerves** emerge directly from the brain and control many sensory and motor functions, primarily in the head and neck.

+ When assessing maxillofacial emergencies, cranial nerve function should be examined using the tests below.

Table 9.1. Cranial Nerve Function and Assessment

Cranial Nerve	Assessment
I. Olfactory: controls sense of smell	Have patient identify a smell with eyes closed using each nostril individually.
II. Optic: central and peripheral vision	Have patient read something; assess peripheral vision.
III. Oculomotor: constriction of pupils	Test pupil response with penlight.
IV. Trochlear: downward eye movement	Have patient follow your finger moving toward their nose.
V. Trigeminal: face	Check sensation on forehead, cheeks, and jaw; test jaw strength; have patient clench teeth.
VI. Abducens: sideways eye movement	Have patient look toward each ear and complete cardinal fields.
VII. Facial: movement and expression	Assess facial symmetry; have patient puff cheeks, pucker, raise eyebrows, and smile.
VIII. Vestibulocochlear: controls hearing	Assess patient's gait; have patient close their eyes, hold watch by their ear, and ask what they hear.
IX. Glossopharyngeal: tongue and throat	Assess sweet and sour on back of tongue; assess gag reflex.
X. Vagus: sensory and motor	Have patient swallow while speaking; have patient say "ah."
XI. Accessory: head and shoulder movement	Have patient shrug shoulder and turn head against resistance.
XII. Hypoglossal: tongue position	Have patient stick tongue out midline and then side to side.

Acute Vestibular Dysfunction

LABYRINTHITIS

Pathophysiology

Labyrinthitis occurs in the inner ear when the vestibulocochlear nerve (eighth cranial nerve) becomes inflamed as the result of either bacterial or viral infection. The inflammation affects hearing, balance, and spatial navigation.

Viral cause is most common. Bacterial cause is rare if the patient is on antibiotics but may occur if a middle ear infection (otitis media) breaches both the tympanic membrane and the oval window of the inner ear. Onset is characterized as acute, sudden, and painless. The initial episode is most severe, with subsequent episodes showing less intensity. Labyrinthitis symptoms can extend from several weeks to several months.

Risk Factors

+ bacterial cause most common in pediatrics < 2
+ upper respiratory infections
+ otitis media
+ viral cause most common in adults ages 30 – 60:
    ⋄ herpes viruses
    ⋄ Epstein-Barr virus
    ⋄ Ramsay Hunt syndrome
    ⋄ rubeola (measles)
    ⋄ mumps
    ⋄ rubella
    ⋄ influenza
    ⋄ coxsackievirus
    ⋄ cytomegalovirus
    ⋄ polio
+ Lyme disease
+ allergic rhinitis
+ use of some medications:
    ⋄ aspirin
    ⋄ beta-blockers
    ⋄ ACE inhibitors
    ⋄ furosemide and loop diuretics
    ⋄ phenytoin
+ smoking
+ increased alcohol consumption
+ stress

Signs and Symptoms

+ dizziness
+ vertigo
+ nausea and vomiting
+ loss of balance
+ loss of equilibrium
+ tinnitus
+ hearing loss
+ fever
+ irritability or lethargy in children

Diagnostic Tests and Findings

+ No specific tests exist to diagnose; use process of elimination.

+ Rule out:
    ⬦ cerebrovascular accident
    ⬦ meningitis
    ⬦ subarachnoid hemorrhage
    ⬦ head injury
    ⬦ tumors
    ⬦ Ménière's disease

Treatment and Management

+ antihistamines
+ antiemetics
+ benzodiazepines
+ meclizine (Antivert)
+ antibiotics (if bacterial cause suspected)
+ antiviral (if viral cause suspected)
+ corticosteroids
+ bedrest until symptoms subside
+ no driving with dizziness or vertigo

QUICK REVIEW QUESTION

1. A 40-year-old female is diagnosed with labyrinthitis in the ED after all other potential neurological causes for sudden onset of vertigo, nausea, and tinnitus have been ruled out. While the nurse is preparing the patient for discharge, the patient asks if she can return to work tomorrow. What should the nurse anticipate discussing with the patient about the course of this disease?

MÉNIÈRE'S DISEASE
Pathophysiology

Ménière's disease is the result of chronic excess fluid in the inner ear. Fluid accumulation is the result of malabsorption in the endolymphatic sac or blockage of the endolymphatic duct. The excess fluid causes the endolymphatic space to enlarge, increasing inner ear pressure and possibly rupturing the inner membrane (not to be confused with rupture of the tympanic membrane in the middle ear as seen with otitis media).

While typically only one ear is affected, it does occur bilaterally in about 20% of cases. Onset may be minor with subtle symptoms, with subsequent episodes manifesting with more severe symptoms. Attacks can occur frequently, up to several times per week, or infrequently, several months or years apart. Attacks typically last anywhere from 20 minutes to 24 hours. Ménière's is also referred to as *idiopathic syndrome of endolymphatic hydrops*.

Risk Factors

+ most common in adults 40 – 60
+ cause unknown
+ suspected contributing risk factors:
    ⬦ family history (around 50% of patients)
    ⬦ excess fluid/endolymph accumulation from increased localized potassium
    ⬦ anatomical abnormality of inner membrane
    ⬦ excess dietary sodium
+ triggers for attacks:
    ⬦ changes in atmospheric pressure and elevation
    ⬦ fatigue
    ⬦ stress
    ⬦ emotional distress

Signs and Symptoms

+ dependent on stage of disease and progress of attack
+ classic triad of symptoms:
    ⬦ fluctuations in hearing/hearing loss
    ⬦ tinnitus
    ⬦ vertigo
+ pre-attack (aura):
    ⬦ loss of balance
    ⬦ dizziness or lightheadedness
    ⬦ pressure in ear
    ⬦ hearing loss or tinnitus
    ⬦ headache
+ mid-attack:
    ⬦ sudden severe vertigo
    ⬦ loss of balance
    ⬦ loss of equilibrium
    ⬦ anxiety
    ⬦ nausea and vomiting
    ⬦ diarrhea
    ⬦ blurred vision
    ⬦ nystagmus
    ⬦ cold sweat
    ⬦ shivering
    ⬦ palpitations
    ⬦ tachycardia
+ post-attack:
    ⬦ extreme exhaustion
    ⬦ need for sleep
+ late-stage disease:
    ⬦ permanent hearing loss
    ⬦ increased, constant tinnitus and/or ear pressure
    ⬦ decrease in episodes of vertigo
    ⬦ increase in balance disturbances
    ⬦ increase in visual disturbances
    ⬦ Tumarkin's otolithic crisis (drop attacks)

Diagnostic Tests and Findings

+ No specific tests exist to diagnose; use process of elimination.
+ Rule out:
    ⬦ cerebrovascular accident
    ⬦ meningitis
    ⬦ subarachnoid hemorrhage
    ⬦ head injury
    ⬦ tumors
    ⬦ labyrinthitis
+ Key findings are history of symptoms lasting 20 minutes to 24 hours.
    ⬦ vertigo
    ⬦ tinnitus
    ⬦ hearing loss

Treatment and Management

+ reduced sodium diet
+ diuretics (non-potassium-sparing)
+ antiemetics
+ benzodiazepines
+ meclizine
+ intratympanic gentamicin (injected by ENT)
+ intratympanic steroids (injected by ENT)
+ referral to otolaryngology

Dental Conditions

Pathophysiology

Emergency dental conditions commonly seen in the ED are dental traumas, abscessed teeth, and acute dental pain.

Risk Factors

+ trauma:
    ◇ motorized vehicle accident
    ◇ sports injuries
    ◇ childhood play
    ◇ physical assault
    ◇ falls
    ◇ biting on hard objects
+ abscess/infection:
    ◇ homelessness
    ◇ malnutrition
    ◇ poor dentation
    ◇ dental caries

+ dental pain:
    ◇ poor dentation
    ◇ dental caries
    ◇ dry socket
    ◇ exposed root

Signs and Symptoms

+ trauma:
    ◇ fractured or cracked tooth
    ◇ dental avulsion
    ◇ lacerations
+ abscess/infection:
    ◇ orofacial edema
    ◇ halitosis
    ◇ visible pus or exudate
    ◇ taste of pus or exudate in mouth
    ◇ fever

+ dental pain:
    ◇ visible signs may be absent
    ◇ presence of dental caries
    ◇ edentulousness

Diagnostic Tests and Findings

- trauma:
  - avulsion
  - visible fracture/crack in tooth
  - radiology/X-ray
- abscess/infection:
  - CBC with elevated WBC; increase in neutrophils with acute bacterial infection
  - fever
  - wound culture
  - blood cultures if sepsis is suspected
- dental pain:
  - diagnostics limited
  - diagnosis based on patient's subjective data

Treatment and Management

- trauma:
  - Place avulsed tooth in Hank's balanced salt solution (HBSS) or milk.
  - Reinsert tooth if viable.
  - Stabilize fracture to prevent aspiration.
  - Suture repair oral lacerations as warranted.
  - Dental/oral surgery consult as warranted.
  - Administer analgesics for pain management.
  - Apply ice to the face for pain management and vasoconstriction.
  - Avoid oral ice.
- abscess/infection:
  - Incise and drain.
  - Administer antibiotics.
  - Administer analgesics for pain management.
  - Dental/oral surgery consult as warranted.
- dental pain:
  - Administer analgesics for pain management.
  - Dental/oral surgery consult as warranted.

QUICK REVIEW QUESTION

3. A patient arrives at the ED with a complaint of severe mouth pain for the past three days. Assessment findings include edematous gingivitis, an enlarged spongy nodule with purulent yellow exudate along the bottom left molars, facial edema, and tender lymph nodes. What is the diagnosis and why is medical care important?

Epistaxis

Pathophysiology

Epistaxis is hemorrhage or bleeding in the nasal passages caused by rupture of vasodilated vessels in the mucous membranes. Rupture can occur in one or more vessels and more commonly presents unilaterally. Emergency treatment should be considered if bleeding cannot be self-controlled or compromises the airway. Epistaxis can occur frequently in some individuals and rarely requires emergency management.

Risk Factors

+ coagulation disorders
+ common cold
+ deviated septum
+ nasal surgery
+ allergic rhinitis
+ facial trauma

+ forceful sneezing
+ rhinotillexomania
+ dry, un-humidified environmental air
+ use of anticoagulant medications
+ inhalation of chemical irritants
+ intranasal substance abuse

Signs and Symptoms

+ visible frank bleeding from nares
+ presence of clotting
    ✧ may range in size from tiny to as large as a golf ball
+ presence of blood in nasopharyngeal and oral airways
+ emergency care needed if:
    ✧ patient has difficulty breathing or airway is compromised
    ✧ bleeding exceeds 30 minutes with compression applied
    ✧ patient is under the age of 2
    ✧ bleeding initiated subsequent to an injury
    ✧ bleeding appears excessive (greater than standard nosebleeds)

Diagnostic Tests and Findings

+ visualization of bleeding with use of a nasal speculum, headlight, or penlight
+ facial X-ray warranted for injury

Treatment and Management

+ Sit upright and lean forward to prevent aspiration (do not tilt head backward).
+ Use suction to maintain patent airway if warranted.
+ Apply continuous pressure to midline septum by pinching with fingers for up to 15 minutes.
+ Apply ice for pain management and vasoconstriction.
+ Use nasal decongestant spray to assist with vasoconstriction.

- ✦ Cauterize affected vessels.
- ✦ Use nasal tampon.
- ✦ Pack the nose.
- ✦ Refer to otolaryngology.

QUICK REVIEW QUESTION

4. A patient arrives in the ED with acute epistaxis after being hit with a football in the face during a high school game. The patient suddenly goes into respiratory distress. What actions should the nurse take immediately?

Facial Nerve Disorders

BELL'S PALSY

Pathophysiology

Bell's palsy is a unilateral facial paralysis or weakness caused by inflammation of the facial nerve (seventh cranial nerve). Onset is sudden and facial droop is similar in appearance to droop present with a cerebrovascular accident. In most cases the weakness will resolve over weeks to months; occasionally, it may recur. Bell's palsy typically occurs in younger adults and children. Cause is unknown but may be related to viral infections, autoimmune disease, or vascular ischemia.

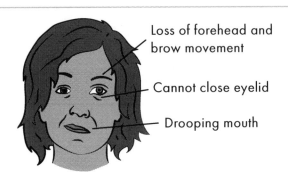

Loss of forehead and brow movement

Cannot close eyelid

Drooping mouth

Figure 9.1. Bell's Palsy

Risk Factors

- ✦ pregnancy
- ✦ diabetes
- ✦ herpes simplex virus
- ✦ herpes zoster
- ✦ coxsackievirus
- ✦ Epstein-Barr virus
- ✦ influenza B
- ✦ adenovirus
- ✦ rubella
- ✦ cytomegalovirus
- ✦ Lyme disease

Signs and Symptoms

- ✦ mild to total unilateral paralysis of facial muscles
- ✦ characteristic facial droop
- ✦ asymmetrical facial features and smile
- ✦ painful sensations on affected side
- ✦ difficulty speaking
- ✦ dysphagia

Diagnostic Tests and Findings

- ✦ initial diagnostics to rule out cerebrovascular accident
- ✦ history of recent viral infection and/or autoimmune disease

- laboratory tests for specific viral and autoimmune conditions, including:
  - EBV panel
  - Lyme disease
  - influenza swab
  - ESR
  - ANA
- elevated WBC with identified increase in lymphocytes in acute viral infection

Treatment and Management

- corticosteroids
- antivirals if indicated
- patch on affected eye if diminished blink reflex to limit risk for corneal abrasion
- oral glycerin swabs for dry mouth
- Yankauer suction for excess saliva
- referral to neurology if warranted

QUICK REVIEW QUESTION

5. A 14-year-old patient arrives at the ED with sudden onset of right-sided facial droop. The patient reveals a recent influenza infection, and Bell's palsy is the suspected diagnosis. What treatment should the nurse anticipate giving this patient?

TRIGEMINAL NEURALGIA

Pathophysiology

Trigeminal neuralgia—or tic douloureux—is a condition of the trigeminal nerve (fifth cranial nerve) that causes unilateral stabbing, shooting pain and burning sensations along the nerve branches. Paroxysms can affect any or all of the three nerve branches: ophthalmic, maxillary, and mandibular, and painful spasms both start and end abruptly. The cause is unknown, but pressure and compression of the vascular vessels near the trigeminal nerve root is suspected.

Trigeminal neuralgia is chronic, and the slightest touch or stimulation may precipitate a painful episode. The initial attacks may be short; however, it can progress to longer and more frequent attacks.

Risk Factors

- age-related anatomical changes of the cerebral artery and veins:
  - most common in ages 50 – 60
- more common in women
- multiple sclerosis
- facial trauma
- triggers:
  - washing or shaving face
  - wind or other environmental pressure
  - brushing teeth
  - consuming food and fluids

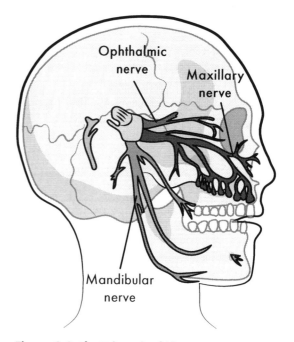

Figure 9.2. The Trigeminal Nerve

Signs and Symptoms

+ characteristic unilateral pain along branches of the fifth cranial nerve

+ abrupt onset and ending of pain lasting several minutes to several days

+ pain-free intervals ranging from several minutes to several days

+ trigger points associated with onset of pain (described previously)

+ facial muscle contractions causing eye to close and mouth to twitch on affected side

Diagnostic Tests and Findings

+ diagnosis based on description of pain including:
   ✧ type
   ✧ location
   ✧ triggers

+ diagnostics to rule out cerebrovascular accident and other neurological deficits

Treatment and Management

+ First line of treatment is medication.
   ✧ anti-seizure medications:
      + carbamazepine (Tegretol)
      + gabapentin (Neurontin)
      + phenytoin (Dilantin)
   ✧ baclofen (Lioresal)

+ Neurology consult if warranted.

QUICK REVIEW QUESTION

6. A 50-year-old female patient arrives at the ED with a complaint of excruciating pain when anything touches her face and when eating, brushing her teeth, and putting on makeup. Her symptoms have evolved over the past few weeks. Her medical history includes possible multiple sclerosis. She could not tolerate being touched for the physical assessment and made it partway through the neurological exam. What diagnosis and treatment should the nurse anticipate?

Foreign Bodies in Maxillofacial Region

FOREIGN BODIES IN THE NASAL AND ORAL ORIFICES

Pathophysiology

Non-penetrating foreign bodies may be present in the orifices of the maxillofacial region as a result of aspiration or direct entry. The foreign body can be any type, size, or shape of substance; each incident will be individually assessed and managed.

+ Common foreign bodies in nares: popcorn kernels, beads, batteries, Styrofoam pellets, pebbles, and insects

+ Common foreign bodies in ear: earring backings, beads, pebbles, popcorn kernels, and insects

Risk Factors:

+ common in children < 3
+ cognitive impairment
+ outdoor recreation (insects)

Signs and Symptoms

+ rhinorrhea; may smell foul if present for a prolonged period
+ unilateral edema of alar tissue
+ sensation of foreign body in nasal passage
+ ear pain or pressure
+ headache
+ auditory disturbances

+ hearing loss
+ visible foreign body
+ deviated septum
+ inflammation/edema in turbinates
+ otitis media
+ otitis externa
+ may be asymptomatic

Treatment and Management

+ Airway management is priority to prevent passage of foreign body through nasopharynx.
+ Tilt head of bed 45 – 90 degrees.
+ For objects in the nares:
    ✧ Administer 0.5% phenylephrine to reduce nasal inflammation.
    ✧ Use topical lidocaine for anesthetic effect.
    ✧ Instruct patient to blow nose while blocking unaffected nostril.
    ✧ For small children, parent may assist with positive pressure ventilation by covering the mouth of the child with their own mouth and blowing softly into the airway. The unaffected nostril should be blocked simultaneously.
    ✧ Use forceps or suction catheter for retrieval.
    ✧ Pass a balloon-tip catheter (5 – 6 French) above foreign body and inflate to move foreign body toward distal nares.
    ✧ Do not irrigate vegetative or porous materials.
    ✧ In the case of insects, insert topical lidocaine alcohol or mineral oil to disable movement, or use a flashlight to draw insect out of nares.
+ For objects in the ears:
    ✧ Use caution to avoid pushing foreign body deeper into the ear canal, which poses a risk for tympanic membrane rupture.
    ✧ In the case of insects, insert topical lidocaine alcohol or mineral oil to disable movement, or use a flashlight to draw insect out of ear canal.
+ Refer to otolaryngologist as warranted.

QUICK REVIEW QUESTION

7. What noninvasive technique can be used by the nurse to remove a live insect foreign body from the ear canal?

Pathophysiology

Foreign bodies found in the maxillofacial region vary by type and point of entry. Each incident should be individually assessed and managed.

Risk Factors

+ MVAs
+ occupational accidents
+ falls
+ acts of war and violence
+ physical assault
+ sports-related injuries

Signs and Symptoms

+ entry point
+ bleeding
+ nasal drainage (rule out cerebrospinal fluid)
+ contusions
+ crepitus
+ hematoma
+ tissue edema
+ disfigurement
+ non-healing wounds
+ purulent exudate
+ chronic sinus drainage
+ fever

Diagnostic Tests and Findings

+ palpation or visualization of foreign body
+ facial muscle function assessment
+ X-ray
+ CT scan
+ ultrasonography
+ CBC
+ chemistry panel
+ blood cultures and serum lactate to assess for progression to bacteremia and sepsis
+ fluid volume status

Treatment and Management

+ ABCs are the priority.
+ Maintain patency of airway.
+ Monitor for aspiration.
+ Administer pain medication.
+ Administer IV fluids with hemorrhage.
+ Administer IV antibiotics.
+ Clear mouth of foreign objects and suction blood.
+ Apply direct pressure for hemorrhage.
+ Clean or irrigate wounds, then dress.
+ Remove foreign object(s) as possible.
  ✧ Do not remove object until safe to do so.
+ Administer oxygen as warranted.
+ Immobilize spine and neck as warranted.
+ Prepare to intubate as warranted.
  ✧ nasotracheal intubation
  ✧ orotracheal intubation
+ Surgical consult.
+ Plastic surgery consult.

Infections

LUDWIG'S ANGINA

Pathophysiology

Ludwig's angina is a gangrenous cellulitis that attacks the soft tissue of the neck and the floor of the mouth, generally following an abscess of the second and third molars or other dental infection. The bacterial infection is fast moving and causes extensive edema of the neck and mouth, which can place the patient at high risk for airway obstruction and death. Although it generally starts in the submandibular space, it will spread to nearby tissues and can encircle the airway, resulting in constriction.

Risk Factors

+ more than 90% of cases caused by dental infections, which can result from:
  + tooth extraction
  + mouth injury
  + poor oral hygiene
  + jaw fractures
+ acute glomerulonephritis
+ systemic lupus erythematous
+ aplastic anemia
+ neutropenia
+ diabetes
+ staphylococcus
+ streptococcus
+ immunosuppressive diseases
+ tongue piercing
+ alcoholism

Signs and Symptoms

+ tongue enlargement and protrusion
+ sublingual pain and tenderness
+ compromised breathing
+ difficulty swallowing
+ drooling
+ neck pain, edema, and erythema
+ fever
+ weakness
+ fatigue
+ chills
+ confusion
+ chest pain
+ sepsis

Diagnostic Tests and Findings

+ visible tongue enlargement and displacement
+ elevated core temperature

+ CBC with elevated WBC; increase in neutrophils with acute bacterial infection

+ blood cultures and serum lactate to assess for progression to bacteremia and sepsis

+ dental exudate culture if present

+ CT scan for edema and inflammation in the submandibular and sublingual spaces

Treatment and Management

+ ABCs are the priority.

+ Administer oxygen as warranted.

+ Prepare to intubate as warranted.

+ Emergent tracheotomy.

+ Administer IV antibiotics.

+ Incise and drain.

+ Surgical/dental consult if warranted.

QUICK REVIEW QUESTION

9. A male patient is admitted to the ED one week after oral surgery with pain and swelling to the left side of his face and neck, which has progressed through the day. He states he has had difficulty swallowing and is drooling. He rates the pain 7/10 and vital signs reveal a temperature of 100.0°F (37.8°C) and pulse of 114 bpm. The oral cavity is tender and painful upon palpation. What diagnosis is appropriate for these signs and symptoms, and what test can be ordered to confirm?

OTITIS

Pathophysiology

Acute otitis media (AOM) is inflammation of the middle ear that usually results from inflammation in the mucous membranes of the nasopharynx. The middle ear fills with fluid and that fluid may also become infected. Otitis media is a recurrent disease; many children may experience six or more episodes.

Otitis media with effusion (OME) occurs when uninfected fluid remains in the middle ear. It usually results when the Eustachian tube is blocked, which prevents the fluid from draining.

Risk Factors

+ most common in children < 3

+ upper respiratory infection

+ allergic rhinitis

+ Down syndrome

+ craniofacial anomalies

Signs and Symptoms

+ acute otitis media:
  + otalgia
  + otorrhea
  + tugging on ear
  + headache
  + fever
  + irritability
  + loss of appetite
  + vomiting
  + diarrhea
  + loss of balance

- otitis media with effusion:
  - hearing loss
  - tinnitus
  - vertigo
  - otalgia

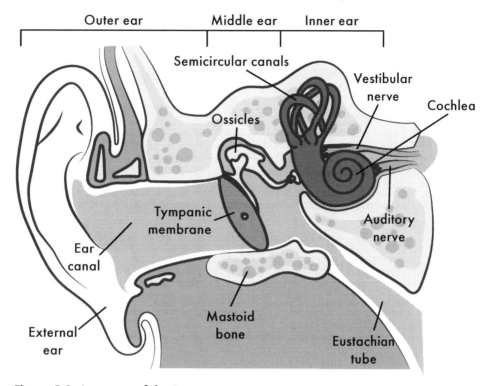

Figure 9.3. Anatomy of the Ear

Diagnostic Tests and Findings

- abnormal otoscope findings:
  - perforated tympanic membrane
  - opaque tympanic membrane
  - bulging tympanic membrane
  - erythema of tympanic membrane
  - middle ear effusion
  - decreased mobility with pneumatic otoscopy
- enlarged lymph nodes

Treatment and Management

- can heal spontaneously
- antibiotics
  - oral antibiotics if membrane is intact
  - antibiotic drops directly in affected ear if tympanic membrane is ruptured
- analgesics for pain management
- referral to otolaryngology

QUICK REVIEW QUESTION

10. A 2-year-old child is brought to the ED crying inconsolably and rubbing the left ear. The parents state that the child has had a mild cold and runny nose for the past week that progressed to irritable behavior and onset of fever a few hours ago. An otoscope exam reveals an intact erythemic tympanic membrane with visible bulging and striation of vessels. What does the nurse anticipate for pain management for this child?

SINUSITIS

Pathophysiology

Sinusitis is caused by inflammation and edema of the membranes lining the sinus cavities. Normally the sinuses contain air; however, when blocked by edematous membranes they fill with fluid and bacteria, leading to infection.

Risk Factors

+ common cold
+ allergic rhinitis
+ nasal polyps
+ immune deficiencies
+ deviated septum
+ nasal edema
+ smoking

Signs and Symptoms

+ facial pressure and pain
+ headaches
+ nasal congestion and blockage
+ green or yellow nasal discharge
+ decreased sense of smell
+ cough
+ fever
+ fatigue
+ halitosis
+ tooth pain

Diagnostic Tests and Findings

+ tenderness with palpation over sinus cavity
+ presence of nasal symptoms
+ presence of headache
+ CT scan if serious infection is suspected

Treatment and Management

+ decongestant
+ antihistamine
+ analgesics for pain management
+ antibiotics
+ humidified air
+ warm compress
+ saline nasal drops
+ corticosteroids

QUICK REVIEW QUESTION

11. A 27-year-old male is admitted to the ED with a complaint of facial pressure, rhinorrhea, and nasal congestion. Yellow discharge is seen on tissue when he blows his nose, and he states the presence of a nasty taste in his mouth. His nose deviates to his right and appears swollen. He has a low-grade fever of 100.1°F (37.8°C); otherwise vital signs are stable. He states he was drinking and play-fighting with his brother a week ago and was punched in the nose. He did not seek treatment although it felt like his nose was broken. What diagnosis is appropriate, and what may have triggered the signs and symptoms?

MASTOIDITIS

Pathophysiology

Mastoiditis is a bacterial infection of the mastoid air cells within the mastoid bone. The infection typically occurs after acute otitis media for which treatment was either not provided or was ineffective in resolving the infection. Fluid takes over the air-filled spaces; left untreated, mastoiditis can erode the bone, leading to life-threatening abscesses or septic thrombosis.

Risk Factors

+ recent middle ear infection
+ recurrent ear infections

Signs and Symptoms

+ otitis media
+ tympanic membrane rupture
+ fever
+ papilledema
+ erythema and edema over mastoid process

Diagnostic Tests and Findings

+ diagnosis based on physical findings
+ laboratory values and CT scan not indicated

Treatment and Management

+ antibiotics
+ analgesics for pain management
+ referral to otolaryngology

QUICK REVIEW QUESTION

12. A patient arrives at the ED with a complaint of earache, drainage, headache, and fever for the past three days. History reveals recurrent ear infections, and eventually mastoiditis is diagnosed. What will be the treatment plan for this patient?

Maxillofacial Fractures

Pathophysiology

Maxillofacial fractures occur from both blunt and penetrating traumas. Fractures may involve one or more structures, may be open or closed, and may require surgical reduction. Emergency management focuses on maintaining a patent airway and stabilizing the patient for surgical intervention. Most fractures will involve the integrity of surrounding tissues, requiring complex repair to muscular, vascular, and dermal structures as well as the reduction and fixation of the affected bone.

Types of maxillofacial fractures:

+ nasal: most common of all facial fractures and least likely to need specialist consultation
+ orbital rim and blowout fractures: fractures of orbital floor or lateral and medial orbital walls; occur from direct blow to the orbit such as from a baseball or fist

- mandibular: fractures of the lower jaw; may be singular or multiple
- maxillary: fractures of the upper jaw
  - Le Fort I: horizontal fracture; separates teeth from upper structures—"floating palate"
  - Le Fort II: pyramidal fracture; teeth are the base of the pyramid, fracture passes diagonally along the lateral wall of the maxillary sinuses, apex of pyramid is the nasofrontal junction—"floating maxilla"
  - Le Fort III: craniofacial disjunction transverse fracture line passes through the nasofrontal junction, maxillofrontal suture, orbital wall, zygomatic arch, and zygomaticofrontal suture—"floating face"

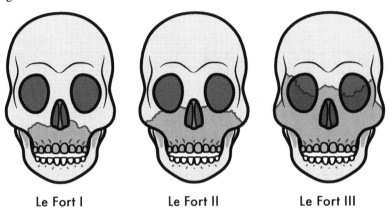

Le Fort I   Le Fort II   Le Fort III

Figure 9.4. Types of Maxillary Fractures

- Zygomaticomaxillary complex (tripod) fracture: simultaneous fracture of the lateral and inferior orbital rim, the zygomatic arch, and lateral maxillary sinus wall; occurs from direct blow to the lateral cheek

Risk Factors

- more common in men
- MVAs
- acts of war and violence
- physical altercations

- sports injuries
- domestic violence

Signs and Symptoms

- visible facial injury or deformity
- pain, tenderness, or paresthesia over affected area
- epistaxis
- ecchymosis
- dark discoloration under eyes
- asymmetrical appearance

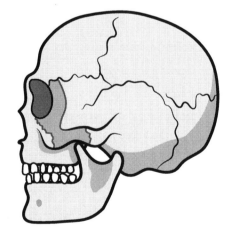

Figure 9.5. Zygomaticomaxillary Complex (Tripod) Fracture

- ocular:
  - diplopia
  - restricted extraocular movements
  - decreased vision or loss of vision
  - enophthalmos
  - periorbital hematoma
  - periorbital edema
  - subconjunctival hemorrhage
  - chemosis
- dental/oral:
  - visible dental fractures or avulsions
  - impaired mastication
  - malocclusion
- subcutaneous emphysema/crepitus over sinus cavities
- trismus
- tympanic membrane rupture
- rhinorrhea of cerebrospinal fluid

Diagnostic Tests and Findings

- facial X-ray
- CT scan (head and neck)
- if dental avulsions, chest X-ray in case of aspiration of avulsed teeth/bone

Treatment and Management

- Maintain airway patency.
- Maintain cervical spine precautions.
- Reduction and fixation:
  - Ranges from manual setting as with a simple nasal fracture to surgical intervention for complex fractures.
- Repair of open structures:
  - Ranges from simple laceration suturing to complex neurovascular and muscle reattachment.
- Goal of all treatments is to preserve function and minimize disfigurement.
- Consult as warranted:
  - oral/maxillofacial surgery
  - neurology
  - ophthalmology
  - otolaryngology

QUICK REVIEW QUESTION

13. What diagnostic test needs to be performed stat on a patient with a suspected mandibular fracture that presents with dental avulsions?

Peritonsillar Abscess

Pathophysiology

Peritonsillar abscess is an acute medical emergency that compromises the airway. Purulent exudate accumulates between the tonsillar capsule and the pharyngeal constrictor muscle causing cellutis and edema. This is a life-threatening condition that can quickly advance to mediastinitis, intracranial abscess, necrotizing fasciitis, streptococcal toxic shock syndrome, and empyema if the infection is not aggressively managed.

Risk Factors

+ most common in teenagers and young adults ages 20 – 40
+ acute tonsillitis
+ smoking
+ poor oral hygiene

Signs and Symptoms

+ visible abscess on soft palate
+ severe sore throat
+ enlarged lymph nodes
+ fever
+ trismus
+ drooling
+ dysphagia
+ halitosis

Diagnostic Tests and Findings

+ visualization of abscess
+ ultrasound
+ CBC with elevated WBC; increase in neutrophils with acute bacterial infection
+ blood cultures and serum lactate to assess for progression to bacteremia and sepsis

Treatment and Management

+ ABCs:
  + airway patency
+ incision and drainage
+ needle aspiration
+ surgical consult
+ antibiotics
+ analgesics for pain management
+ corticosteroids
+ suction to manage secretions

QUICK REVIEW QUESTION

14. An 18-year-old patient arrives at the ED with a complaint of sore throat, drooling, and severe halitosis that the nurse can detect from several feet away. In the triage setting, what can the nurse immediately assess for to determine the level of acuity for this patient?

Ruptured Tympanic Membrane

Pathophysiology

The **tympanic membrane** (eardrum) is a stiff yet flexible structure that separates the ear canal from the middle ear. Any tear or perforation in this membrane is termed a rupture. In uncomplicated cases a ruptured eardrum heals without treatment in a few weeks; complicated cases may require specialized procedures and/or surgery.

Risk Factors

+ middle ear infections
+ barotrauma
+ air bag impact

+ acoustic trauma
+ skull fracture
+ inserting foreign objects (e.g., cotton swabs)

Signs and Symptoms

+ severe pain upon rupture, which quickly subsides
+ fluid drainage:
  ⬦ clear (effusion)
  ⬦ purulent (infection)
  ⬦ sanguineous (trauma)
  ⬦ serous (suspect cerebrospinal)— emergent

+ hearing loss or reduction
+ tinnitus
+ vertigo with nausea and vomiting
+ whistling sound or crepitus with blowing nose

Diagnostic Tests and Findings

+ visible findings upon otoscope exam

+ CT scan or X-ray if trauma is initiating cause

Treatment and Management

+ dependent on root cause of rupture
+ emergent treatment not always warranted
+ trauma protocols
+ antibiotic ear drops for infection

+ analgesic ear drops for pain management
+ foreign body removal
+ referral to otolaryngology

QUICK REVIEW QUESTION

15. A patient presents to the ED with a complaint of left ear pain following her first time scuba diving. Her medical history is unremarkable and vital signs are stable. The patient states there was an episode of severe pain just as she surfaced. The pain got better, but now she has difficulty hearing. What tool will be used for initial evaluation and what would be the most basic treatment?

Temporomandibular Joint Dislocation

Pathophysiology

Temporomandibular joint (TMJ) dislocation is a painful condition that can occur related to trauma, excessive opening of the mandible, or force applied to a partially opened mouth. The jaw can dislocate into several positions, including anterior, posterior, superior, and lateral. Anterior displacements are very common and are classified as acute, chronic recurrent, or chronic.

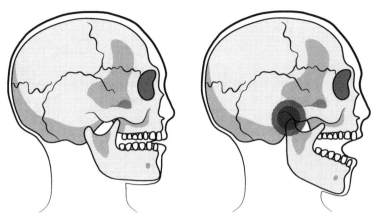

Figure 9.6. Temporomandibular Joint (TMJ) Dislocation

Risk Factors

+ history of dislocations
+ thin mandibular fossa
+ dystonic reactions
+ seizures
+ Marfan syndrome
+ ligament injury
+ dental extractions

+ vomiting
+ anesthesia
+ after endoscopic procedures
+ intubation
+ spasms
+ direct blow to chin

Signs and Symptoms

+ palpable displacement of joint
+ jaw pain
+ malocclusion
+ speech difficulties

+ drooling
+ dysphagia
+ trismus

Diagnostic Tests and Findings

+ X-ray to rule out fractures
+ gingival lacerations related to fracture

+ bilateral tongue blade testing
+ CT scan

Treatment and Management

+ ABCs
+ manual reduction (closed):
  ⋄ analgesia (pre-reduction)
  ⋄ muscle relaxer (pre-reduction)

+ surgical treatment or reduction (open)
+ X-ray after reduction
+ oral/maxillofacial surgery consult

16. A patient presents to the ED with an anterior TMJ dislocation. The patient states he has jaw pain and trouble swallowing and talking and can feel that his jaw is crooked. What is the nurse's primary assessment and what will be the treatment?

ANSWER KEY

1. Labyrinthitis runs a course of several weeks to several months. The nurse should educate the patient that bedrest is essential and that use of prescribed medications will manage symptoms. It is likely that additional episodes will occur, although they may be less severe than the onset of disease.

2. Ménière's disease presents suddenly with vertigo and tinnitus. While hearing loss can be present, it is common that early attacks lack the typical triad of symptoms. A history of less severe episodes of vertigo is consistent with progressive chronic disease. A patient who is afebrile and denies cold or flu symptoms is likely to have Ménière's disease and not labyrinthitis.

3. An abscess is an emergent situation because the infection can spread to the bone and vascular system, causing sepsis and potential death.

4. Suction immediately to maintain patent airway. Sit the patient upright and lean the head forward to prevent aspiration. Ensure pressure is applied to the midline septum to slow the progress of bleeding.

5. The nurse should provide comfort measures to assist with dry eyes, which could include moisture/saline drops and patching to prevent dryness and potential for corneal abrasion. Oral glycerin swabs could be used for dry mouth symptoms, and Yankauer suction can control excess pooling of saliva secretions. Corticosteroids and antiviral medication may be prescribed.

6. Based on signs and symptoms, the patient is suffering from trigeminal neuralgia. The nurse should anticipate pharmacotherapy as a first line of treatment.

7. Some live insects, such as moths, are naturally drawn to light. The nurse can direct a flashlight or exam light into the ear canal to draw the insect outward. This technique may not work if the insect is injured or is trapped in wax or fluid.

8. This is a traumatic injury with the risk of death. The nurse should start with the ABCs: stabilizing the airway is priority. Prepare for intubation before the airway is lost and administer oxygen or bag patient until airway is secured. Suction oral cavity and start large-bore IVs and fluids for blood loss. Apply direct pressure or pressure bandages to bleeding wounds and administer IV pain medication and sedative. Once the patient is stable, evaluation and removal of buckshot can follow.

9. Signs and symptoms are consistent with early onset of Ludwig's angina. A CT scan to evaluate the soft tissue would be appropriate.

10. Pain from otitis media is caused by the pressure exerted on the tympanic membrane by fluid or exudate. Initial treatment with acetaminophen or ibuprofen is beneficial in reducing pain and fever if present. Antibiotic therapy will assist with pain management by reducing the bacterial count and subsequent pressure. If the pressure causes the tympanic membrane to rupture, pain will immediately subside, but scar tissue can result, greatly impacting future hearing.

11. Sinusitis is an appropriate diagnosis. The deviated septum and possible broken nose most likely prompted it. The deviated septum and edema would block the sinus cavity, allowing bacteria to grow and start the infection.

12. Mastoiditis requires hospitalization and antibiotics to stop the infection before irreversible damage occurs. If treatment is unsuccessful, surgery may be required.

13. The patient should receive a chest X-ray to assess for aspiration of avulsed teeth and bone fragments.

14. The nurse can use a penlight to assess the tonsillar tissue and soft palate for presence of a peritonsillar abscess. Peritonsillar abscess is an emergent finding and requires rapid evaluation by a medical provider.

15. An otoscope will be used to assess the tympanic membrane for a tear or hole. For a minor rupture of the eardrum no treatment would be necessary.

16. With facial trauma, the ABCs are priority. A manual reduction is most likely if fractures are ruled out first.

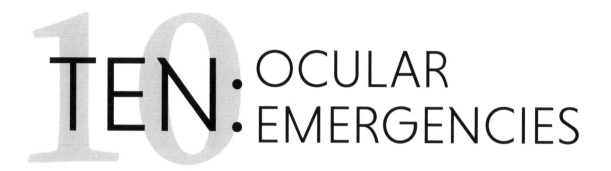

TEN: OCULAR EMERGENCIES

Foreign Bodies in Ocular Region

Pathophysiology

Ocular foreign bodies are any substance or object that does not belong in the eye. Foreign bodies are described based upon their location.

✦ extraocular (lid, sclera, conjunctiva, and cornea)

✦ intraocular (anterior chamber, iris, lens, vitreous, retina, and intraorbital)

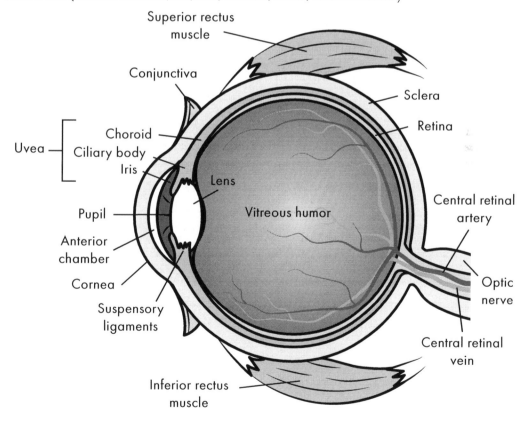

Figure 10.1. Anatomy of the Eye

Size, shape, substance, impact velocity, and location will greatly impact severity of symptoms and ultimate outcome.

Risk Factors

+ occupational (wood, metal debris)
+ failure to use safety glasses
+ environmental (wind, sand, insects, vegetative materials)
+ landscaping (lawnmower, weed-whacker, yard debris)
+ high-velocity machinery
+ welding
+ explosives, fireworks
+ shrapnel
+ acts of violence

Signs and Symptoms

+ painful pressure or burning sensation
+ penetrating injury
+ bleeding
  ⬦ dependent on location of foreign body
+ increased lacrimation that is clear upon initial injury
+ discharge possibly thick or yellow if infection is present
+ erythema
+ inflammation
+ edema of palpebra
+ blepharospasm
+ photosensitivity
+ decrease in visual acuity
+ headache

Diagnostic Tests and Findings

+ fluorescein staining
  ⬦ Abrasion will appear yellow in normal light.
  ⬦ Abrasion will appear green in cobalt blue light.
+ slit lamp or Woods lamp exam to identify the degree of injury or illness
+ X-ray, CT scan, or ultrasound for open globe injuries
+ decreased visual acuity (measured with Snellen chart)
+ Seidel test to confirm vitreous leakage from intraocular foreign body

Treatment and Management

+ Irrigate with normal saline or eye wash solution.
+ May use Morgan Lens for extraocular foreign bodies, or if sensation of foreign body is present but foreign body is not visible.
+ Evert upper lid to confirm absence/presence of foreign body.
+ Remove foreign body using cotton-tipped applicator, metal spud, or 25-gauge needle (extraocular only).
+ Administer topical anesthetic (caines).
+ Administer topical antibiotics.

- Administer topical NSAIDs.
  - Steroids containing ophthalmic solutions are not indicted for emergency use.
- Administer ophthalmic lubricating solution (artificial tears).
- Patch only if foreign body is retained, pending ophthalmology referral.

- Instruct patient to avoid wearing contact lenses until eye has healed.
- Refer to ophthalmology.
  - Refer for all intraocular foreign bodies immediately to ophthalmology.
  - Refer within 24 hours for retained extraoccular foreign body, or after complicated extraocular removal.

QUICK REVIEW QUESTION

1. A patient in a small community hospital is diagnosed with a retained foreign body to the left lens with vitreous leakage present. The patient will require transfer to a larger hospital for emergent ophthalmology consult. How will the nurse prepare this patient for transport?

Glaucoma

Pathophysiology

Glaucoma is a group of eye diseases that cause an increase in intraocular pressure and compression of the optic nerve. These include:

- primary open-angle glaucoma
- normal tension (low-pressure) glaucoma
- secondary glaucoma related to diabetes or cataracts
- angle-closure glaucoma

The compression causes degeneration of the optic nerve fibers and apoptosis of the retinal ganglion cells, resulting in permanent vision loss. Most glaucomas are chronic in nature and develop slowly and painlessly over time. The emergency nurse should be familiar with the visual impact of these chronic glaucomas as the patient may have a deficit of peripheral vision that can impact communication methods.

Acute angle-closure glaucoma is a medical emergency that occurs when the intraocular pressure increases rapidly to 30 mm Hg or higher (normal pressure is 8 – 21 mm Hg). Permanent vision loss from compression of the optic nerve can occur in as little as a few hours if not rapidly treated. Additionally, scarring of the trabecular meshwork can lead to chronic forms of glaucoma, and cataracts can develop as latent complications. Acute onset commonly occurs in conjunction with pupil dilation, such as when transitioning from light to dark environments.

The following information is for acute angle-closure glaucoma.

Risk Factors

- family history
- being of Asian descent
- more common in women
- age > 60

- hyperopic vision
- shallow anterior chamber
- thickened lens

Signs and Symptoms

- abrupt onset of pain
- visual changes
  - described as blurry, cloudy, or halos of light
- headache
- nausea and vomiting
- erythema

Diagnostic Tests and Findings

- corneal edema with clouding
- fixed pupil, mid-dilated (5 – 6 mm)
- Tono-Pen (increased intraocular pressure)
- fundoscopic exam (pale, cupped optic disc)
- slit lamp exam (shallow anterior chamber)

Treatment and Management

- topical miotic ophthalmic drops to constrict pupil (pilocarpine)
- topical beta blockers
- topical alpha-adrenergic agents (clonidine)
- IV administration of acetazolamide
- IV administration of mannitol
- immediate ophthalmology referral and consult

QUICK REVIEW QUESTION

2. Two patients arrive at the ED separately complaining of acute onset of eye pain. The first patient, a 35-year-old Asian male, describes pain to his left eye as burning, with onset occurring while he was outside in his yard. Clear tearing and erythema are present. The second patient is a 65-year-old Caucasian female who describes her pain as deep and sharp with onset occurring as she was exiting the matinee show at the local movie theater. Which patient does the nurse recognize as needing emergent medical evaluation?

Infections

CONJUNCTIVITIS

Pathophysiology

Conjunctivitis is the inflammation of the thin connective tissue that covers the outer surface of the sclera (bulbar conjunctiva) and lines the inner layers of the eyelids (palpebral conjunctiva). Conjunctivitis is one of the most common nontraumatic eye complaints, and is commonly referred to as pink eye. Noninfectious conjunctivitis can result from environmental allergies or chemical irritants. Infectious conjunctivitis results from bacterial or viral causes and is highly contagious.

Risk Factors

- contact with infected individual or surface areas
- young age
- attendance at daycare, school, camps
- environmental allergies
- contact lens use

Signs and Symptoms

+ burning or itching sensation
+ increased lacrimation
    ◇ clear if noninfectious
    ◇ thick or yellow if bacterial or viral
+ erythema of sclera and inner eyelids

+ edema of palpebra
    ◇ periorbital edema if severe
+ sensation of foreign body or grit
+ typically no decrease in visual acuity

Diagnostic Tests and Findings

+ based solely on physical exam findings and history

Treatment and Management

+ warm or cool compress for comfort
+ topical antibiotics (if bacterial cause is suspected)
+ topical steroid if severe periorbital edema is present
+ ophthalmic lubricating solution

+ discharge teaching:
    ◇ Do not wear contact lenses until infection has resolved.
    ◇ Do not touch any surface area after touching eyes.
    ◇ Do not share makeup or facecloths.
    ◇ Wash hands frequently.

> ### QUICK REVIEW QUESTION
>
> **3.** Parents bring their 4-year-old and 13-month-old children to the ED for evaluation of their eyes. The parents state that a few days ago the older child returned from daycare with signs and symptoms consistent with conjunctivitis. Now the younger sibling has the same signs and symptoms but does not go to daycare. What would the nurse tell the parents about infectious eye conditions and how the sibling can avoid further spread of the infection?

UVEITIS AND IRITIS

Pathophysiology

Uveitis is the inflammation of any of the structures in the uvea. Inflammation can occur in:

+ the iris (iritis or anterior uveitis)
+ the ciliary body (intermediate uveitis)
+ the choroid (choroiditis or posterior uveitis)

Panuveitis describes inflammation that occurs throughout all three structures. Uveitis may occur unilaterally (most common acute cause is infectious) or bilaterally (most commonly related to autoimmune conditions).

There are two types of uveitis: granulomatous and non-granulomatous. **Non-granulomatous iritis** is the most common type of uveitis seen in the ED. Acute iritis may take several weeks to resolve. If left untreated it may result in chronic uveitis, which can lead to secondary formation of cataracts, glaucoma, macular edema, and permanent vision loss.

Risk Factors

+ typically occurs in adults ages 20 – 50
+ genetic alteration of gene HLA-B27
+ trauma
+ Lyme disease
+ toxoplasmosis
+ herpes simplex virus
+ varicella zoster virus
+ cytomegalovirus
+ tuberculosis
+ syphilis
+ HIV/AIDS
+ sarcoiditis
+ rheumatoid arthritis
+ ankylosing spondylitis
+ systemic lupus erythematosus
+ Behcet's disease
+ smoking

Signs and Symptoms

+ pain described as global aching or tenderness
+ cilliary spasm
+ conjunctival erythema
+ photophobia
+ vision changes
+ vitreous floaters
+ keratitis

Diagnostic Tests and Findings

+ based on physical findings and medical history
+ slit lamp exam (inflammation in anterior chamber)
+ Tono-Pen (increased intraocular pressure)
+ small, irregularly shaped pupil
+ accumulation of white blood cells behind the cornea
+ outpatient laboratory testing to identify specific cause of disease

Treatment and Management

+ topical mydriatic ophthalmic drops to dilate the pupil
+ topical corticosteroids
+ referral to ophthalmology within 24 hours

QUICK REVIEW QUESTION

4. A 35-year-old female with a known history of HIV is diagnosed in the ED with iritis following an acute onset of erythema, tenderness, and photophobia. Clinically, the left pupil is small and irregular in shape. The patient asks the nurse when her eye will "return to normal." What patient education should the nurse anticipate delivering?

Ocular Burns

Pathophysiology

Ocular burns are classified as chemical (subdivided as alkali- or acid-based) or radiant energy (thermal or ultraviolet). Chemical burns occur through transference of the chemical substance to the eye by way of splash, spray, or direct touch. Alkali burns penetrate deep into the eye, causing liquefactive necrosis, while acidic burns cause a coagulated necrosis closer to the surface of the injury. Radiant energy burns occur from exposure to intense heat, explosions, hot cooking oils, electrical arc, lasers, and direct gaze into ultraviolet light.

Ocular burns commonly involve multiple structures, including the palpebra, conjunctiva, sclera, corneal layers, anterior chamber, and retina. The outcome varies based on the agent of exposure, time length of exposure, and ocular structures involved, but usually involves some degree of vision loss. Ocular burns tend to occur bilaterally and often in combination with other injuries such as dermal burns, penetrating objects, and compromised airways.

Risk Factors

+ common in males ages 18 – 64 (industrial/ employment related)
+ common in pediatrics ages < 3 (accidental exposure in the home environment)
+ chemical exposure (industrial, household cleaners)
+ failure to use protective eyewear
+ occupation (laboratory, mechanic, welding)
+ fireworks
+ e-cigarette use
+ direct visualization of the sun, eclipse

Signs and Symptoms

+ extreme pain or burning sensation
+ erythema
+ inflammation
+ periorbital edema
+ copious lacrimation
+ photosensitivity
+ blepharospasm
+ decrease in visual acuity
+ penetrating injury may be present

Diagnostic Tests and Findings

+ conjunctival hyperemia
+ subconjunctival hemorrhage
+ chemosis
+ corneal opacification
+ inflammatory reaction of the anterior chamber
+ ocular hypertonia
+ fluorescein staining
+ slit lamp exam to identify the degree of injury
+ Tono-Pen (secondary acute angle-closure glaucoma)

Treatment and Management

+ Stabilize airway if compromised.
+ Assess for concurrent injury such as dermal burns or penetrating objects.

+ Irrigate for minimum of 30 minutes with isotonic solution.
  ⋄ Assess pH level after irrigation; if > 7.4, continue with additional irrigation.
  ⋄ Severe burns may require up to 10 L of isotonic solution.
  ⋄ Topical anesthetics (caines) may be added to irrigant solution.
  ⋄ Consider use of Morgan Lens to assist with irrigation.
  ⋄ Only defer irrigation if globe rupture is suspected.
+ Apply topical corticosteroids.
+ Apply topical antibiotics.
+ Apply topical cycloplegics.
+ Consider applying an occlusive dressing.
+ Obtain copy of chemical safety data sheet if applicable.
+ Consider consultation with regional poison control center.
+ Refer to ophthalmology.

Ocular Trauma

CORNEAL ABRASION

Pathophysiology

The cornea is the transparent outer covering of the anterior eye. A **corneal abrasion** is a scratch or abrasive friction on the outer surface of the epithelium (the cornea's outer layer). Symptoms, severity, and outcome are variable based on the layers of the cornea involved and the size of the area affected. Corneal abrasions typically heal within 24 – 72 hours without complications, but in some cases may progress to infection, keratitis, or ulceration.

Risk Factors

+ occupational (wood, metal debris)
+ non-use of safety glasses
+ external trauma
+ dry eye
+ trichiasis
+ presence of a foreign body
+ environmental (wind, sand, insects, vegetative materials)
+ self-injury (poke in the eye with a fingernail or makeup applicator)
+ after surgery/anesthesia or unconsciousness (complaint of painful sensation in eye[s] within 1 – 3 hours of awakened state)
+ lagophthalmos
+ facial palsy
+ diabetes
+ contact lens use

Signs and Symptoms

+ painful pressure or burning sensation
+ increased lacrimation that is clear upon initial injury
+ discharge possibly thick or yellow if infection is present
+ erythema
+ inflammation
+ edema of palpebra
+ blepharospasm

+ photosensitivity
+ sensation of foreign body or grit
+ headache
+ decrease in visual acuity
  ⋄ may be described as blurred, dull, or foggy such as with looking out a dirty or scratched window
  ⋄ varies based on extent of affected area and layers involved

Diagnostic Tests and Findings

+ fluorescein staining
  ⋄ Abrasion will appear yellow in normal light.
  ⋄ Abrasion will appear green in cobalt blue light.
+ slit lamp or Woods lamp exam to identify the degree of injury or illness

+ eversion of upper eyelid to assess for presence of foreign bodies
+ decreased visual acuity (measured with Snellen chart)

Treatment and Management

+ Do not patch.
  ⋄ Patching was once considered a standard of care for corneal abrasions.
  ⋄ Patching decreases oxygen delivery to the cornea and increases risk of infection.
+ Irrigate to remove foreign body, if present.
+ Apply topical anesthetic (caines).
+ Apply topical antibiotics.

+ Apply topical NSAIDs.
  ⋄ Steroids containing ophthalmic solutions are not indicted for emergency use.
+ Administer ophthalmic lubricating solution.
+ Refer to ophthalmology if warranted.
+ Give discharge instructions:
  ⋄ Do not wear contact lenses until abrasion is healed.

QUICK REVIEW QUESTION

6. A patient arrives in the ED complaining of a burning sensation in both eyes with increased tearing. The patient states he had "day surgery" for oral tooth extraction about 8 hours ago and noticed the pain shortly after being discharged. The nurse identifies that the pain is bilateral, making the presence of a foreign body unlikely. What diagnostics should the nurse anticipate for this patient?

HYPHEMA

Pathophysiology

Hyphema is a collection of blood inside the anterior chamber between the cornea and iris. Blood accumulates as a result of a traumatic tear in the vascular structure of the iris or pupil, and it may rise to a level that fully occludes all vision.

Hyphema bleeding differs in appearance from bleeding that is seen with a subconjunctival hemorrhage. Hyphema is dependent; the blood rises in a horizontal fashion in front of the iris as it accumulates, similar to how water levels rise in a closed chamber. A **subconjunctival hemorrhage** is painless and occurs from rupture of localized surface vessels in the sclera. A subconjunctival hemorrhage is irregularly shaped, covers the white portion of the eye, and does not result in visual deficit or loss.

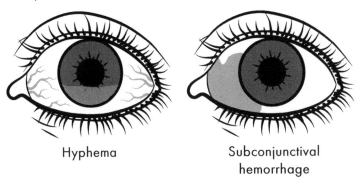

Hyphema

Subconjunctival hemorrhage

Figure 10.2. Hyphema versus Subconjunctival Hemorrhage

Risk Factors

+ blunt trauma injury
+ lacerating injury
+ post intraocular surgery
+ bleeding disorders (hemophilia, von Willebrand)
+ ocular neoplasms
+ inflammatory herpes simplex virus
+ retinal microvascular disease (often diabetes-induced)
+ varicella zoster virus
+ anticoagulant use
+ spontaneous
+ alcohol consumption

Signs and Symptoms

+ visible accumulation of blood
+ decreased visual acuity
+ pain
+ headache
+ photophobia

Diagnostic Tests and Findings

+ slit lamp or Woods lamp exam to identify the degree of injury or illness
+ Tono-Pen (increased intraocular pressure)
+ for severe bleeding, laboratory coagulation studies

Treatment and Management

- head of bed elevated ≥ 45 degrees
- bed rest
  - Increased activity will increase risk for bleeding.
- topical corticosteroids
- topical cycloplegics
- topical beta blockers
- topical alpha-adrenergic agents (clonidine)
- IV administration of acetazolamide
- IV administration of mannitol
- immediate ophthalmology referral and consult
- Discharge teaching:
  - Avoid alcohol.
  - Do not take anticoagulants.
  - Avoid strenuous activities.
  - Elevate head of bed.

QUICK REVIEW QUESTION

7. A patient is admitted to the ED with severe inflammation around the right eye. He stated he was hit with a baseball and complains of severe pain, pressure, sensitivity to light, and blurred vision. As the nurse's assessment progresses she notes blood filling the area over the iris under the cornea. What potential diagnosis will this patient receive and what treatment should the nurse anticipate?

LACERATION

Pathophysiology

Corneal lacerations extend into the deeper layers of the cornea and are more symptomatic and painful than corneal abrasions. Lacerations are considered partial thickness (closed globe) and do not penetrate the globe structure of the eye.

Lacerations involving other external structures of the eye such as the palpebra, sclera, lacrimal system, and conjunctiva may result in bleeding and require sutures for repair. These lacerations are always considered potential penetrating eye injuries until proven otherwise.

Risk Factors

- occupational (wood, metal debris, fragments)
- non-use of safety glasses
- external trauma
- environmental (wood splinters, tree branch)
- self-injury (poke in the eye with a fingernail or makeup applicator)
- motorized vehicle accidents (often involving glass)

Signs and Symptoms

- extreme pain or burning sensation
- copious lacrimation
- erythema
- inflammation
- edema (localized or periorbital)
- misshapen palpebra, conjunctiva, or external structures
- blepharospasm
- photosensitivity
- decrease in visual acuity

- bleeding if vascular structures are involved
- subconjunctival hemorrhage
- headache

Diagnostic Tests and Findings

- fluorescein staining
  - Laceration will appear yellow in normal light.
  - Laceration will appear green in cobalt blue light.
- slit lamp or Woods lamp exam to identify the degree of injury or illness
- decreased visual acuity (measured with Snellen chart)
- radiology/X-ray or CT scan if foreign body retention is suspected

Treatment and Management

- foreign body removal/irrigation
- eye shield for protection
  - Do not use pressure or absorbent dressings.
- topical anesthetic (caines)
- topical antibiotics
- topical NSAIDs
  - Steroids containing ophthalmic solutions are not indicted for emergency use.
- ophthalmic lubricating solution
- suture repair if warranted
  - Use injectable anesthetics for suture repair; epinephrine will aid in vasoconstriction.
- immunization status (tetanus)
- ophthalmology or occuloplastics referral if warranted
- discharge teaching:
  - Do not wear contact lenses until abrasion is healed.

QUICK REVIEW QUESTION

8. A patient with a closed globe injury is observed holding a facecloth over the affected eye "for comfort" but has removed the protective eye shield to do so. What complication of introducing external pressure to this eye does the nurse need to monitor for?

GLOBE RUPTURE

Pathophysiology

A **global rupture** (open globe) occurs from a full thickness laceration or tearing of the cornea and sclera. Rupture may occur as the result of blunt trauma, penetrating injury (entry wound without exit), or a perforating injury (entry and exit wounds present). Rupture can also occur post-trauma due to a rapid rise in intraocular pressure.

Risk Factors

- pediatrics (trip and fall with sharp objects in hand)
- males 18 – 64 (occupational hazards)
- age > 65 with history of ocular surgery (trip and fall)

Signs and Symptoms

+ eccentric or teardrop-shaped pupil
+ sunken eye appearance and loss of volume
+ gross deformity or misshapen eye
+ pain
+ subconjunctival hemorrhage
+ laceration or penetrating object

+ bleeding at site of injury
+ decreased visual acuity
+ edema
+ erythema
+ ecchymosis
+ decreased visual acuity

Diagnostic Tests and Findings

+ reactive afferent pupillary defect
+ external prolapse of the uvea (iris, ciliary body, or choroid)
+ iridodialysis
+ tenting of the sclera or cornea at the site of globe puncture
+ extrusion of vitreous

+ positive Seidel test (vitreous leakage)
+ slit lamp or Woods lamp exam to identify the degree of injury or illness
+ fluorescein strips
+ ultrasound, X-ray, or CT scan to assess for ocular hemorrhage, muscular or nerve damage, and fractures

Treatment and Management

+ Use an eye shield for protection.
    ✧ Do not use pressure or absorbent dressings.
+ Maintain bedrest.
+ Elevate head of bed 30 degrees.
+ Do NOT:
    ✧ remove foreign body or penetrating objects.
    ✧ measure intraocular pressure.
    ✧ irrigate.
+ Apply topical anesthetics.

+ Initiate NPO status (patient is immediate surgical candidate).
+ Administer IV analgesics and antiemetic medications.
+ Avoid Valsalva maneuvers.
+ Avoid eye manipulation or extraoccular movements.
+ Young children may require sedation.
+ Refer for immediate ophthalmology consult.

QUICK REVIEW QUESTION

9. A 22-year-old male patient arrives at the ED after sustaining injury to his left eye during a bar fight. The eye is edematous, there is visual prolapse of the uvea, and vitreous extrusion is present. The patient exhibits signs of pain and is unable to tolerate visual acuity testing at this time. What nursing interventions does the nurse anticipate?

Retinal Artery Occlusion

Pathophysiology

Retinal artery occlusion occurs when there is a blockage of vascular flow through the retinal arteries, resulting in a lack of oxygen delivery to the nerve cells in the retina. Blockage may occur from thrombi or emboli, and is sometimes referred to as an ocular stroke.

Risk Factors

+ carotid artery stenosis
+ coronary artery disease
+ atherosclerosis
+ artificial heart valves
+ A-fib
+ diabetes

+ hypertension
+ sickle cell disease
+ pregnancy
+ giant cell arteritis
+ use of oral contraceptives
+ IV substance abuse

Signs and Symptoms

+ unilateral, sudden, painless loss of vision

Diagnostic Tests and Findings

+ dilated fundoscopic exam
+ red fovea (cherry-red spot)
+ optic disc pallor and edema
+ relative afferent pupillary defect
+ fluorescein angiography

+ Tono-Pen (increased intraocular pressure)
+ additional diagnostics for thrombotic and embolic risk factors after confirmation of retinal artery occlusion

Treatment and Management

+ topical beta blockers
+ IV administration of acetazolamide
+ IV administration of mannitol

+ IV administration of methylprednisolone
+ ocular massage
+ referral to ophthalmology

QUICK REVIEW QUESTION

10. A patient is diagnosed with a central retinal artery occlusion of the right eye after experiencing a sudden loss of sight while outside gardening 60 minutes before arrival. The nurse obtains the following medication list from the patient: metformin 500 mg twice daily, chewable aspirin 81 mg daily, warfarin (Coumadin) 5 mg daily, diltiazem (Cardizem) 60 mg three times daily, cetirizine (Zyrtec) 10 mg daily, metoprolol (Lopressor) 25 mg twice daily, and pravastatin 40 mg daily. What risk factors can the nurse identify based upon the diagnosis and medication history?

Retinal Detachment

Pathophysiology

The retina is a thin tissue composed of nerve cells that lines the back wall of the ocular cavity. **Retinal detachment** occurs when the pigmented epithelial layer of the retina separates from the choroid layer (visualize how thin layers of an onion peel can separate from each other) either by tension, trauma, or fluid accumulation between the layers. Vision loss results from lack of available oxygen and deterioration of photoreceptor cells. Retinal detachments may be preceded by retinal tears or breaks and occur at any age.

Risk Factors

+ age > 65
+ family history of retinal detachment
+ history of retinal detachment of opposite eye
+ history of cataract surgery
+ traumatic injury
+ high myopia (nearsightedness)
+ diabetes mellitus
+ lattice degeneration (thinning in the peripheral retina)
+ Marfan syndrome
+ retinopathy of prematurity
+ uveitis inflammation
+ malignant hypertension
+ neovascular ("wet") macular degeneration

Signs and Symptoms

+ painless onset of visual changes
  ⋄ Loss of vision is not immediate (unlike retinal artery occlusions).
+ reduction in peripheral vision
+ curtain-like shadow over visual field
+ photopsia
+ sudden or gradual increase of multiple floaters
  ⋄ Floaters appear as wispy spider web-like formations that "float "across the visual field.
  ⋄ Floaters are more obvious when looking at white walls or areas covered in snow.

Diagnostic Tests and Findings:

+ visual acuity measured with Snellen chart to establish baseline
+ fundoscopic exam to assess for Schafer's sign, vitreous hemorrhage, and scleral depression
+ red reflex
+ mild relative afferent pupillary defect
+ bedside ultrasound

Treatment and Management

+ if traumatic cause, treat underlying injury
+ bedrest
+ quiet environment
+ immediate referral to ophthalmology
+ surgical treatment by ophthalmology/ retinal specialist

11. A 25-year-old female patient arrives at the ED with complaint of "a curtain" shading her peripheral vision and "hazy strings" floating across her visual field. Onset was yesterday but is becoming progressively worse. Medical history is nonsignificant except for tonsillectomy at age 8. The nurse conducts a visual acuity test and the patient states results are consistent with her baseline sight of 20/100 without glasses. Explain how this patient may be at risk for retinal detachment.

Ulcerative Keratitis

Pathophysiology

Ulcerative keratitis is characterized by crescent-shaped inflammation of the epithelial layer that progresses to necrosis of the corneal stroma. Ulcers may occur from infectious or noninfectious causes, and they form scar issue when healing. Without treatment, ulcers may infiltrate deeper structures of the eye, causing secondary uveitis, prolapse of the iris or cilliary body, hypopyon, and endophthalmitis/panophthalmitis.

Risk Factors

+ traumatic injury
+ diabetes mellitus
+ immunodeficiency
+ autoimmune disease (rheumatoid arthritis, Sjogren's syndrome)
+ varicella zoster virus
+ herpes simplex virus
+ syphilis
+ systemic side effects of medications such as amiodarone, flouroquinilones, antimetabolites/neoplastic agents, tamoxifen, NSAIDs, thorazine
  ✧ Damages may be irreversible.
+ side effects of topical medications
  ✧ Any ophthalmic solution may cause an allergic ulcerative keratitis.
+ use of contact lenses

Signs and Symptoms

+ painful pressure, severe pain, or burning sensation
+ increased lacrimation
+ erythema
+ inflammation
+ edema of the palpebra
+ white or cloudy spot on cornea
+ blepharospasm
+ photosensitivity
+ sensation of foreign body or grit
+ decrease in visual acuity
  ✧ may be described as blurred, dull, or foggy such as with looking out a dirty or scratched window
  ✧ varies based on extent of affected area and layers involved
+ headache

Diagnostic Tests and Findings

+ visual acuity (measured with Snellen chart)
+ slit lamp or Woods lamp exam to identify the degree of injury or illness
+ fluorescein strips
+ culture of ulcer

Treatment and Management

+ Do not patch.
  ◇ Patching was once considered a standard of care for corneal abrasions.
  ◇ Patching decreases oxygen delivery to the cornea and increases risk of infection.
+ Apply nonocclusive eye shield for protection.
+ Apply topical anesthetic (caines).
+ Apply topical antibiotics.
+ Apply topical NSAIDs.
  ◇ Steroids containing ophthalmic solutions are not indicted for emergency use.
+ Administer ophthalmic lubricating solution.
+ Refer to ophthalmology.
+ Give discharge instructions:
  ◇ Do not wear contact lenses until abrasion is healed.

QUICK REVIEW QUESTION

12. A patient was seen in the ED and diagnosed with a corneal abrasion. The patient returns 6 days later stating that pain has become significantly worse and that the front of his eye appears white in color, impacting his central vision. The patient admits to not completing the course of prescribed antibiotic ophthalmic drops and reinserting his contact lenses the following day. The contact lens remains in the affected eye as the patient was unable to remove it before returning to the ED. How would the nurse explain to the patient how the corneal abrasion progressed to ulcerative keratitis?

ANSWER KEY

1. Because the patient has an intraocular foreign body, patching the affected eye is appropriate pending exam by ophthalmology. Avoid use of Morgan Lens for irrigation. Apply topical anesthetics and topical NSAIDs for pain management. Apply topical antibiotics for infection prophylaxis.

2. The second patient, the 65-year-old female, has identified risk factors for acute angle-closure glaucoma and presents with an onset of pain that occurred when transitioning from a dark to a light environment. The first patient's symptoms are more consistent with a corneal abrasion or foreign body.

3. Bacterial conjunctivitis is highly contagious and commonly occurs in young children who attend daycare or school. Bacteria is transferred from the infected eye to the hands when touched, and easily contaminates all touched surfaces. When another individual touches the contaminated surface, then touches their eyes, the bacteria spreads, causing a new infection. The parents should be advised to have their children wash their hands frequently and avoid sharing items like facecloths until the infection has cleared.

4. Acute iritis can take several weeks to resolve. The patient will require use of topical steroids to decrease inflammation and mydriatic ophthalmic drops to prevent the onset of secondary glaucoma. The mydriatic drops will alter the appearance of the pupil, making it larger. Follow-up with ophthalmology is essential to monitor for secondary complications that can lead to permanent vision loss.

5. Assess pH level with litmus paper or pH indicator strips. (In a pinch, a urinalysis test strip may be used after cutting off test areas above the pH level.) Touch the paper or test strip to the conjunctival fornix. If results are > 7.4, additional irrigation is warranted.

6. Determine extent of injury with a slit lamp or Woods lamp exam and use fluorescein staining to assess for presence of corneal abrasions. The cause of the abrasion(s) for this patient is potentially related to use of general anesthesia during recent oral surgery. Anesthesia diminishes the corneal reflexes and decreases basal tear production.

7. Hyphema is a collection of blood inside the anterior space of the eye between the cornea and iris. There will be a resultant increase in intraocular pressure that must be monitored closely and treated if applicable. Bedrest, keeping the head of bed elevated ≥ 45 degrees, and avoiding use of anticoagulant medications and alcohol are standards of care.

8. This patient is at risk for developing an open globe rupture. External pressure can elicit an increase in intraocular pressure, causing strain at the weakest point of the sclera at the insertion point of the extraocular muscles. Eye shield protection is essential during the healing process of corneal lacerations.

9. This patient exhibits signs consistent with an open global rupture. The nurse should initiate NPO status and obtain intravenous access. Pain and nausea should be managed to avoid vagal stimulus. Eye shield may be placed to discourage eye manipulation or movements. Head of bed should be elevated to 30 degrees and bedrest status maintained.

10. This patient appears to have risk factors of diabetes, hypertension, hyperlipidemia, and possible A-fib or vascular disease. These conditions increase risks for development of thrombolytic and atheroembolisms, which can occlude the retinal, cerebral, coronary, or pulmonary arteries.

11. High myopia, or nearsightedness, is a risk factor for retinal detachment. High myopia occurs when the shape of the eye is elongated from front to back, causing tension and stretching of the retinal structure. The stretching can cause a hole or break in the retinal tissue, allowing fluid to enter between the layers, ultimately causing the retina to detach.

12. This patient's symptoms and history are consistent with an infectious corneal ulcer related to contact use. Contact lenses can transfer bacteria to the surface of the eye and essentially trap it under the contact for a prolonged period of time. The patient already had a breach in surface integrity from the preexisting abrasion.

ELEVEN: ORTHOPEDIC EMERGENCIES

Achilles Tendon Rupture

Pathophysiology

The **Achilles tendon** links the calf muscle to the heel bone. When this tendon is overstretched it may partially or completely tear, resulting in the inability to walk.

Risk Factors

+ male gender
+ aging causing a decrease in blood supply
+ rheumatoid arthritis
+ gout
+ obesity
+ crepitus when moving ankle
+ previous injury

+ corticosteroid injections
+ use of fluoroquinolone antibiotics
+ repeated physical activity or overuse
+ sports
+ failure to warm up before sports
+ worn-out shoes

Signs and Symptoms

+ pain
+ swelling
+ tenderness
+ stiffness before activity
+ decreased strength

+ hearing or feeling a pop on occurrence
+ unable to flex foot or push off on toes when walking
+ fever

Diagnostic Tests and Findings

+ gap felt on palpation of area of rupture
+ ultrasound

+ MRI

Treatment and Management:

+ Apply ice.
+ Administer analgesics (ibuprofen).
+ Rupture may require surgery.
+ Stabilize ankle flexed downward.
  - walking boot
  - cast
+ Suggest crutches.

Amputation

Pathophysiology

Amputation is the total or partial removal of an extremity, including arms, legs, fingers, and toes, either by surgery or trauma or due to illness.

Traumatic amputations may be complete or partial and can occur spontaneously in an uncontrolled (non-surgical) setting. Particular care needs to be taken to assess for concurrent injury such as fractures, crush injuries, wounds, and vascular compromise.

Surgical amputation is the controlled removal of a limb or limbs, usually to prevent the progression of a disease or infection (such as gangrene), to prevent pain, or to remove a malignancy. The above-knee amputation (AKA) and below-knee amputation (BKA) are the most common amputation surgeries.

Risk Factors

+ traumatic
  - motorized vehicle accidents
  - self-removal
  - severe trauma (e.g., snowblower, mechanical, industrial)
+ surgical
  - burns
  - cancer of bone and/or tissue
  - serious infection
  - neuroma
  - neoplasm
  - frostbite
  - sepsis with necrosis
  - peripheral arterial diseases or disorders
  - diabetes
  - birth deformities

Signs and Symptoms

+ traumatic amputation
  - intense pain
  - hemorrhage
  - anxiety
  - absent or weak distal pulses (if amputation is partial)
+ special consideration for all amputees
  - phantom nerve pain after amputation
+ surgical amputation indicated for:
  - non-healing or slow-healing wounds
  - gangrene
  - dry, smooth, shiny skin on affected limb
  - ineffective antibiotic treatment

Treatment and Management (traumatic amputation)

- ✦ ABCs are the priority.
- ✦ Preserve detached limb.
  - ✧ Gently replace attached tissue and maintain normal positioning.
- ✦ Administer IV fluids.
- ✦ Administer pain medication.
- ✦ Prepare for blood transfusion.
- ✦ Cover patient to prevent shock.
- ✦ Surgery may be required for reattachment or removal.

- ✦ Prevent further injury to wound.
  - ✧ Apply direct pressure for bleeding.
  - ✧ Cleanse area with sterile saline solution.
  - ✧ Cover with thick material.
- ✦ Monitor for:
  - ✧ cardiogenic shock
  - ✧ hypovolemic shock
  - ✧ septic shock
  - ✧ neurogenic shock

QUICK REVIEW QUESTION

2. A homeless patient arrives in the ED with a complaint of pain in the lower left extremity. The medical history includes untreated diabetes and an infected laceration on the affected leg from a month-old cut. On assessment, the lower leg is pale, cold, and covered in blisters oozing a foul-smelling fluid. What is the nurse's primary concern and what will come next for the patient?

Blast Injury

Pathophysiology

Blast injuries result from proximity to an explosion, and the severity of the injury will vary with the type and size of the explosion and its distance from the body. There are two types of blast injuries: primary and secondary.

Primary injuries are caused by the wave of increased pressure (the blast wave) created by the explosion. These injuries are usually internal, often in the ears, lungs, and gastrointestinal tract. **Blast lung injury (BLI)** is a primary injury seen after an explosion and is characterized by respiratory difficulties with no external signs of injury.

Secondary injuries are caused by debris set in motion by the explosion. These are usually penetrating wounds and skeletal fractures.

Risk Factors

- ✦ working with explosives
- ✦ working around volatile substances
- ✦ fireworks
- ✦ pressure cookers
- ✦ gas leaks
- ✦ acts of war or violence

Signs and Symptoms

- ✦ primary injuries
  - ✧ blast lung injuries (BLI) clinical triad:
    - ✦ apnea
    - ✦ hypotension
    - ✦ bradycardia

- ⋄ ruptured tympanic membrane
  - • possible predictor of BLI
- ⋄ air embolism
- ⋄ sensory damage
- ⋄ brain trauma
+ secondary injuries
  - ⋄ lacerations
  - ⋄ penetrating injuries
  - ⋄ crush injuries
- ⋄ evisceration
- ⋄ fractures
- ⋄ eye injuries
- ⋄ partial or total amputation
- ⋄ hemorrhage
- ⋄ hypovolemia
- ⋄ shock
- ⋄ burns

Diagnostic Tests and Findings

+ X-ray
+ CT scan
+ bedside ultrasound

+ CBC, chemistry panel, coagulation studies (PT, INR, aPTT)
  - ⋄ Results will vary based on type and severity of injury.

Treatment and Management

+ Treatment and management will vary based upon extent of injury. May include care of traumatic amputation, fractures, burns, or wounds.
+ ABCs are the priority.
+ Administer IV fluids.
+ Administer pain medication.
+ Prepare for blood transfusion.
+ Cover patient to prevent shock.
+ Preserve tissue from partial/complete amputations.

+ Prevent further injury to wound.
  - ⋄ Apply direct pressure for bleeding.
  - ⋄ Cleanse area with sterile saline solution.
  - ⋄ Cover with thick material.
+ Monitor for:
  - ⋄ cardiogenic shock
  - ⋄ hypovolemic shock
  - ⋄ septic shock
  - ⋄ neurogenic shock

QUICK REVIEW QUESTION

3. A patient arrives at the ED after an explosion at a fireworks factory. Witnesses stated the patient was placing a wick when the explosion occurred. Assessment findings include second- and third-degree burns to face, neck, bilateral hands, and arms. The patient's blood pressure is 90/76 mm Hg, HR is 42 bpm, and RR is 5 with episodes of apnea. Tympanic membranes are ruptured and a butterfly pattern is seen on X-ray. IV fluids and high-flow oxygen were started on arrival and labs are pending. What should the nurse prepare for next?

Compartment Syndrome

Pathophysiology

Compartment syndrome is the result of increased pressure within a muscle compartment, usually as a result of a fracture or crush injury. When the increased pressure in the closed compartment exceeds the pressure of perfusion, blood circulation is impaired, resulting in ischemia of the nerves and muscle tissue. Oxygen deficiency and the buildup of waste produce nerve irritation, resulting in pain and a decrease in sensation. With progression of ischemia, muscles become necrotic, which can lead to rhabdomyolysis, hyperkalemia, infection, amputation, and death if left untreated. Lower legs and arms are the most common areas; however, compartment syndrome can also occur in the abdomen.

Risk Factors

+ most commonly caused by extremity fractures
+ crush injuries
+ muscle tears or sprains
+ sepsis
+ casting or compression bandage
+ burns
+ snakebites

+ severe contusions
+ blood clots
+ prolonged periods of unconsciousness
+ after abdominal surgery
+ after repair of a vascular injury
+ anabolic steroid use
+ drug overdose (gluteal muscles)

Signs and Symptoms

+ the 6 P's
  ◇ pain
    + not proportional to extent of injury
    + does not respond to opioid medications
  ◇ paresthesia
  ◇ pallor
  ◇ paralysis
  ◇ pulselessness
  ◇ poikilothermia

+ increased pain with stretching affected muscles
+ decreased urine output
+ hypotension
+ tissue tight on palpation
+ edema
+ tight, shiny skin

Diagnostic Tests and Findings

+ compartment pressure within 20 to 30 mm Hg of the mean arterial pressure
+ radiology/X-ray
+ ultrasound

+ CT scan with or without contrast
+ MRI
+ CK if rhabdomyolysis is suspected

Treatment and Management

+ Administer analgesics.
+ Surgical consult ASAP.
+ Prepare for fasciotomy.

+ Administer continuous IV fluids.
+ Measure compartment pressure.
+ Monitor for hypovolemia after release.

- ✦ Monitor for hypotension after release.
- ✦ Maintain fluid volume status.
- ✦ Maintain urine output > 30 cc/hr.

QUICK REVIEW QUESTION

4. A patient with an existing Salter-Harris fracture of the right wrist arrives at the ED with acute onset of paresthesia and pain in the distal fingers. The patient states they had a new cast applied yesterday in the outpatient setting. The nurse observes pallor in the extremities and is unable to obtain a radial pulse. What immediate action should the nurse take?

Contusions

Pathophysiology

Contusions appear as ecchymosis and/or hematomas. They are caused by broken blood vessels and the accumulating blood, leakage, or hemorrhage into the soft tissue of the injured area. Most often these injuries are caused by blunt force or mechanical trauma such as a kick, blow, or fall, and occur internally without disrupting the outer skin integrity. Generally, symptoms start to resolve in days. However, serious complications can result from infection, blood clots, calcification, and development of cysts that may require surgery.

Risk Factors

- ✦ age > 65
- ✦ common in pediatrics (active play consistent with normal growth and development)
- ✦ bleeding disorders
- ✦ vitamin K deficiency
- ✦ low platelet count
- ✦ vascular defects
- ✦ falls
- ✦ use of anticoagulants
- ✦ sports injuries

Signs and Symptoms

- ✦ intact skin
- ✦ discoloration (blue, purple, ecchymotic)
- ✦ edema
- ✦ pain
- ✦ tenderness

Diagnostic Tests and Findings

- ✦ visual examination
- ✦ coagulation studies
- ✦ platelet count
- ✦ ultrasound or CT scan if clot is suspected

Treatment and Management

- ✦ Elevate severe contusions.
- ✦ Use heat for older injuries.
- ✦ Wrap with elastic bandage compress.
- ✦ Rest.
- ✦ Apply cold compress for new injuries at 10-minute intervals.

+ Follow up if:
  ⬧ lump on the bruised area
  ⬧ abnormal bleeding (urine, nose, or gums)
  ⬧ severe pain in the area
  ⬧ pain lasting longer than three days
  ⬧ large or frequent contusions

QUICK REVIEW QUESTION

5. A 10-year-old patient presents to the ED with several small contusions and one large contusion on the thigh following a bicycle wreck. The patient was wearing a helmet and denies hitting her head. What can the nurse implement to reduce the pain and swelling of the larger contusion?

Costochondritis

Pathophysiology

Costochondritis is the inflammation of the costal cartilage, which joins the ribs to the sternum. It usually affects the fourth, fifth, and sixth ribs. The inflammation causes the chest wall to be tender and painful upon palpation. There is no known definite cause, and the condition will generally resolve without treatment.

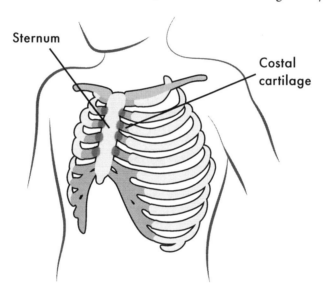

Figure 11.1. Costochondritis

Risk Factors

+ more common in women
+ ages 12 – 14
+ viral respiratory infections from coughing
+ fibromyalgia
+ ankylosing spondylitis
+ psoriatic arthritis
+ repeated minor trauma to chest
+ bacterial infection after chest surgery
+ IV drug use

Signs and Symptoms

- tenderness on palpation of rib joints
- sharp pain at chest wall
- exacerbation with exercise, minor injury, or URI
- radiation of pain from chest to abdomen and back

- rib pain increases with deep breathing and movement of the trunk
- can cause breathing problems
- may cause anxiety
- signs of postsurgical infection

Diagnostic Tests and Findings

- history

- physical exam

Treatment and Management

- rest
- application of heat or ice
- anti-inflammatories

- avoidance of sports and exercise
- steroid injection with local anesthetic if anti-inflammatory is ineffective

QUICK REVIEW QUESTION

6. What clinical findings would lead the nurse to suspect costochondritis in a 13-year-old girl with a complaint of chest pain?

Dislocations

Pathophysiology

Dislocations occur when the two bones of a joint are separated and it no longer functions as a single unit. Deformity of the joint will remain until it is realigned and put back in place. The most common joints dislocated include the shoulder and fingers. However, dislocations of the knees, hips, and elbows can occur.

Risk Factors

- tendency to fall
- MVA
- sports participation

- genetic disorders such as Ehlers-Danlos syndrome, Larsen syndrome, Weill-Marchesani syndrome, spondyloepiphyseal dysplasia, and congenital hip disorders

Signs and Symptoms

- joint noticeably deformed or displaced
- edema
- contusions

- extreme pain
- decreased or no ROM

Diagnostic Tests and Findings

+ physical exam
+ X-ray

+ MRI

Treatment and Management

+ Administer analgesics.
+ Treat based on site and severity.
+ Reduce or maneuver bones into position with anesthetic.
+ Immobilize joint with splint or sling.

+ Refer to physiotherapy.
+ Surgery if:
  ⋄ unable to reduce nerve, vascular, or ligament damage

QUICK REVIEW QUESTION

7. A woman over the age of 65 is admitted to the ED after falling from a ladder. She reports severe pain and tenderness in her right shoulder and is unable to move it. Following the physical exam, the nurse determines there is a dislocation. What signs and symptoms would the nurse likely have observed on assessment?

Fractures

Pathophysiology

A **fracture** is any break in a bone. Fractures can be open or closed. Open fractures include a break in the skin; with a closed fracture, the skin is intact. Open fractures create the potential for infection via bacteria entering through the open skin.

Further classifications of fractures are made based on the configuration of the fracture.

+ Non-displaced: Broken area of the bone remains in alignment; this is the optimal condition for reduction and healing.
+ Displaced: Broken areas of bone are not aligned. It may require manual or surgical reduction including hardware for fixation.
+ Transverse: A horizontal break in a straight line across the bone occurs from a force perpendicular to the break.
+ Oblique: A diagonal break occurs from a force higher or lower than the break.
+ Spiral: A torsion or twisting break around the circumference of the bone is common in sports injuries.
+ Comminuted: The break is fragmented into 3 or more pieces. This is more common in people older than 65 and those with brittle bones.
+ Compression: The break is crushed or compressed, creating a wide, flattened appearance. It frequently occurs with crush injuries.
+ Segmental: Two or more areas of the bone are fractured, creating a segmented area of "floating" bone.

+ Greenstick: In this type of incomplete break, the bone is not completely separated and bends to one side; it is common in children.

+ Avulsed: A "chip" fracture displaces small segments of bone from the main bone at the area of tendon/ligament attachment. It results from tension/pulling of the tendons/ligaments away from the bone.

+ Torus/buckle fracture: This is an incomplete fracture with bulging of the cortex, common in children.

+ Impacted: The ends of the bone are impacted or "jammed" into each other from forceful impact.

+ Salter-Harris: This is a growth plate fracture, classified as I – V.

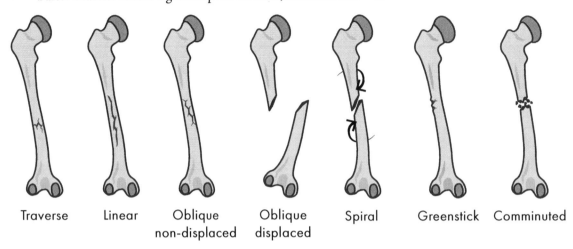

Traverse   Linear   Oblique non-displaced   Oblique displaced   Spiral   Greenstick   Comminuted

Figure 11.2. Types of Fractures

Risk Factors

+ age > 65
+ female (hip fracture)
+ comorbidities
  ◇ cancers
  ◇ osteoporosis
  ◇ cognitive or balance impairments
  ◇ cardiovascular disease (syncope and pre-syncope)
+ calcium and vitamin D deficiency
+ nutritional disorders (anorexia)
+ obesity
+ loss of muscle mass
+ decrease in bone density

+ vision loss
+ unsteady gait
+ decreased activity
+ trauma
+ MVA
+ falls
+ pharmacological use of corticosteroids and antihypertensive medications
+ childhood play activities
+ sports injuries
+ alcohol and drug abuse
+ tobacco use

Signs and Symptoms

+ pain increasing with movement

+ tenderness

- swelling
- visual or palpated deformity
- crepitus
- abnormal movement
- decreased ROM
- inability to bear weight

- contusions
- nausea and/or vomiting
- bleeding
- pallor
- dizziness

Diagnostic Tests and Findings

- history of injury occurrence
- physical exam
- X-ray for each injury as dictated

- CT scan
- MRI

Treatment and Management

- Administer analgesics.
- Cleanse open wounds.
- Monitor for hemorrhage and hypovolemic shock.
  - external or internal
  - estimated blood loss
    - pelvic fracture: 1.5 – 4.5 L
    - hip fracture: 1.5 – 2.5 L
    - femur fracture: 1 – 2 L
    - humerus fracture: 1 – 2 L
- Monitor for fat embolism syndrome.
  - comminuted fractures of the femur or tibia
  - fractures of the ribs or pelvis
- Reduce (manual or surgical as indicated).
- Immobilize (casting or splint as indicated).
  - Splints: non-circumferential, applied for acute care, and allow space for swelling while awaiting orthopedic consult
  - Casts: circumferential, more effective with immobilization, and more permanent
  - Hand/phalanges
    - thumb spica
    - finger splint
    - ulnar gutter
    - radial gutter
  - Forearm/wrist
    - volar
    - single sugar tong
  - Elbow/forearm
    - long arm posterior
    - double sugar tong
  - Knee
    - posterior knee
    - knee immobilizer
  - Tibula/fibula
    - bulky Jones
    - posterior ankle
  - Ankle
    - bulky Jones
    - posterior ankle
    - stirrup
    - walking boot
  - Foot
    - walking boot
    - posterior ankle with or without toe box
- Refer to physiotherapy.
- Refer to orthopedic.

8. A teenage male was admitted to the ED following a fall on outstretched hand (FOOSH) that occurred while skateboarding. The patient denied hitting his head and complains of nausea and pain increasing with movement. The physical assessment findings are tenderness, slight deformity, lateral and medial bruising, and progressive swelling to the affected (left) hand. Radial pulse is strong and palpable and capillary refill time is brisk. No pallor of the extremity is present. What should the nurse do next?

Inflammatory Conditions

Pathophysiology

Inflammatory conditions occur from the immune system attacking the body's own cells or tissues or from accumulation of chemical byproducts causing acute inflammation in the connective tissues. Inflammation causes a thickening of the synovial membrane and leads to irreversible damage to the joint capsule and cartilage from scarring. Both acute and chronic conditions result in pain, erythema, swelling, stiffness.

Common inflammatory conditions include:

+ rheumatoid arthritis
+ psoriatic arthritis
+ osteoarthritis
+ ankylosing spondylitis
+ scleroderma
+ gout
+ Sjogren's syndrome
+ systemic lupus erythematosus

Risk Factors

+ hereditary
+ past injury at site of inflammation
+ obesity
+ autoimmune disease
+ renal/liver failure related to decreased excretion (as with uric acid)

Signs and Symptoms

+ erythema
+ joint symptoms
  ⋄ pain
  ⋄ edema
  ⋄ stiffness
  ⋄ deformity
  ⋄ loss of function
+ weakness
+ fever
+ chills
+ headache
+ decrease in energy
+ decreased appetite
+ muscle pain and stiffness

Diagnostic Tests and Findings

+ history including joints involved
+ X-rays
+ ESR
+ CRP
+ CBC

Treatment and Management

+ Treatment is based on disease type, age, health, history, and severity of disease.

+ Treat underlying disease.

+ Administer topical or oral analgesics (NSAIDs).

+ Administer corticosteroids.

+ Patient should either rest or exercise, depending on the underlying disease and characteristics of symptoms.

+ Patient may require assistive devices.

+ Refer to physiotherapy.

QUICK REVIEW QUESTION

9. A 75-year-old woman arrives at the ED complaining of severe pain in both hands. She has limited income and has not sought prior treatment. She states the pain has increased recently, she is progressively losing function of her hands, and her knees have recently started hurting as well. On assessment the nurse finds the joints in both hands to be reddened, swollen, and disfigured, and the patient's knees slightly swollen. What condition should the patient's symptoms lead the nurse to suspect?

Joint Effusion

Pathophysiology

Joint effusion, or a swollen joint, occurs when the normally small amount of fluid in the synovial compartment of a joint increases. The additional fluid can be the result of infection, inflammation (often from an autoimmune condition), or trauma.

Risk Factors

+ rheumatoid arthritis

+ psoriatic arthritis

+ osteoarthritis

+ ankylosing spondylitis

+ infectious arthritis

+ joint injuries

+ gout

Signs and Symptoms

+ deep, throbbing pain in joints

+ skin warm on palpation

+ stiffness in joints

+ decreased ROM

+ edema

+ erythema

Diagnostic Tests and Findings

+ history

+ arthrocentesis

+ joint fluid analysis

+ X-ray

+ MRI

+ blood tests (WBC, CRP, ESR, uric acid)

Treatment and Management

+ Administer analgesics.
+ Treat for inflammation.
  ⬦ NSAIDs
  ⬦ steroids
  ⬦ anti-inflammatory or steroid injections
+ Remove fluid.

+ Administer colchicine for gout.
+ Administer disease-modifying anti-rheumatic drugs (DMARDs).
+ Treat for infection.
  ⬦ antibiotics
  ⬦ surgery to drain infection

QUICK REVIEW QUESTION

10. A patient with a history of osteoarthritis comes to the ED with complaints of knee pain that is progressively getting worse. The X-ray results show joint effusion. What should the nurse expect to find on the physical assessment?

Low Back Pain

Pathophysiology

Low back pain can arise from any of the anatomical structures of the back, including vertebrae, intervertebral discs, spinal nerves, or any of the muscles, tendons, and ligaments found in the lower back. The pain can be classified as either radiating or non-radiating. Pathology of non-radiating lower back pain is typically unknown or idiopathic in nature, but the pathology of radiating lower back pain is usually more apparent.

Causes of lower back pain include:

+ sprains and strains: acute injuries to muscles, tendons, or ligaments, often from rapid lifting or twisting motions
+ disc hernia, rupture, or degeneration: intervertebral discs bulging, rupturing, or degenerating with age
+ cauda equina syndrome: a complication of a ruptured disc in which compression causes an onset of bowel, bladder, and sexual dysfunction that can become permanent if not quickly treated

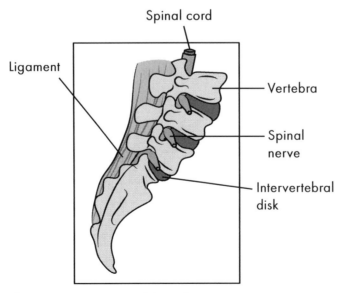

Figure 11.3. Anatomy of the Spine

- compression fractures: weakening and breaking of the vertebrae (often due to osteoporosis)
- radiculopathy: compression, inflammation, or injury of spinal nerve roots
- sciatica: compression of the sciatic nerve that produces radiating pain that travels the nerve path from the buttock through the posterior leg
- spondylolisthesis: occurs when a vertebra of the lower spine slips out of place, pinching a spinal nerve
- spinal stenosis: narrowing of the spinal column that can compress the spinal cord and spinal nerves
- infections: infection of the vertebrae (osteomyelitis), discs (discitis), or sacroiliac joints (sacroiliitis)
- tumors and cysts: rare cause of back pain, but may occur from metastasis of cancer from elsewhere in the body
- other conditions that present with lower back pain as a symptom:
  - kidney stones
  - abdominal aortic aneurysm
  - osteoporosis
  - endometriosis
  - fibromyalgia

Risk Factors

- age > 65
- occupational (heavy lifting, motion)
- sports injury (twisting motions)
- trauma
- falls
- MVA
- existing disease (osteoporosis, arthritis, infection, cancer)

Signs and Symptoms

- pain
  - localized or radiating
  - acute or chronic
  - described as shooting, dull, throbbing, etc.
  - exacerbated by movement of upper extremities, lower extremities, or torso
- paresthesia and weakness, varying in intensity from back through lower extremities
- if nerve root compressed
  - bowel and bladder incontinence
  - sexual dysfunction

Diagnostic Tests and Findings

- history
  - trigger activities
  - alleviating actions
- neurologic exam
- EMG
- CT scan
- MRI
- X-ray
- physical exam
  - spine alignment
  - ROM
  - tenderness
  - overlying skin irregularities
  - Lasègue's sign
  - Patrick's test
  - muscle strength

Treatment and Management

- Treatment is based on injury type and severity.
- Administer topical and oral analgesics.
- Administer corticosteroids.
- Administer muscle relaxers.
- Administer nerve block.
- Offer patient a lumbar support brace or pillow.

- Refer patient to:
  - physiotherapy
  - chiropractor
  - neurologist
- Educate patient:
  - no heavy lifting
  - massage and exercise as warranted

QUICK REVIEW QUESTION

11. A retired nurse is admitted to the emergency room with complaints of severe lower back pain. The patient states he has bulging disks; however, the pain has progressed over the past month and now pain has been radiating down his left leg since he lifted a heavy box at home. The nurse's assessment finds tenderness on the lower spine and the patient cannot straight-lift his legs. What is the most likely cause of the current condition?

Osteomyelitis

Pathophysiology

Osteomyelitis is an infection in the bone that can occur directly (after a traumatic bone injury) or indirectly (via the vascular system or other infected tissues). In children, osteomyelitis is most commonly found in the long bones of the upper and lower extremities, while in adults it is most common in the spine.

Risk Factors

- compound fractures
- deep puncture wounds
- necrotic wounds or ulcers
- uncontrolled diabetes
- pneumonia
- upper tibial osteotomy
- sickle cell disease

- peripheral artery disease
- after joint replacement
- orthopedic hardware
- central lines
- Foley catheter
- dialysis tubing
- IV substance abuse

Signs and Symptoms

- may be absent
- fever
- chills

- pain at site of infection
- lethargy in children
- presence of infection (warmth, exudate)

Diagnostic Tests and Findings

- CBC (elevated WBC and a left shift in neutrophils)
- culture and sensitivity
- surgery for bone biopsy
- probe (dull) through foot ulcer to vicinity of bone
- CT
- MRI

Treatment and Management

- Debride bone and tissue.
- Administer long course of IV antibiotics.
- Incise and drain.
- Re-vascularize affected area (bypass grafts).
- Tissue or bone graft may be necessary.
- Remove foreign objects (plates or screws).
- Administer hyperbaric oxygen therapy.
- Patient may require hospitalization.
- Surgery may be required.
- Amputation should be a last resort.
- Educate patient on wound care and nutrition.

QUICK REVIEW QUESTION

12. A noncompliant patient with diabetes who has peripheral neuropathy admits to the ED complaining of sudden severe pain on the plantar surface of their right foot. The patient is obese, lives alone, and admits to not doing foot checks. The nurse's assessment finds a temperature of 100.9°F (38.3°C), with vital signs otherwise stable. A foot ulcer is noted to be errythemic surrounding the perimeter of the wound and has a necrotic wound bed with foul-smelling purulent discharge. The nurse believes this patient has osteomyelitis. What is the best test to confirm this diagnosis?

Strains and Sprains

Pathophysiology

Both strains and sprains are very common injuries and share similar signs and symptoms. **Sprains** involve the tearing or stretching of ligaments, whereas **strains** involve the tearing or stretching of muscle or tendons. Acute strains are from pulling or stretching the muscle abruptly. Chronic strains occur from repeated movements of a muscle.

Risk Factors

- sprains
  - overextension with severe stress applied
  - knee affected by pivoting, usually involving sports
  - ankle affected by switching surfaces when walking or running
  - wrist affected by open-handed falls
  - thumb affected by overextension during sports
- acute strains
  - falling on icy surfaces
  - throwing objects when running or jumping
  - heavy lifting
  - awkward position when lifting

- chronic strains
  - racket sports
  - exercise
  - aerobics
  - gymnastics
  - golfing
- sprains and strains
  - lack of exercise
  - fatigue or exhaustion
  - inadequate or no warmup of muscles
  - poorly fitting footwear

Signs and Symptoms

- sprains
  - pain
  - edema
  - contusions
  - decreased ROM
  - hear or feel a pop on incident
- strains
  - pain
  - edema
  - spasms
  - decreased ability to move muscle

Diagnostic Tests and Findings

- ROM
- X-ray to rule out fracture
- MRI

Treatment and Management

- Treatment is based on type and severity of injury.
- Mild sprains or strains are typically treated at home.
- Apply ice immediately after injury.
- Apply compress to affected area.
- Elevate extremity.
- Administer analgesics for pain (ibuprofen, NSAIDs).
- Immobilize area if injury is severe.
- In some cases, surgery is necessary.
- Refer patient to physiotherapy if necessary.

QUICK REVIEW QUESTION

13. A patient arrives at the ED with a complaint of lower back pain occurring when shoveling 6 inches of snow. There is no prior history of back issues and the patient is 25 years old. The nurse determines it is most likely a strain. What brought the nurse to this conclusion?

ANSWER KEY

1. The nurse should ask the patient if they heard or felt a pop when the pain occurred. The nurse should also evaluate the patient's ability to flex the toes downward and assess for swelling, tenderness, and/or a gap on palpation.

2. The patient exhibits signs and symptoms of gangrene associated with the infected laceration, possible sepsis, and untreated diabetes. The nurse should begin preparing the patient for surgery for removal of the affected leg.

3. Patient is exhibiting symptoms of blast lung injury. Intubation will be essential and tracheotomy may be considered if airway damage and swelling prohibits advancement of ET tube.

4. Remove the cast ASAP, reassess circulation, sensation, movement, and neurovascular status. If compartment syndrome is suspected, prepare for emergent fasciotomy or surgical consult.

5. The nurse should administer an analgesic, elevate the extremity above heart level as possible, and apply ice packs at 10-minute intervals to decrease internal bleeding.

6. Chest pain with tenderness on palpation of the fourth, fifth, and sixth ribs is the classic sign of costochondritis. Myocardial chest pain is less common in young patients.

7. Signs and symptoms of dislocation would include reported severe pain, deformity, bruising, decreased or no ROM, and swelling.

8. The patient has signs and symptoms consistent with a left wrist fracture. X-rays will be required to assess the extent of injury and bone(s) involved. The nurse should anticipate administering analgesic medication and assisting with orthocasting or splinting of the hand until orthopedic referral can be arranged.

9. The nurse should suspect the patient has rheumatoid arthritis. The patient exhibits several physical findings relating to this disease: it is progressive, affects bilateral joints, and causes disfigurement.

10. Findings could include deep, throbbing pain; warm, reddened skin; stiffness; decreased ROM; and swelling.

11. A herniated disk or disks has applied pressure to the spinal nerves, causing shooting pain and the inability to raise her legs. The heavy lifting at home most likely caused the disk to herniate.

12. A bone biopsy is considered the gold standard for diagnosing. The patient will require a surgical procedure to obtain the bone specimen. In the interim, broad-spectrum IV antibiotics should be initiated.

13. The diagnosis is based on the patient's statement of activity when the injury occurred. Risks for strains include lifting heavy objects (snow) and awkward positioning (shoveling).

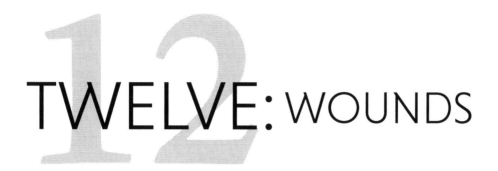

TWELVE: WOUNDS

General Wound Notes

+ Wound healing is impacted by underlying comorbidities and risk factors including:
    ⋄ diabetes
    ⋄ renal disease
    ⋄ immunosuppressive diseases
    ⋄ anemia
    ⋄ malnutrition
    ⋄ alcohol consumption
    ⋄ hypoxia to localized tissue
    ⋄ peripheral vascular disease
    ⋄ advanced age
    ⋄ pharmacological use of:
        + anticoagulants
        + corticosteroids
        + antineoplastics
        + colchicine
        + NSAIDs

+ Use the following tetanus guidelines for all open wounds.
    ⋄ Children ages 7 and under receive:
        + DT vaccine
        + DTaP vaccine
    ⋄ Children over 7 and adults receive:
        + Td vaccine
        + Tdap vaccine
    ⋄ Recommended adult immunization schedule:
        + 1 dose of Tdap if not previously received
        + Td booster every 10 years
        + 1 dose of Tdap during every pregnancy
    ⋄ Recommended childhood standard immunization schedule:
        + DTaP at 2 months, 4 months, 6 months, 15 months, and 4 – 6 years of age
        + Tdap at 11 – 12 years of age

Abrasions

Pathophysiology

First degree (or stage 1) abrasions are minor injuries resulting from superficial damage to the epidermis. Injury occurs from mechanical forces such as trauma, shearing, or friction that scrapes or rubs away the epidermal layers. Since the epidermis is avascular, bleeding does not occur, but moist serous drainage may be present.

Second degree (stage 2) abrasions extend into the upper dermal layers. Scant bleeding can occur and risk for infection and scarring increases with deeper tissue involvement. These are also known as partial-thickness wounds.

Risk Factors

+ advanced age (frail skin)
+ common in pediatrics (age-appropriate injuries from play)
+ falls onto rough surfaces
+ recreational sports (biking, skateboarding, running)
+ MVAs (road rash)
+ friction on fibers (rug burn)

Signs and Symptoms

+ noticeable breach in skin barrier
+ surface debris from area of injury (dirt, tar, grass, cloth fibers)
+ pain
+ inflammation
+ erythema
+ serous drainage or scant bleeding
+ most common surfaces:
  ⋄ elbows
  ⋄ knees
  ⋄ chin

Treatment and Management

+ Irrigate wound.
+ Cleanse area with saline solution or mild soap and water.
+ Apply topical antibiotic.
+ Apply topical anesthetic or ice.
+ Cover using:
  ⋄ clean, moist dressing
  ⋄ nonstick/non-adherent dressing
+ Stage 1 abrasions heal in 3 – 5 days.
+ Stage 2 abrasions may take up to 5 – 10 days.

> ### QUICK REVIEW QUESTION
>
> 1. A patient is treated in the ED following a bicycle accident. The patient has a large area of "road rash" along the right outer leg and across both palms. The wounds present with scant bleeding and serous drainage mixed with copious amounts of dirt and debris. Fractures and vascular injury have been ruled out, and full range of motion is intact. What should the nurse anticipate for wound care for this patient?

Abscess

Abscesses are soft skin and tissue injuries characterized as a localized collection of pus, exudate, and lymphocytes in the deep dermal layers of the skin. The most common cause is bacterial—*Staphylococcus aureus* or *Streptococcus pyogenes*.

Risk Factors

+ immunosuppression
+ diabetes mellitus
+ being a MRSA+ or staphylococcal carrier
+ IV drug use
+ poor hygiene
+ crowded living conditions

Signs and Symptoms

+ raised focal area of induration (hardened mass)
+ pustule "head"
+ erythema of overlying epidermis
+ warm to touch
+ tender/painful to touch
+ spongy/fluid-filled
+ nonmobile and non-firm to palpation

Diagnostic Tests and Findings

+ ultrasound
+ CBC with differential
+ wound culture

Treatment and Management

+ Incise and drain.
+ Perform needle aspiration.
+ Administer prescribed antibiotic therapy.
+ Wound may be packed for wicking effect.
+ Request surgical consult if:
  ◇ abscess overlies area of vascularization
  ◇ fistula is suspected
  ◇ affected area is on face, hands, or breasts

> QUICK REVIEW QUESTION
>
> 2. A patient diagnosed with an infectious abscess is being admitted for antibiotic therapy. What precautions should the nurse ensure are taken by clinicians?

Avulsions

Pathophysiology

An **avulsion** is a wound in which the skin is separated from the body by an external force tearing or pulling the tissue. Avulsions may occur in small localized areas or cover a vast area. These wounds are full thickness, involve injury to the deep tissue layers, and are irregularly shaped. The separated skin may or may not be attached. The skin edges do not approximate, and skin flaps and fragments can remain. Exposed ligaments, tendons, muscle fibers, and bone may be visible. Scarring is generally more prevalent with these types of wounds, and skin grafting or cosmetic repair may be necessary.

A **degloving injury** is an avulsion where the skin is completely separated from the underlying structures. (Visualize peeling off a glove or a sock: all skin is completely absent distal to the injury.)

Risk Factors

- advanced age (skin tears)
- falls
- industrial accidents
- MVAs
- traumatic injury
- animal bites

Signs and Symptoms

- noticeable breach in skin barrier and underlying structures
- severe pain
- bleeding (moderate to severe)
- edema
- inflammation
- burning sensation

Diagnostic Tests and Findings

- Assess circulation.
- Assess sensory and motor function.
- Assess peripheral and distal pulses.
- Assess for underlying fracture via radiology/X-ray.

Treatment and Management

- Control bleeding.
- Prepare local anesthetic (e.g. xylocaine [Lidocaine]).
  - Avoid using anesthetic containing epinephrine for avulsions of face, phalanges, or male genitalia.
- Apply topical anesthetic.
- Administer analgesics.
- Debride wound as necessary.
  - Irregularly shaped, detached tissue may be removed to aid in the healing process.
- Irrigate wound with saline solution.
  - Avoid application of soap, hydrogen peroxide, or alcohol directly on wound.
- Cover wound.
  - Apply an absorbent, non-adhering bandage or dressing.
  - Apply compression bandage if warranted.
- Provide ice to assist with vasoconstriction and pain relief.
- Administer antibiotics as prescribed (may require IV access).
- Elevate extremity.
- Provide crutches or sling as necessary.
- Arrange surgical consults or referrals.
  - Prepare patient for surgery if warranted.
- Verify immunization status.

3. Paramedics report that a patient arriving at the ED is stable and was involved in a motorcycle accident. He was thrown on impact and slid across a gravel road. A large flap of skin from the thigh to the knee is still attached, and the area was covered with compression dressings and a gauze wrap. Bleeding is currently controlled. What assessment(s) should the nurse prepare to do?

Crush Injuries

Pathophysiology

Crush injuries are caused by compressing or crushing forces damaging underlying vascular and musculoskeletal structures. External laceration and injury may or may not be present. Vascular leakage and increases in venous pressure can advance to compartment syndrome (discussed in detail in chapter 11). Neurovascular compression results in ischemia and decreased perfusion; no oxygen is present for aerobic metabolism, so compromised cells revert to anaerobic metabolism. The resulting increase in lactic acid leads to metabolic acidosis, reducing coagulopathy, and can advance to disseminated intravascular coagulation. Prolonged compression of muscle tissue rapidly releases myoglobin, potassium, uric acid, and phosphorus, resulting in rhabdomyolysis.

Risk Factors

+ common in pediatrics (slamming fingers in doors)
+ homelessness
+ industrial accidents
+ MVAs (especially with prolonged extraction)
+ prolonged pressure on affected side
  ⋄ passing out from substance and alcohol abuse
  ⋄ unattended injury such as CVA or fall
+ natural disasters; extraction from debris and building collapse

Signs and Symptoms

+ 6 P's
  ⋄ pain
  ⋄ paresthesia
  ⋄ pallor
  ⋄ paralysis
  ⋄ pulselessness
  ⋄ poikilothermia
+ inflammation/edema
+ decreased urine output
+ decreased circulation, sensation, and movement
+ dark, tea-colored urine
+ vasodilation
+ hypovolemic shock
+ tachycardia
+ hypotension

Diagnostic Tests and Findings

+ X-ray to rule out underlying fractures
+ CT scan
+ urinalysis to assess for presence of myoglobin/heme

- ♦ CPK
- ♦ chemistry panel to assess for hyperkalemia and hypocalcemia
- ♦ ABGs
- ♦ lactate
- ♦ platelets
- ♦ compartment pressure measurement

Treatment and Management

- ♦ Administer IV fluids.
- ♦ Monitor for cardiac arrhythmias.
- ♦ Administer oxygen.
- ♦ Do NOT elevate extremity.
- ♦ Prepare patient for fasciotomy if signs of compartment syndrome present.
- ♦ The reduction/fixation of fractures and laceration repair are secondary treatments in acute injuries where rhabdomyolysis and/or compartment syndrome are suspected.

QUICK REVIEW QUESTION

4. A nonverbal child sustained a crush injury to the second, third, and fourth fingers from a slamming car door. The mother tells the nurse that the child's hand feels cold and is pale. What should the nurse assess for?

Foreign Bodies

Pathophysiology

Wounds can contain foreign bodies that may not be visible to the naked eye. Depending on the mechanism and severity of the injury, the possibility of foreign bodies should be a consideration. The key indicator of a foreign body is inflammation triggered by the body's immune response to the invader(s). The timing of the reaction and the amount of inflammation depends on the composition of the foreign body. Smoother objects such as glass, metals, and plastics may not initiate an inflammatory response.

Risk Factors

- ♦ penetrating injury or punctures to the skin

Signs and Symptoms

- ♦ visually observed foreign body
- ♦ painful pressure sensation in or around affected area
- ♦ possible bleeding
- ♦ inflammation of wound
- ♦ pain with light palpation around object

Diagnostic Tests and Findings

- ♦ Avoid deep tissue palpation using fingers to eliminate risk of injury to clinician.
- ♦ Assess peripheral circulation.

- Assess for neurovascular status.

- Assess sensory and motor function.

- CBC results showing an elevation in total WBC and monocytes are consistent with inflammation.

- Depending on the type of object, various methods of imaging may be used to find foreign objects in deep tissue.
    - CT scan
    - X-ray
    - ultrasound

Treatment and Management

- Remove foreign object(s).

- Cleanse area thoroughly by irrigating with saline solution.

- Administer prophylactic antibiotics as necessary.

- Dress wound as applicable.

- Verify immunization status.

QUICK REVIEW QUESTION

5. The patient presents to the ED following a motor vehicle accident. Following the visual assessment, removal of debris, and dressing of the wounds, the patient complains of discomfort in her right palm. What action should the nurse take?

Injection Injuries

Pathophysiology

High-pressure equipment allows for various substances, such as paint, grease, fuel, and industrial chemicals, to be injected into the body through an almost unseen point of entry. The force of injury can range from 3,000 to 10,000 psi with a velocity of up to 400 mph. Although these injuries may seem small, they often result in amputation, tissue necrosis, compartment syndrome, multiple surgeries, contractures, and can eventually progress to acute renal failure, septic infection, and death. Delay in seeking treatment will result in higher acuity.

Risk Factors

- working with or around high-pressure equipment
    - careless use of high-pressure equipment
    - faulty equipment

- occupational fields such as roofing, painting, and mechanics

- fatigue or impairment due to substance abuse

Signs and Symptoms

- small puncture wound

- edema of involved extremity

+ ischemia

+ ecchymosis

+ localized edema

+ most common site of injury: index finger of the nondominant hand

Diagnostic Tests and Findings

+ Assess circulation and distal pulses.

+ Assess sensory and motor function.

+ Assess neurovascular status.

+ Order X-ray or CT scan (with or without contrast).

Treatment and Management

+ Request surgical consult and exploration ASAP.

+ Administer prophylactic antibiotics.

+ Measure girth to monitor for compartment syndrome.

+ Debride wound.

+ Irrigate wound.

+ Dress wound as applicable.

+ Verify immunization status.

QUICK REVIEW QUESTION

6. A patient returned to the ED a day after treatment for an injection injury to his left arm. He stated that the previous day he started experiencing deep aching, electrical-like pain, and numbness in his arm. On assessment the nurse notes edema, tight skin, and some ecchymosis. The nurse starts an IV, applies oxygen, administers pain medication, and maintains the arm lower than the heart. What is the nurse preparing for?

Lacerations

Pathophysiology

A **laceration** is a tear of the soft tissue inside or outside the body. External lacerations may be straight with approximated edges or irregularly shaped with jagged edges. They can be caused by broken glass or sharp-edged items. External lacerations that involve full thickness of the skin layers into the subcutaneous tissue are at high risk for infection due to bacteria or debris from the object causing the injury.

Internal lacerations occur from compression or movement of internal organs by internal and external forces. Friction, shear, or puncture from fractures of the ribs or pelvic structures can cause internal lacerations to the spleen and liver, resulting in hemorrhagic shock. Traumatic rape or use of foreign objects for sexual stimulation can result in both external and internal lacerations to the female genitalia, male genitalia, anus, and rectum.

Risk Factors

+ MVAs

+ industrial accidents

+ acts of violence

+ cooking injuries (typically knives)

+ falls:

  ◇ adults from heights > 15 feet

  ◇ pediatric from > 2 – 3 times body height

Signs and Symptoms

+ external
    + bleeding (moderate to severe)
    + pain (slight to moderate)
    + edges jagged or approximated
    + localized edema
    + may occur in conjunction with foreign body, avulsion, or abrasions
    + surface debris from object of injury

+ internal
    + hemorrhagic shock
    + hypotension
    + cardiac arrest
    + abdominal pain
    + abdominal guarding
    + rectal bleeding
    + vaginal bleeding
    + diffuse ecchymosis across lower abdomen and back
    + scrotal edema or ecchymosis

Diagnostic Tests and Findings

+ external
    + Conduct a visual exam.
    + Assess circulation and distal pulses.
    + Assess sensory and motor function.
    + Assess neurovascular status.
    + Rule out foreign body or underlying fracture with radiology/X-ray.

+ internal
    + Request a CT scan with or without contrast.
    + Conduct stool guaiac test.
    + Order CBC, chemistry panel, and coagulation studies (PT, INR, aPTT).
    + Perform a chest X-ray.
    + Perform a pelvic exam.

Treatment and Management

+ external
    + Control bleeding.
    + Irrigate with normal saline.
    + Prepare for closure with suturing, stapling, Dermabond adhesive, or Steri Strips as appropriate.
    + Dress wound as appropriate.
    + Apply topical anesthetic.
    + Ice to assist with vasoconstriction and pain relief.
    + Prepare local anesthetic such as xylocaine.
        + Avoid use of anesthetic containing epinephrine for lacerations of face, phalanges, or male genitalia.
    + Administer antibiotics as prescribed (may require IV access).
    + Administer analgesics.

+ internal
    + Request surgical consult ASAP.
    + Administer vasopressors.
    + Administer IV fluid bolus.
    + Begin ACLS protocol.
    + Administer prophylactic antibiotics.
    + Administer analgesics.
        + Avoid use of NSAIDs and aspirin.
    + Maintain NPO status.
    + Request SANE consult if appropriate.

7. A 2-year-old child is brought to the ED by her parents after tumbling down a flight of stairs at home. The patient is conscious, ambulating independently, and has full range of motion. Upon preparing for discharge the mother observes blood-tinged stool in the patient's diaper. What should the nurse suspect is the cause?

Missile Injuries

Pathophysiology

The severity of damage from a bullet (missile, projectile) injury is dependent on the type, trajectory, and velocity of the bullet and on the characteristics of the tissue or organs involved. Regardless of the area of entry, the bullet will crush any structure it passes through, and shearing, compression, and tearing of the tissues will occur. The soft tissue may collapse upon recoil, resulting in development of a cavity. Possible complications of missile injuries include peritonitis, hemodynamic shock, and amputation.

Signs and Symptoms

+ visually observable entry and/or exit wound(s)
+ unstable vital signs
+ bleeding (internal or external)
+ hematuria
+ rectal bleeding
+ evisceration

Diagnostic Tests and Findings

+ Conduct a primary survey for entry/exit wounds.
    ⟡ Remove all clothing.
+ Conduct a secondary survey to diagnose all injuries.
+ Assess extremity pulses, capillary refill time, and skin temperature and color.
+ Assess vascular system for trauma (hard/soft signs).
+ Perform neurologic and sensory exams.
+ Order CT angiogram with oral, rectal, and IV contrast.
+ Perform bedside ultrasound (eFAST exam).
+ Order X-ray.
+ Order MRI.

Treatment and Management

+ Follow trauma protocols.
+ Administer IV fluids.
+ Apply pressure/tourniquet to bleeding injuries.
+ Administer blood as warranted.
+ Administer analgesics.
+ Administer broad spectrum IV antibiotics with suspected peritonitis.
+ Request surgical consult.

Pilonidal Cyst

Pathophysiology

A **pilonidal cyst** is an inflammation of the hair follicles that run along the crease of the buttock from sacrum to anus. Pus, skin debris, and leukocytes collect, forming an abscess, most commonly present at the cleft of the buttocks near the tailbone. Emergency treatment is geared toward symptomatic relief; pilonidal cyst formation is chronic in nature.

Risk Factors

+ male gender, ages 30 – 45
+ occupation with prolonged sitting
+ prolonged sitting without ergonomic support (e.g., stadium seating, air travel, car rides)
+ obesity
+ coarse hair
+ large amount of body hair
+ hyperhidrosis

Signs and Symptoms

+ palpable abscess or "bump" at base of tailbone or upper cleft of buttocks
+ pain with palpation
+ inability to sit comfortably

Diagnostic Tests and Findings

+ ultrasound

Treatment and Management

+ Incise and drain.
+ Perform needle aspiration.
+ Administer prescribed antibiotic therapy.
+ Wound may be packed for wicking effect.
+ Request surgical consult for recurring events or excision of sinus tract.

Pressure Ulcers

Pathophysiology

Pressure ulcers (also known as pressure injuries, decubitus ulcers, or bedsores) are wounds occurring secondary to tissue ischemia. Unrelieved pressure is the most common cause, with the majority of wounds occurring over a bony prominence. Unrelieved pressure compromises the blood flow to the skin and underlying tissue, which deprives the tissue of oxygen and nutrients and also limits waste removal. Pressure ulcers are described as stage 1 through stage 4; they can also be labeled as a deep tissue injury or unstageable (criteria are given below).

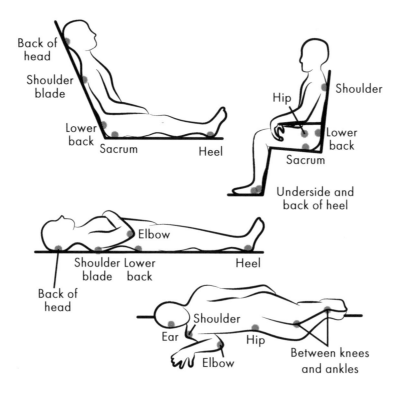

Figure 12.1. Common Sites of Pressure Ulcers

Risk Factors

+ advanced age
+ being nonambulatory, paraplegic, quadriplegic, or having decreased mobility
+ anemia
+ malnutrition or improper nutrition
+ incontinence of bowel or bladder
+ mental deficits
+ decreased subcutaneous fat layers
+ decreased sensation
+ dehydration

+ use of durable medical equipment, brace/support, or prosthetic
+ comorbidities:
  ✧ diabetes
  ✧ peripheral vascular disease
  ✧ peripheral artery disease
  ✧ hypoxia
  ✧ COPD
  ✧ spinal cord injury
  ✧ CVA
  ✧ failure to thrive

Signs and Symptoms

- stage 1: intact skin
  - area of localized erythema in patients with light-pigmented skin
  - area of localized blue, purple, or dark red hue in patients with dark-pigmented skin
  - non-blanchable
  - firm, boggy, or spongy compared to surrounding tissue
  - warmer or cooler than surrounding tissue
  - pain present as itching or burning sensation
- stage 2: partial-thickness tissue loss
  - dermis exposed, shallow open ulcer
  - pink wound bed without slough
  - intact blisters (serum or serosanguinous filled)
  - ruptured blisters
  - pain present as a deeper itching or burning sensation
- stage 3: full thickness; tissue loss up to, but not including the fascia
  - subcutaneous tissue exposed
  - slough
  - eschar
  - pain lessened as nerve damage occurs
  - bone, tendon, muscle not exposed
  - potential for undermining
  - potential for tunneling
- stage 4: full-thickness tissue loss extending through the fascia
  - visibly exposed bone, tendons, and muscle
  - slough
  - eschar
  - potential for undermining
  - potential for tunneling
  - pain may not be present because of complete damage to nerve endings and eschar tissue
- unstageable: unable to measure depth because of obscured view
  - full-thickness skin
  - tissue loss is covered with slough/eschar
- deep tissue injury (DTI)
  - intact or non-intact skin
  - non-blanching dark red, maroon, or purple discoloration
  - separated blister with dark wound bed
  - blood-filled blister
  - ecchymosis
  - may resolve without further injury

Diagnostic Tests and Findings

- angiogram/venography
- X-ray to rule out osteomyelitis
- wound culture
- HgbA1c

- protein level
- elevated ESR
- CBC, BUN, creatinine

Treatment and Management

- Treat per facility policy and stage of wound.
- Reduce pressure on affected area.
- Control pain.
- Monitor for signs of infection.
  - Administer antibiotics as warranted.
- Cleanse per wound consult instructions.
  - Use saline solution or commercial wound prep.
  - Saline solution should never be used if the patient is prescribed a sulfonamide topical agent.

- Do not remove eschar.
- Do not rupture blister.
- Do not remove top layer of blister if ruptured.
- Possibly refer to:
  - wound clinic
  - surgeon (for debridement)
  - physical therapy
  - dietitian

QUICK REVIEW QUESTION

10. An elderly patient is admitted to the ED from an extended care facility. On assessment the nurse finds a 10 × 10 cm full-thickness wound on the coccyx. Upon further assessment there is undermining and adipose tissue present; however, no bone or tendon is observed. What stage will the nurse assign to this wound?

Puncture Wounds

Pathophysiology

Puncture wounds are caused by an object entering through soft tissue, resulting in hemorrhage and damage to the skin and underlying tissues. The penetrating object also deposits organisms or foreign bodies into the deeper tissue, increasing the risk for infection. Unresolved infection may indicate a retained foreign body and requires further medical attention.

Puncture wounds commonly occur on extremities, in particular the plantar area of the foot. These wounds can be difficult to visualize and clean due to the size and depth of the injuries.

Risk Factors

- industrial work (high-pressure injection equipment)
- work with or exposure to needles

- animal bites

Signs and Symptoms

+ visually observed entry hole (usually small)
+ bleeding
+ decreased ROM
+ patient perception of debris

+ signs of infection
  ⋄ pain
  ⋄ erythema
  ⋄ warmth
  ⋄ edema
  ⋄ drainage

Diagnostic Tests and Findings

+ Check for elevated ESR and C-reactive protein.
+ Order radiology/X-ray or CT scan.
+ Perform visual exam.

+ Assess circulation and distal pulses.
+ Assess sensory and motor function.
+ Assess neurovascular status.

Treatment and Management

+ Administer analgesics.
+ Apply topical anesthetic.
+ Irrigate with saline solution.
+ Dress wound as warranted.

+ Administer prophylactic antibiotics.
+ Verify immunization status.
+ Order surgical consult if warranted.

QUICK REVIEW QUESTION

11. A patient arrived at the ED following a dog attack. There are several abrasions on her arms and hands and two puncture wounds on her foot. The patient states that when she tried to kick at the dog, it bit through her shoe and punctured the plantar surface of her foot. Should prophylactic antibiotics be administered to this patient? Why or why not?

Subungual Hematoma

Pathophysiology

In a **subungual hematoma**, vascular leakage of blood and serous fluid accumulates under the nail bed of the upper or lower phalanges. The hematoma results from trauma or compression to the affected nail bed and is transient in nature. Most subungual hematomas will resolve without medical intervention. Emergency treatment is appropriate for injuries where fracture is suspected, laceration is present, or there is severe pain.

Risk Factors

+ industrial/occupational
+ common in pediatrics (age-appropriate injuries from play)

+ dyspraxia

Signs and Symptoms

+ visible ecchymosis or frank bleeding under nail bed

+ pain pressure in affected phalanges

+ purulent drainage if infection is present

Diagnostic Tests and Findings

+ X-ray to rule out underlying fracture

Treatment and Management

+ trephination: boring of hole into the nail bed to relieve the underlying pressure
    + Choose preferred method of trephination: cautery, scalpel, or large-bore needle.
    + Immobilize patient during procedure.
    + Ice pre-procedure for anesthetic affect.
    + The goal is to bore through the nail only, and not into the underlying nail bed.
    + Pain relief is achieved immediately.

QUICK REVIEW QUESTION

12. A patient is being prepared for trephination of a subungual hematoma in the left second finger. What pain management should the nurse prepare to provide after the procedure?

ANSWER KEY

1. The nurse should identify that the patient has a mix of stage 1 and stage 2 abrasions. The nurse should prepare to irrigate with saline solution or assist the patient in cleansing with mild soap and water. The nurse will apply topical antibiotic ointment if ordered, and cover the wounds with nonstick or moist dressings. Ice can be applied over the dressing to assist with vasoconstriction and pain relief.

2. An infectious abscess requires contact precautions. Abscesses are most commonly caused by *Staphylococcus aureus*. Wound cultures to determine if the infectious agent is MRSA+ may take up to 48 hours, and care needs to be taken immediately to prevent the transmission of disease.

3. Because the patient is stable and bleeding is controlled, circulation would be priority, including distal pulses. The nurse should then assess the wound.

4. The nurse should assess for the 6 P's. Poikilothermia (coolness surrounding the injury) and pallor are both present. In a nonverbal child a Wong-Baker or FACES scale can be used to assess for pain. Paresthesia can be assessed by response to light and firm touch, and the radial peripheral pulses should be assessed for perfusion status.

5. The nurse should suggest the doctor order an X-ray. Foreign bodies are not always visible and may be located in the deeper tissue of the wound. An X-ray would confirm or rule out the possibility of debris in the deep tissue and decrease the risk for infection or complications.

6. The patient presented with signs and symptoms of compartment syndrome following an injection injury. The patient is being prepared for surgical intervention for decompression.

7. Lacerations to the internal organs can present latently, and the first observable signs may be rectal bleeding or diffuse ecchymosis. The nurse should elevate this patient's status to emergent and notify the medical provider immediately of the change in condition.

8. Start IV fluids and order a surgical consult and a CT angiogram with contrast. Rectal bleeding may indicate internal bleeding or hemorrhage.

9. The nurse should prepare the patient to have the pilonidal cyst incised and drained. The nurse will then need to pack the wound.

10. Stage III is defined as full-thickness skin and tissue loss no deeper than adipose tissue. Tunneling and undermining may or may not be present.

11. This is a high-risk patient, so antibiotics should be administered. When puncture wounds occur through a shoe, the existing bacteria from the sole will be introduced deep into the tissue of the foot, substantially increasing the risk of infection.

12. Once the pressure of the hematoma is released, pain relief is almost immediate. The patient may continue to place ice on the affected area but there is no need for prescribed pain medications.

THIRTEEN: 13 ENVIRONMENTAL EMERGENCIES

Burns

Pathophysiology

Burns are trauma to the skin or underlying tissue caused by heat, radiation, electricity, or chemical exposure. The heat causes protein denaturation of the cells that leads to coagulative necrosis, platelet aggregation, and vessel constriction. The damage leaves the dermis open to bacterial infections and fluid loss.

Burns are classified by depth as first degree, second degree, and third degree (described below). Burns are also described by the **total body surface area (TBSA)** involved. TBSA is calculated by assigning a numerical value to the areas that are burned; the rule of 9s is the most commonly used method.

Risk Factors

+ more common in people > 65
+ poverty
+ occupational exposure to fire or steam
+ children cooking
+ alcohol or drug use

Signs and Symptoms

+ first degree:
    ✧ affects only the dermis
    ✧ reddened area
    ✧ blanches easily with light pressure
    ✧ pain
    ✧ swelling

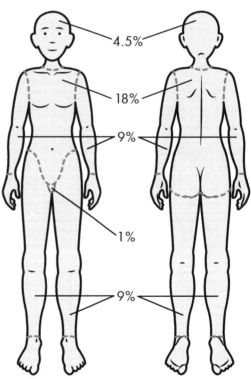

Figure 13.1. Rule of 9s for Calculating Total Body Surface Area (TBSA) of Burns

- second degree (superficial partial-thickness burns):
  - blanches with pressure
  - pain
  - swelling
  - development of vesicles or bullae in 24 hours
  - often appear wet
- second degree (deep partial-thickness burns):
  - color is white or red
  - does not blanch
  - development of vesicles or bullae
  - often appear dry
- third degree:
  - vary in appearance:
    - white
    - red
    - black and charred
    - brown and leathery
  - no pain or reduced pain (due to nerve damage)
  - no development of vesicles or bullae
  - hypovolemia
    - hypotension
    - whole-body edema
  - metabolic acidosis
  - rhabdomyolysis
  - hemolysis
  - acute kidney injury

Diagnostic Tests and Findings

- Assess wound.
  - Document location and depth on burn diagram.
- Check for indications of hypovolemia:
  - increased sodium
  - increased BUN
  - increased specific gravity
  - increased hematocrit
  - decreased potassium
  - increased osmolality
- Check for indications of kidney failure:
  - increased BUN
  - increased creatinine
- Draw CBC with differential to diagnose infections.

Treatment and Management

- Calculate TBSA.
  - for partial- and full-thickness burns
  - used to correct hypovolemia
- Administer IV fluids.
- Administer IV lactated Ringer's per Parkland formula:
  - 4 ml × TBSA (%) × body weight (kg)
  - Give 50% in first 8 hours; then 50% in next 16 hours.
  - Formula time starts at the time the burn happens.
  - Expected urine output is 0.5 ml/kg/hr in adults and 0.5 – 1.0 ml/kg/hr in children < 30 kg.
- Analgesics may be administered.
- Colloids, usually albumin, are administered 12 hours post-burn.

- Escharotomy may be needed for constricting areas of eschar.
  - Clean wounds and apply sterile dressing.
    - Dressings should be changed every day.
    - Use silver salve.
  - Surgery may be necessary for deeper burns that are not expected to heal within 2 weeks.
    - Remove eschar within 3 days.
    - Grafting may be necessary.
  - Administer antibiotics as needed for infection.
  - Watch for signs and symptoms of hypothermia.
  - Physical therapy will help prevent contraction and minimize scarring.

QUICK REVIEW QUESTION

1. A patient presents to the ED with second degree burns on their legs. The nurse establishes that the patient is breathing and has a pulse. What should the nurse prepare to do next?

Chemical Exposure

Pathophysiology

Chemical exposure can result from inhaling, eating or drinking, or otherwise coming in contact with chemical agents. The injury will depend on the how the patient was exposed, what chemical they were exposed to, and the length of time of the exposure.

In 2012 the hazard communication standard (HCS), which is overseen by OSHA, was revised and now requires all chemical manufacturers, distributers, and importers to provide safety data sheets (SDS), for all chemical agents. The SDS (formally known as material safety data sheets [MSDS]) for a chemical agent will include information on toxicology, first aid, and exposure control.

Risk Factors

- more common in infants and people > 65
- mental disabilities
- occupational exposure to chemicals
- alcohol or drug use

Signs and Symptoms

- ingestion:
  - burns, irritation, or redness around the mouth
  - breath that smells like chemicals
  - nausea and vomiting
  - abdominal pain
  - difficulty breathing
  - confusion or altered LOC
  - seizures
- inhalation:
  - burning sensation
  - increased secretions
  - coughing
  - wheezing
  - dyspnea
  - edema
  - laryngospasm
  - confusion or altered LOC

+ contact:
  ✧ erythema
  ✧ burning or itching
  ✧ visible burns
  ✧ edema of the area
  ✧ blisters
  ✧ hives
  ✧ skin that is darkened in color or looks leathery
  ✧ pain or numbness of skin

Diagnostic Tests and Findings

+ ingestion:
  ✧ EGD may show damage.
+ inhalation:
  ✧ EGD may show damage.
  ✧ Chest X-ray may show infiltrates, bronchiolar thickening, and a patchy mosaic of hyperinflation, pneumonia, or pulmonary fibrosis.
  ✧ Spirometry will show decreased lung capacity.
  ✧ Pulse oximetry may show decreased oxygen saturation.
+ contact:
  ✧ Diagnosis is based on signs and symptoms.

Treatment and Management

+ Consult poison control.
+ Consult SDS for specific chemical agents.
+ For ingestion:
  ✧ Monitor airway and establish if compromised.
    • Avoid nasotracheal intubation.
    • Be prepared for a cricothyrotomy or percutaneous needle cricothyrotomy.
  ✧ Administer activated charcoal or antidote.
  ✧ Perform EGD to determine level of damage.
  ✧ Surgery may be needed for perforation.
  ✧ Do not administer emetics or gastric lavage.
+ For inhalation:
  ✧ Monitor airway and establish if compromised.
    • Avoid nasotracheal intubation.
    • Be prepared for a cricothyrotomy or percutaneous needle cricothyrotomy.
  ✧ Perform EGD to determine level of damage.
  ✧ Monitor for ARDS.
  ✧ Administer oxygen.
  ✧ Administer bronchodilators.
  ✧ Perform chest X-ray.
  ✧ Administer spirometry test.

- For contact:
  - Decontaminate the affected areas.
    - Remove patient's clothing if necessary.
    - Rinse skin with water for 15 – 20 minutes.
  - Treat wounds.
  - Administer IV fluids for exposure that produces burns.
  - Manage pain.
  - Administer antibiotics if needed to prevent infection.

QUICK REVIEW QUESTION
2. Why is inducing vomiting or gastric lavage contraindicated when a patient has swallowed a chemical?

Electrical Injuries

Pathophysiology

Generated electrical energy causes external and internal injury from the electrical current running through the body. Injuries will vary depending on the intensity of the current, voltage, resistance, the length of time exposed, entry and exit locations, and the tissue and organs affected by the electrical current. Generated electrical injury can result in skin burns, damage to internal organs or tissue, respiratory arrest, or cardiac arrhythmias/arrest.

Risk Factors

- exposure to generated electrical energy
  - common in utility workers

Signs and Symptoms

- skin:
  - burns with a clean line of demarcation
  - burns at the entry and exit points
  - subcutaneous or deeper tissue injury possibly greater than the areas indicated by the line of demarcation
- muscular system:
  - pain
  - involuntary contractions
  - injury/trauma possible secondary to involuntary contractions (such as falls)
  - rhabdomyolysis in severe cases
- respiratory:
  - difficulty breathing
  - arrest

- nervous system:
  - seizures
  - confusion or loss of consciousness
  - paralysis
- cardiac:
  - A-fib
  - asystole
- compartment syndrome in severe cases:
  - massive edema
  - hypovolemia
  - hypotension

Diagnostic Tests and Findings

+ history of being exposed to generated electrical energy
+ ECG showing arrhythmias; most severe include:
    ⬦ asystole
    ⬦ V-tach
    ⬦ V-fib
    ⬦ increased PVCs
+ cardiac enzymes positive for tissue damage if cardiac involvement

Treatment and Management

+ Assess the unresponsive patient to see if CPR needs to be initiated.
+ Following resuscitation, do a head-to-toe assessment for injuries secondary to falls.
+ Administer IV fluids.
    ⬦ Standard burn fluid-resuscitation protocols are not used as there is usually more damage than is seen on surface burns.
    ⬦ IV fluid treatment goal is to maintain urine output of 75 – 100 ml/hr.
+ Surgical debridement of wound areas.
+ Treat pain with IV opioids.
+ Head CT or MRI for patients with impaired cognitive function.
+ Monitor cardiac function.
+ Monitor kidney function.

> ### QUICK REVIEW QUESTION
>
> **3.** A conscious patient comes into the ED and states that he touched a live electrical wire. He has a small injury on his left hand and a small exit injury on the bottom of his left foot, but reports he feels no other symptoms. Why would the nurse proceed with a full electrical injury workup?

Envenomation Emergencies

SNAKEBITE

Signs and Symptoms

+ increased permeability of capillary membranes (local and systemic)
+ clinically significant thrombocytopenia
+ nausea and vomiting
+ diarrhea
+ shortness of breath
+ paresthesia
+ anaphylaxis
+ shock

Treatment and Management

+ Loosely wrap and immobilize bitten extremity at or above heart level.
+ Measure the affected area.
+ Secure airway.

- Administer oxygen.
- Draw labs and collect urine.
- Administer antivenom.

- Blood product should not be administered before antivenom.

SPIDER BITE

Signs and Symptoms

- Brown spider bites:
    - delayed pain
    - ecchymosis
    - erythema
    - bleb formation
- Widow spider bites:
    - immediate pain
    - muscle cramping and weakness
    - diaphoresis
    - hypertension
    - tachycardia

- Venom:
    - neurotoxic
    - necrotizing

Treatment and Management

- Treatment of venomous bites is local wound care and treatment of local symptoms.
- Brown spider bites may require surgical excision.
    - typically delayed to allow the completion of necrosis
- Widow spider bites sometimes require pain treatment and administration of an antivenom.
- Tetanus prophylaxis may be given.

SCORPION STING

Signs and Symptoms

- immediate pain
- possible numbness or stinging
- no edema
- significant symptoms in children:
    - muscle spasms or irregular movements
    - restlessness or anxiety
    - diaphoresis

- significant symptoms in adults:
    - tachycardia
    - hypertension
    - increased respiration
    - muscle spasms
    - weakness
- respiratory issues rare in both children and adults

Treatment and Management

- Provide supportive treatment.

- NPO for 8 – 12 hours after bite.

- Encourage the patient to rest.
- Administer benzodiazepines if muscle spasms are present.
- Administer IV drugs for hypertension or pain.

- Only administer antivenom to patients with severe symptoms who are not responding to supportive care.
- Tetanus prophylaxis may be given.

BEE, WASP, HORNET, AND FIRE ANT STINGS

Signs and Symptoms

- Bee, wasp, and hornet stings have a local reaction that is characterized by immediate pain, burning, and itching.
  - The affected area will have erythema and edema and possibly local cellulitis.
- Ant stings have a local reaction that is characterized by immediate pain and a flare or wheal lesion that usually resolves in about 45 minutes, giving way to a pustule.
  - Systemic reactions may occur in those with allergic reactions to the venom:
    - angioedema
    - bronchospasms
    - urticaria
    - possible refractory hypotension
    - anaphylaxis

Treatment and Management

- Remove stinger if still in place.
- Offer ice, antihistamines, or NSAIDs to reduce pain, burning, and itching.
- Assess airways for signs of an allergic reaction.
  - Allergic reactions can be treated with IV antihistamines.
  - Anaphylaxis is treated with parenteral epinephrine and IV fluids.
  - Vasopressors may be needed.

QUICK REVIEW QUESTION

4. Why is compression of the area of most bites contraindicated?

Food Poisoning

Pathophysiology

Food poisoning is an acute infection in the GI system cause by the ingestion of infectious organisms or noninfectious substances. The organism or substance enters through the mouth and produces a toxin or irritant that causes mild to severe acute gastroenteritis in the small intestine.

The CDC identifies *Norovirus, Salmonella, Clostridium perfringens, Campylobacter,* and *Staphylococcus aureus* as the top five infectious foodborne agents. Other infectious agents that can lead to life-threatening illness include *Clostridium botulinum, Listeria, Escherichia coli,* and *Vibrio.*

Risk Factors

+ increased risk of severe/life threatening symptoms:
  - children ≤ 5
  - adults > 65
  - immunocompromised people
  - pregnant people

+ eating contaminated meat not stored and/or cooked at proper temperature
+ eating food from unsafe sources
+ drinking contaminated water

Signs and Symptoms

+ onset of symptoms 6 – 24 hours after ingestion
+ watery diarrhea
+ nausea and vomiting
+ dehydration secondary to diarrhea and vomiting
+ abdominal pain and cramping
+ chills and/or fever

+ generalized weakness and fatigue
+ severe symptoms:
  - fever > 101.5°F (38.6°C)
  - diarrhea with hematochezia
  - intractable vomiting
  - diarrhea for > 3 days
  - hypovolemia

Diagnostic Tests and Findings

+ stool culture positive for presence of bacteria, toxins, endotoxins, or parasites
+ CBC with differential (to determine whether bacterial or viral)

Treatment and Management

+ Provide supportive treatment.
  - oral or IV hydration if patient is dehydrated
  - electrolyte replacement if needed
+ Antibiotics are not usually given for a diagnosis of food poisoning.

QUICK REVIEW QUESTION

5. A patient is being discharged with a diagnosis of food poisoning. The patient asks if she can get a prescription or take something OTC to stop the diarrhea. What instructions should the nurse provide?

Lightning Strikes

Pathophysiology

When a person is struck by lightning, the electrical energy can result in cardiac arrest, neurological deficits (both acute and long term), and changes in the level of consciousness. It differs from generated electrical energy in that it does not usually cause burns, rhabdomyolysis, or internal organ or tissue damage.

Risk Factors

+ being outside during a lightning storm

Signs and Symptoms

+ cardiac:
    ◇ asystole
    ◇ varied arrhythmias
+ neurological:
    ◇ confusion
    ◇ amnesia
    ◇ loss of consciousness
    ◇ sleep disturbances
    ◇ attention deficit issues
    ◇ keraunoparalysis (weakness in limbs following a lightning strike):
        + paralysis featuring cold and mottled skin
        + temporary; lasts a few hours (possible residual long-term effects)
        + most often in the lower extremities
        + loss of sensation in affected limbs
+ hearing loss due to tympanic membrane perforation

Diagnostic Tests and Findings

+ positive report of being struck by lightning
+ patient with amnesia found outdoors on the ground during or after a storm
+ abnormal ECG:
    ◇ asystole
    ◇ V-tach
    ◇ V-fib
    ◇ prolonged QTc
    ◇ abnormal cardiac enzymes:
    ◇ elevated CK
    ◇ elevated CK-MB
    ◇ elevated troponin

Treatment and Management

+ for chest pain:
    ◇ Administer ECG.
    ◇ Draw cardiac enzyme labs.
+ for neurological symptoms:
    ◇ Perform head CT.
+ tympanoplasty

QUICK REVIEW QUESTION

6. A patient who has been stuck by lightning is admitted. What diagnostic test(s) should the nurse prepare to perform?

Parasite and Fungal Infestations

GIARDIASIS

Pathophysiology

Giardiasis is the common name for the parasitic infection cause by *Giardia lamblia*, a flagellated protozoan that attaches itself to the mucosa of the small intestine. Once attached to the mucosa, the protozoan releases spores into the fecal material, allowing the infection to spread. The infection disturbs the normal flora in the GI tract, leading to GI upset.

Risk Factors

+ waterborne
    ⋄ drinking water contaminated with feces
    ⋄ eating food, most often porous fruit, washed in contaminated water
    ⋄ drinking from contaminated streams
+ transferred person-to-person:
    ⋄ fecal to oral (seen most commonly in mental health and day care facilities)
    ⋄ sexual intercourse

Signs and Symptoms

+ mostly asymptomatic
+ if symptoms appear (1 – 14 days):
    ⋄ watery stools
    ⋄ abdominal cramping and pain
    ⋄ flatulence
    ⋄ weight loss
+ chronic infection in children:
    ⋄ failure to thrive
+ chronic infection in adults > 65
    ⋄ anorexia
    ⋄ IBS
    ⋄ impaired cognitive function

Diagnostic Tests and Findings

+ stool sample:
    ⋄ Positive enzyme immunoassay is most accurate and comprehensive.
    ⋄ Presence of parasite and spores (visible under microscope) determines if infection is present.
    ⋄ Presence of parasite excretion determines if infection is acute or chronic.

Treatment and Management

+ IV fluids if needed for dehydration
+ IV push antiemetic for vomiting
+ oral antibiotics for symptomatic patients:
    ⋄ metronidazole (Flagyl)
    ⋄ tinidazole (Tindamax)
+ oral anti-parasite medication for symptomatic patients:
    ⋄ nitazoxanide (Alinia)

QUICK REVIEW QUESTION

7. A 23-year-old woman presents to the ED with symptoms of giardiasis. Before administering the antibiotics tinidazole or metronidazole to the patient, what part of the patient's medical history should the nurse check?

RINGWORM

Pathophysiology

Ringworm is a superficial fungal infection (not actually caused by worms) that only affects the skin. The fungus penetrates the skin superficially to feed on organic material. Ringworm is known by several different names based on the affected area.

+ tinea capitis: scalp, eyelashes, or eyebrows

+ tinea corporis: skin of the trunk or extremities

+ tinea pedis or athlete's foot: feet

+ tinea cruris or jock itch: groin

+ tinea unguium: toenail bed

Risk Factors

+ live in a warm, humid climate

+ direct contact with ringworm:
  ✦ touching another person or animal infected with ringworm
  ✦ sharing showers, towels, clothes, or bedding with someone infected with ringworm

Signs and Symptoms

+ tinea capitis:
  ✦ scaling and erythematous patches on the scalp
  ✦ papules or pustules on the scalp

+ tinea corporis:
  ✦ characteristic bull's-eye–shaped pink or red skin lesion

+ tinea pedis:
  ✦ scaling in between toes or on soles of both feet
  ✦ red areas between toes (possible maceration)

+ tinea cruris:
  ✦ small red scaling patches in groin area

+ tinea unguium:
  ✦ thick nail beds that crumble easily
  ✦ loss of entire nail

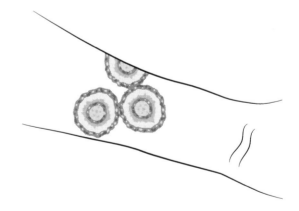

Figure 13.2. Tinea Corporis Bull's-Eye Rash

Diagnostic Tests and Findings

+ positive potassium hydroxide wet mount:
  ⬥ To obtain specimen, use scalpel or glass slide to remove skin from the lesion area.

Treatment and Management

+ tinea capitis:
  ⬥ oral griseofulvin for 6 weeks
  ⬥ shampoo hair 2 – 3 times with ketoconazole (Nizoral) or selenium sulfide shampoo
+ tinea corporis:
  ⬥ mild cases: topical antifungal cream
  ⬥ severe cases: oral griseofulvin or terbinafine
+ tinea pedis:
  ⬥ mild cases: vinegar-and-water soak
  ⬥ severe cases: griseofulvin or terbinafine

+ tinea cruris:
  ⬥ mild cases: topical antifungal cream
  ⬥ severe cases: oral griseofulvin or terbinafine
+ tinea unguium:
  ⬥ itraconazole
  ⬥ terbinafine

QUICK REVIEW QUESTION

8. The nurse is providing discharge instructions to a patient who has been prescribed griseofulvin for ringworm. What should the nurse tell the patient to ensure the medication is effective?

SCABIES
Pathophysiology

Scabies is an infection of the skin cause by a mite, *Sarcoptes scabiei*. When the mite burrows into the skin, it causes irritation, redness, and itching.

Risk Factors

+ living or long stays in densely populated areas (e.g., schools, shelters, long-term care facilities)
+ transmitted person-to-person with direct contact

Signs and Symptoms

+ red, itchy area on the skin that looks like a pinhole
+ usually seen between fingers, axillary folds, and the waistband area
+ intense itching in the affected area that is more pronounced overnight

Diagnostic Tests and Findings

+ skin scraping of affected area on microscope slide
+ positive detection of organism on microscope slide

Treatment and Management

+ Contact precautions are needed during treatment of patients with scabies.

+ Bag clothing and bed linens.

+ Try topical treatment first.
    + Patient should be washed with warm soapy water and allowed to cool and fully dry.
    + Topical scabicide is applied to the entire body from the neck down.
    + If an area of skin is missed, the scabies will move to the untreated area.
    + Topical cream should be left on for 12 – 24 hours.
    + Patient should wash or be washed after 24 hours.
    + Second application of topical treatment may be administered.
    + Patient's linens and clothing should be washed and new linens and clothes provided.

+ If topical treatment is ineffective, oral ivermectin is prescribed.
    + It is important to get a proper weight for patients being prescribed ivermectin.

QUICK REVIEW QUESTION

9. What instructions should a nurse give to patients who are applying topical cream for scabies?

Radiation Exposure

Pathophysiology

Radiation is high-energy waves or particles that can damage human cells. Radiation is classified as either **ionizing**—which damages tissue—or **nonionizing**. Sources of ionizing radiation include X-rays and radioactive substances (e.g., uranium). Radiation exposure is measured in units called **grays** (Gy); 1 gray is equal to 1 joule of radiation per kilogram.

Radiation results in tissue damage that can be local (such as burns) or systemic. The degree of tissue injury resulting from radiation exposure depends on several factors, including the dose of radiation, the length of exposure, the type of radiation, and the area and amount of the body that was exposed.

Risk Factors

+ working in an environment where radiation is used (e.g., hospitals, imaging centers, nuclear reactors)

+ contact with unsecured food irradiators

+ being treated with radiation

Signs and Symptoms

+ acute radiation syndromes (ARS) from intense exposure of the whole body to radiation
    + 3 stages:
        + prodromal: minutes to 2 days after exposure
        + latent asymptomatic: hours to 21 days after exposure
        + overt systemic illness: hours to > 60 days after exposure

- cerebrovascular syndrome
  - after whole-body exposure to high amounts of ionizing radiation (> 30 Gy)
  - seizures
  - tremors
  - ataxia
  - cerebral edema
  - always fatal within hours to 2 days
- gastrointestinal syndrome
  - after whole-body exposure to ionizing radiation of 6 – 30 Gy
  - intractable nausea and vomiting
  - diarrhea
  - fluid imbalance/dehydration
  - hypovolemia
  - vascular collapse
  - necrosis of intestinal tissue leading to:
    - intestinal perforation
    - sepsis
    - bacteremia
  - mostly fatal if exposure > 10 Gy
  - survivors will develop hematopoietic syndrome
- hematopoietic syndrome
  - after whole-body exposure to ionizing radiation of 1 – 6 Gy
  - bone marrow cell depletion
  - lymphopenia
  - pancytopenia
  - infections from neutropenia and decreased antibodies
  - petechiae
  - mucosal lining bleeding
  - anemia
  - high risk for cancer and leukemia for survivors
- focal radiation injury
  - brain: headache, nausea and vomiting, drowsiness, Lhermitte's sign, memory loss
  - heart: chest pain, pericarditis, myocarditis
  - gonads: decreased libido, amenorrhea, decreased spermatogenesis
  - lungs: acute pneumonitis, pulmonary fibrosis
  - kidneys: decreased GFR, kidney failure, fibrosis
  - spinal cord: myelopathy
  - fetus: growth retardation, congenital malformation, higher risk for cancer, death
- cutaneous radiation injury (CRI)
- can occur with ARS or focal radiation injury
- injury to the skin or directly underlying tissue due to radiation
  - erythema
  - hyperpigmentation
  - fibrosis
  - necrosis
  - increased risk for squamous cell carcinoma

Diagnostic Tests and Findings

- history of exposure to radiation
- serial absolute lymphocytes:
  - typically decreased
  - can initially be elevated with trauma; increase will last 24 – 48 hours

- serum amylase levels elevated; related to the amount of exposure
- CRP elevated
- decreased blood citrulline levels if GI involvement
- blood FLT3 ligand level to determine hematopoietic damage

Treatment and Management

- It is important during treatment to decrease health care worker exposure and be mindful of radiation contamination.
- If there are physical injuries, trauma is to be treated before radiation poisoning.
- Decontaminate patient.
    - Use radiation meter to monitor progress.
    - Remove clothing and debris.
    - Decontaminate skin.
    - Clean wounds before intact skin.
        - Irrigate wounds with normal saline.
        - Debridement may be done on wound edges.
        - Wash intact skin and hair with lukewarm water and mild detergent.
    - If radiation was swallowed:
        - Induce vomiting or lavage.
        - Rinse mouth.
    - If radiation in eyes:
        - Wash with water or saline.
        - Try to avoid nasolacrimal duct.
- For internal decontamination:
    - potassium iodine (KI)
    - Prussian blue:
        - removes radioactive cesium and thallium from the body
        - radioactive material passed in the feces
        - oral medication
    - diethylenetriamine pentaacetate (DTPA):
        - removes radioactive plutonium, americium, and curium from the body
        - radioactive material passed in the urine
        - can be given IV or as an inhalant for those who have inhaled radiation
- Administer filgrastim (Neupogen).
    - given to stimulate WBC growth
    - for patients with bone marrow damage or low WBC counts
    - helps increase WBC count to reduce risk for infection and bleeding

QUICK REVIEW QUESTION

10. Arriving EMS personnel alert the ED nurse that the patient has been exposed to radiation. What should the ED nurse plan as the first intervention for the patient?

Submersion Injury

Pathophysiology

A **submersion injury** is a respiratory injury or impairment that occurs as a result of being submerged in liquid. The respiratory impairment resulting from submersion leads to hypoxemia, which in turn can lead to organ failure, most notably in the lungs, heart, and brain.

These injuries were previously known as "wet drowning" when water was aspirated or "dry drowning" when the patient had a laryngospasm but did not ingest or aspirate water. The term "near drowning" is another term that is no longer commonly used. Submersion injuries are now classified as **nonfatal** or **fatal**.

Risk Factors

+ most common in children
    ✧ Drowning is the leading cause of trauma mortality in children ages 1 – 4.
+ alcohol or drug use, particularly while swimming or boating
+ participating in dangerous underwater breath-holding behaviors (DUBB), usually teens and young adults

Signs and Symptoms

+ vomiting
+ wheezing
+ change in level of consciousness
+ respiratory failure:
    ✧ tachypnea
    ✧ intercostal retractions
    ✧ cyanosis
+ signs and symptoms not necessarily immediate:
    ✧ Some respiratory damage may take up to 6 hours to produce symptoms.
    ✧ Patient should be taken to the hospital for observation even if asymptomatic.

Diagnostic Tests and Findings

+ patient found in or near water
+ low pulse oximetry reading
+ hypothermia
+ significant metabolic acidosis indicated in ABG results

Treatment and Management

+ Initiate CPR if needed.
    ✧ Resuscitation in drowning victims starts with rescue breathing, not compressions.
+ Treatment of hypoxemia is main concern.
    ✧ Place ET tube and put patient on mechanical ventilation.
    ✧ Start patient on 100% oxygen; titrate down based on serial ABG results.
    ✧ Use positive end-expiratory pressure ventilation.
    ✧ Administer nebulized bronchodilators to relieve bronchospasms or wheezing.

+ Perform chest X-ray.

+ Assess patient for concomitant injuries.

+ Head CT if patient loses consciousness.

Temperature-Related Emergencies

FROSTBITE

Pathophysiology

Frostbite is injury to the dermis and underlying tissue due to cold. The exposure to cold leads to cellular damage, impairment of the vascular system, and an inflammatory response. Frostbite most commonly affects fingers and toes.

Risk Factors

+ exposure to cold weather or wind

+ touching cold material such as ice, metal, or cold packs

+ previous frostbite or other cold injury

Signs and Symptoms

+ early stages:
  ⋄ cold and white skin
  ⋄ numbness or tingling sensation
  ⋄ possible sensation of throbbing in the area

+ mild stage:
  ⋄ skin hard or frozen to the touch
  ⋄ skin red and blistered when warmed and thawed

+ severe stage:
  ⋄ damage to underlying muscle, tendons, and bone
  ⋄ blue, blotchy, or white skin
  ⋄ blood-filled blisters as skin warms
  ⋄ necrotic areas that are black in appearance

Treatment and Management

+ Rewarm affected area.
  ⋄ Use warm water, heated to 104°F – 108°F (40°C – 42°C), in a basin or bath.
  ⋄ Hot water is contraindicated.
  ⋄ Rewarm affected area until it is red in color.

+ Remove necrotic tissue to prevent infection and promote wound healing.

+ Some patients report mild hypersensitivity to cold exposure for months to years after.

QUICK REVIEW QUESTION

12. A patient presents to the ED complaining of both hands being numb. The nurse observes that the patient's hands are blue and establishes that the patient has been outside without gloves for several hours. What intervention should the nurse prepare for?

IMMERSION FOOT

Pathophysiology

Immersion foot is the result of prolonged exposure to a cold and wet environment of a limb that had little or no mobility. The cold causes vasoconstriction of the blood vessels, leading to spasms and ischemia of the vascular system and damage to the vascular and nerve tissue in the affected limb. In severe cases, muscle damage can occur.

Risk Factors

+ prolonged exposure of limb, hand, or foot to cold and wet environment
+ limited or no movement in limbs

Signs and Symptoms

+ The foot or hand is:
  ⋄ numb
  ⋄ cold
  ⋄ pale in color
  ⋄ clammy
  ⋄ swollen
+ In severe cases the area can ulcerate and eschar will develop.

+ If the muscle is affected:
  ⋄ muscle atrophy
+ If the nerve tissue has been affected:
  ⋄ dysesthesia
  ⋄ anesthesia (temporary or permanent)

Diagnostic Tests and Findings

+ Diagnosis is based on signs and symptoms.

Treatment and Management

+ Rewarm by placing hand or foot in water heated to 104°F – 108°F (40°C – 42°C).
+ Limb should be dried.
+ Treat with a sterile dressing if needed.

QUICK REVIEW QUESTION

13. A patient has been diagnosed with a severe immersion injury. During a routine dressing change, the nurse notes that there is dark slough in the wound bed. What should the nurse prepare the patient for?

CHILBLAINS

Pathophysiology

Chilblains is an inflammatory response that occurs in the skin and small blood vessels as a result of repeated exposure to cold but not freezing temperatures. They are most commonly seen in women, underweight patients, and patients with Raynaud's disease.

Risk Factors

+ repeated exposure to cold but not freezing conditions

+ connective tissue disease

Signs and Symptoms

+ red or purple bumps on the skin that can be painful or swollen

+ blistering or ulceration in severe cases

+ complaints of itchy feeling

Treatment and Management

+ Increase circulation in the area by using heating pads.

+ If it is a recurring issue, nifedipine may be taken daily.

+ Apply topical corticosteroids.

QUICK REVIEW QUESTION

14. A patient with a history of Raynaud's disease is complaining of painful red bumps on her hand. What intervention should the nurse prepare for?

HYPOTHERMIA

Pathophysiology

Hypothermia occurs when core body temperature drops below 35°C (95°F), causing a reduction in metabolic rate and in respiratory, cardiac, and neurological functions. When body temperature drops below 30°C (86°F), thermoregulation ceases.

During hypothermia, diuresis and systemic fluid leakage into the interstitial space can lead to hypovolemia. Vasoconstriction due to the cold can mask this hypovolemia. When the patient is rewarmed and the vessels dilate, the patient will go into shock or cardiac arrest if the fluid volume is not replaced.

Risk Factors

+ cold weather

+ immersion in cold water

+ wearing wet clothing in cold or windy climates

+ lying on cold surfaces for prolonged amounts of time (often seen in patients using alcohol or drugs)

Signs and Symptoms

+ intense shivering that lasts until core body temperature drops below 31°C (87.8°F)
  + After the body stops shivering the core body temperature will drop at a faster rate.
+ CNS symptoms:
  + lethargy
  + clumsiness
  + confusion
  + agitation
  + possibly hallucinations
+ hypotension
+ unreactive pupils
+ eventual coma
+ slow and ultimately no respiration
+ decreased cardiac function:
  + initial bradycardia and slow A-fib
  + terminal rhythm of V-fib or asystole

Diagnostic Tests and Findings

+ core body temperature:
  + moderate hypothermia: 28°C – 32°C (82.4°F – 89.6°F)
  + severe hypothermia: less than 28°C (82.4°F)
+ CBC, electrolytes, BUN, and creatinine to show hypovolemia
+ ABGs:
  + Do not correct for low temperatures.
+ ECG readings (very important in hypothermia patients):
  + will show prolonged intervals
  + will read as injury due to myocardial infarction, but will show a J wave or Osborn wave

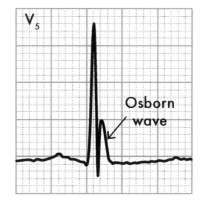

Figure 13.3. Osborn or J Wave

Treatment and Management

+ The first line of treatment is to prevent further heat loss.
  + Remove wet or cold clothing.
  + Insulate patient.
+ The next steps depend on the severity of hypothermia and the amount of cardiac instability.
+ For mild hypothermia:
  + Passively rewarm patients at a rate of 1°C per hour with an insulated blanket and warmed fluids.
  + Use active rewarming with forced hot air in an enclosure.
  + It is better to apply the heat to the core of the body. Heat applied to extremities may increase metabolic demand, which can strain the depressed cardiovascular system.
+ In severe hypothermia, patients should be treated with active core warming.
  + Inhalation: Oxygen should be heated to 40°C – 45°C (104°F – 113°F) and delivered via oxygen mask or ET tube.
  + Infusion: IV fluids or blood products should be heated to 40°C – 42°C (104°F – 107.6°F).

- ❖ Lavage: Closed thoracic lavage can be administered through 2 thoracic tubes; the peritoneal lavage should be heated to 40°C – 45°C (104°F – 113°F).
- ❖ Extracorporeal core rewarming (ECR) is not often performed as it requires a specialist and prearranged protocol.
- ❖ Fluid resuscitation: Administer 1 – 2 L (for adults) or 20 ml/kg (for pediatrics) of 0.9% saline solution heated to 40°C – 42°C (104°F – 107.6°F) via IV.
- ✦ For cardiovascular involvement:
  - ❖ CPR is only administered in patients with a perfusing rhythm when true cardiac arrest is confirmed.
  - ❖ Patients who have V-fib or asystole require CPR.
  - ❖ Defibrillation is only recommended once body temperature reaches about 30°C (86°F).
  - ❖ Administration of advanced cardiac life support drugs should not be expected.

QUICK REVIEW QUESTION

15. A patient is admitted to the ED. The patient fell through ice and was submerged in the water for 20 minutes. The patient is unresponsive and has been intubated. How would the nurse prepare oxygen for administration?

HEAT CRAMPS

Pathophysiology

Heat cramps occur when exercise or physical exertion leads to a profuse loss of fluids and sodium through sweating. When fluids are replaced but sodium is not, the resulting hyponatremia causes muscle cramps.

Risk Factors

- ✦ manual labor jobs
- ✦ exercising or physical exertion in high temperatures and humidity
- ✦ common in athletes and military personnel
- ✦ profuse sweating and drinking large amounts of water with no electrolyte replacement

Signs and Symptoms

- ✦ sudden onset of severe spasmodic muscle cramps:
  - ❖ seen in the extremity muscles
  - ❖ can last from a few minutes to hours
- ✦ may progress to carpopedal spasms, which can incapacitate the hands or the feet

Treatment and Management

- ✦ CMP results are used to determine the need for fluid or electrolyte replacement.
- ✦ Move patient to a cool area and have them rest.
- ✦ Have patient stretch the affected muscle (firm, passive stretching).

- If patient can take fluids by mouth, give a solution of 1 L of water with 10 g of sodium or commercial sports drinks.
- If patient cannot take fluids by mouth, administer an IV of 1 – 2 L of 0.9% saline solution.

QUICK REVIEW QUESTION

16. A patient has been diagnosed with heat cramps and cannot take fluids by mouth. What intervention should the nurse prepare for?

HEAT EXHAUSTION

Pathophysiology

Heat exhaustion occurs when the body is exposed to high temperatures, leading to dehydration. It is not a result of deficits in thermoregulation or the central nervous system.

Risk Factors

- outdoor occupations in high temperatures
- exposure to high temperatures
- physical exertion in high temperatures

Signs and Symptoms

- temperature elevated but < 104°F (40°C)
- sweating
- dizziness
- weakness
- tachycardia
- hypertension
- headache
- nausea and/or vomiting
- syncope
- in severe cases following physical exertion:
  - rhabdomyolysis
  - myoglobinuria
  - acute kidney injury

Diagnostic Tests and Findings

- Diagnosis is based on signs and symptoms.
- Labs will usually indicate dehydration.
  - sodium and potassium elevated
  - BUN and creatinine elevated

Treatment and Management

- Stop physical exertion.
- Move patient to a cool place and have them lie face up.
- If patient is not nauseous or vomiting, give fluids at 1 L/hr.
- If patient is unable to take fluids by mouth, start IV fluids.

17. A patient has been diagnosed with heat exhaustion. Due to nausea and vomiting, the patient is unable to take fluids by mouth and IV fluids have been ordered. At what rate should the nurse anticipate administering the IV fluids?

HEAT STROKE

Pathophysiology

Heat stroke results when the compensatory measures for ridding the body of excess heat fail, leading to an increased core temperature. The resulting inflammatory process can cause multiple organ failure that, if not treated, leads to death.

There are two forms of heat stroke: classic and exertional. **Classic heat stroke** occurs as the result of prolonged exposure to high temperatures with no air conditioning or access to fluids. **Exertional heat stroke** occurs when exercising in extreme heat.

Risk Factors

+ prolonged exposure to high temperatures

+ exercising in high temperatures

+ drugs that lead to hypermetabolic states, such as cocaine

Signs and Symptoms

+ temperature > 104°F (40°C)

+ dysfunction of the CNS:
  ⋄ confusion
  ⋄ delirium
  ⋄ seizures
  ⋄ coma

+ tachycardia

+ tachypnea

Diagnostic Tests and Findings

+ lab findings in CBC, PT, PTT, electrolytes, BUN, creatinine, Ca, CK, and hepatic profile consistent with organ dysfunction

+ irregular values, depending on which organ is affected:
  ⋄ kidney failure: BUN and creatinine elevated
  ⋄ liver failure: ALP and AST elevated
  ⋄ PTT/PT elevated, caused by overall inflammation

Treatment and Management

+ Preferred treatment is aggressive cooling by immersing in cold water.

+ Evaporative cooling may also be used.
  ⋄ Environment must be dry.
  ⋄ Patient must have adequate circulation.

+ CPR can be done while patient is cooling.

+ Treat shivering during cooling to minimize vasoconstriction.
  ⋄ benzodiazepines
  ⋄ chlorpromazine (Thorazine)

- Administer oxygen.
- Hydrate with IV fluids.
    - Administer cooled normal saline.
    - Fluid should be given in bolus doses; monitor central venous pressure, blood pressure, and urine output.
- Treat organ failure as needed.
    - Treat DIC with FFP and platelets.
    - Treat hyperkalemic cardiotoxicity with IV calcium salts.
- Treat and monitor hypotension.
    - Treat with vasoconstrictors.
    - Monitor via pulmonary artery catheter.
- Hemodialysis may be necessary.
- Intubate patients who are comatose to prevent aspiration during seizures and vomiting.

Vector Borne Illnesses

RABIES

Pathophysiology

Rabies is a virus that causes inflammation in the brain. The virus is carried in the saliva of infected animals and is transmitted during animal bites. Once in the body, the virus will travel through the peripheral nervous system to the spinal cord and then to the brain, resulting in encephalitis.

Risk Factors

- being bitten by a bat or other animal that has rabies

Signs and Symptoms

- The closer the bite is to the brain, the faster symptoms will progress.
- Initial symptoms are nonspecific.
    - fatigue
    - fever
    - headache
- Advanced symptoms include:
    - encephalitis:
        - confusion
        - agitation
        - possible bizarre behavior
        - hallucinations
        - insomnia
    - excessive salivation
    - hydrophobia
    - ascending paralysis that progresses to quadriplegia

Diagnostic Tests and Findings

+ confirmed animal bite
+ positive fluorescence antibody test from biopsy of skin near the nape of neck
+ encephalitis
    ⬦ MRI will show inflammation in the brain.
    ⬦ Spinal tap will show virus in CSF.
    ⬦ EEG may indicate encephalitis.
+ normal CT, MRI, or EEG showing no specific changes if no encephalitis

Treatment and Management

+ Clean the wound with soap and water or BZK wipes.
+ Administer rabies vaccine and rabies immune globulin (RIG).
    ⬦ After exposure, vaccines are given: 1.0 ml IM on days 0, 3, 7, and 14.
+ Once rabies has developed, there is no curative treatment.
    ⬦ Supportive care includes heavy sedation and comfort measures until death occurs.

QUICK REVIEW QUESTION

19. A patient has reported being bitten by a bat. How should the nurse clean the wound?

LYME DISEASE
Pathophysiology

Lyme disease is a bacterial infection transmitted through tick bites. The disease is caused by several species of *Borrelia* bacteria, including *B. burgdorferi* and *B. mayonii*. The bacteria enter through the skin and into the blood through a tick bite. Within 3 – 30 days the bacteria will either enter the lymphatic system and cause adenopathy or will continue to circulate in the bloodstream and travel to organs or other skin sites.

Risk Factors

+ prolonged periods of time outdoors in wooded or grassy areas

Signs and Symptoms

+ first stage (early localized stage):
    ⬦ 3 – 30 days post-bite
    ⬦ erythema migrans
    ⬦ will expand and resemble a bull's-eye in appearance
+ second stage (early disseminated stage):
    ⬦ nonspecific flu-like symptoms
    ⬦ may resemble fibromyalgia
    ⬦ symptoms lasting a few weeks

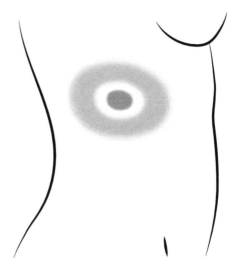

Figure 13.4. Erythema Migrans

- late stage (if left untreated):
  - months to years after infection
  - characterized by arthritis
  - periods of fatigue and low-grade fever followed by flare-ups

Diagnostic Tests and Findings

- positive acute and convalescent serologic testing (ELISA confirmed by Western blot)

Treatment and Management

- oral or IV antibiotics:
  - amoxicillin
  - doxycycline
  - ceftriaxone

QUICK REVIEW QUESTION

20. What type of rash on the skin should prompt the nurse to suspect a patient has Lyme disease? What other tests need to be performed to confirm the diagnosis of Lyme disease?

ROCKY MOUNTAIN SPOTTED FEVER

Pathophysiology

Rocky Mountain spotted fever is an infection caused by *Rickettsia* bacteria, which are carried by hard-shelled ticks. The bacteria lodge themselves in small blood vessels, which become blocked with thrombi, producing vasculitis throughout the body. In extreme cases, DIC can occur.

Risk Factors

- limited to the Western hemisphere
- higher risk for those who live in or near a heavily wooded area

Signs and Symptoms

- fever
- headache
- rash:
  - starts pink and macular, then darkens and becomes maculopapular
  - can become hemorrhagic and ulcerate if untreated
- chills
- muscle pain
- neurological symptoms:
  - restlessness
  - insomnia
  - delirium
  - coma

Diagnostic Tests and Findings

- positive fluorescent antibody staining in skin biopsy from rash areas
- positive PCR

Treatment and Management

+ antibiotics:
    ◇ doxycycline
    ◇ oral or IV chloramphenicol if doxycycline is ineffective

QUICK REVIEW QUESTION

21. An 18-year-old patient presents to the ED with complaints of fever, headache, and muscle pain. The nurse notes a rash consistent with a diagnosis of Rocky Mountain spotted fever. What question should the nurse be sure to ask about the patient's history?

ANSWER KEY

1. The nurse should prepare to establish IV access; 18 is the preferred needle gauge, with 2 accesses if possible.

2. Vomiting or gastric lavage is contraindicated when a patient swallows a chemical because it may cause further damage to the upper airway or throat and mouth.

3. The total amount of internal damage cannot be judged based on external damage. Internal injury or organ dysfunction could still be present even when the patient has little to no external damage and is presenting asymptomatically.

4. Compression may keep the poison in the area, increasing localized damage.

5. Antidiarrheals are contraindicated for patients who have been positively diagnosed with food poisoning. The diarrhea is the body's way of expelling the infectious organism or noninfectious substance. If the diarrhea is stopped, the offending substance will remain in the small intestine, and the patient will remain sick and may worsen.

6. The nurse should prepare for CBC, CMP, cardiac enzymes (CK, CK-MB, troponin levels) and an ECG.

7. The nurse should check the medical record and ask the patient if she is pregnant, for these antibiotics should not be administered to pregnant women.

8. The nurse should make sure to tell the patient to take the medication with a glass of milk or a fatty snack or meal to aid in digestion and absorption of the medication.

9. Scabicide can be a neurotoxin. Topical application after bathing should only be administered when patient is completely dry and has cooled off. Immediately following a warm shower, the skin is likely to absorb a larger amount of the scabicide, which could then lead to percutaneous absorption and possible central nervous system symptoms like seizures.

10. The first nursing intervention/concern is decontamination. The nurse should remove the patient's clothing and wash their skin, hair, and wounds.

11. The nurse should prepare the patient to be intubated.

12. The nurse should gather materials to immerse the patient's hands in warm water.

13. The nurse should prepare the patient to have the area debrided.

14. The nurse should prepare to apply heating pads to the patient's hands.

15. The oxygen needs to be heated to 40°C – 45°C (104°F – 113°F) before being administered to this patient.

16. The nurse should prepare to administer an IV solution of 1 – 2 L of 0.9% saline solution.

17. Fluids should be administered at 1 L/hr.

18. The nurse should gather materials and prepare the patient for insertion of a pulmonary artery catheter.

19. The nurse should prepare to treat the wound with soap and water and then cleanse the wound with BZK wipes.

20. Lyme disease presents with a red, bull's-eye–shaped rash. Other rashes can be similar in appearance to erythema migrans. A positive ELISA test is needed to confirm Lyme disease.

21. The nurse should ask if the patient has recently been in a heavily wooded area.

FOURTEEN: TOXICOLOGICAL EMERGENCIES

Toxidromes

Toxidromes are groups of signs and symptoms present in patients who have large amounts of toxins or poisons in the body. General signs and symptoms are given below, but these may vary based on the specific drug (or combination of drugs) ingested.

Table 14.1. Summary of Toxidrome Symptoms

Toxidrome	HR	BP	RR	Temp	Bowel Sounds	Pupils	Skin	Mental Status
Anticholinergic	↑	↑	—	↑	↓	↑	dry	agitated and delirious
Cholinergic	—	—	—	—	↑	↓	moist	—
Hallucinogenic	↑	↑	↑	—	↑	↑	—	disoriented
Sympathomimetic	↑	↑	↑	↑	↑	↑	moist	agitated and delirious
Sedative-hypnotic	↓	↓	↓	↓	↓	—	dry	lethargic and confused

ANTICHOLINERGIC

Anticholinergic syndrome results from exposure to anticholinergics that inhibit binding of acetylcholine at muscarinic receptor sites.

Most common causes:

+ antihistamines
+ antipsychotics:
    ⬥ chlorpromazine (Thorazine)
    ⬥ droperidol (Inapsine)
    ⬥ haloperidol (Haldol)
    ⬥ quetiapine (Seroquel)
    ⬥ olanzapine (Zyprexa)

- tricyclic antidepressants:
  - amitriptyline
  - imipramine
  - doxepin
- benztropine (Cogentin)
- scopolamine
- atropine
- *Atropa belladonna* (deadly nightshade)

Signs and Symptoms

- "hot as a hare": hyperthermia
- "red as a beet": flushing
- "blind as a bat": mydriasis, blurred vision
- "dry as a bone": dry skin
- "mad as a hatter": agitation, delirium, hallucinations, memory loss
- "full as a flask": urinary retention
- tachycardia
- hypertension
- ileus (immobility of the intestines)
- severe toxicity:
  - seizures
  - rhabdomyolysis
  - dysrhythmia
  - coma

Treatment and Management

- physostigmine salicylate
- Supportive care for symptoms can include:
  - diazepam (Valium) for agitation
  - benzodiazepines for seizures
  - cooling measures for hyperthermia
  - catheter for urinary retention

CHOLINERGIC

A **cholinergic crisis** is the result of excess acetylcholine, which causes overstimulation of muscarinic and nicotinic receptors. Excess acetylcholine is usually the result of inhibition of acetylcholinesterase, the enzyme responsible for breaking down acetylcholine.

Most common causes:

- anticholinesterase:
  - patients with MG
  - patients who have received neostigmine after general anesthesia
- insecticides and pesticides
- nerve agents (e.g., sarin)

General Signs and Symptoms

- HR, BP, and RR may be increased or decreased
- increased bowel sounds
- constricted pupils
- diaphoresis

Muscarinic Signs and Symptoms

- wheezing
- SLUDGE:
    - **Salivation**
    - **Lacrimation**
    - **Urination**
    - **Defecation**
    - **GI cramps**
    - **Emesis**
- DUMBELS:
    - **Diarrhea**
    - **Urination**
    - **Miosis**
    - **Bronchorrhea, bradycardia, bronchoconstriction**
    - **Emesis**
    - **Lacrimation**
    - **Salivation**

Nicotinic Signs and Symptoms

- MTW[T]hFS
    - **Mydriasis**
    - **Tachycardia**
    - **Weakness**
    - **Hypertension, hyperglycemia**
    - **Fasciculations**
    - **Sweating**
- abdominal pain
- paresis

Treatment and Management

- Decontaminate patient if needed.
- Maintain airway and breathing.
- Administer IV fluids.
- Administer antidote:
    - atropine
    - oximes (e.g., pralidoxime)
- Supportive care for symptoms can include:
    - benzodiazepines for seizures

HALLUCINOGENIC

Hallucinogens are substances whose primary effects are to cause hallucinations and changes in mood and sensation. The pharmacology of hallucinogens varies, but they generally act on neurotransmitters, including serotonin and dopamine.

Most common causes:

- LSD
- psilocybin ("magic mushrooms")
- mescaline
- DMT
- salvia divinorum
- dextromethorphan (DXM)
- PCP

Signs and Symptoms

+ psychiatric effects:
  ⋄ feeling of euphoria
  ⋄ heightened sensitivity to sensory input
  ⋄ fear/panic
  ⋄ dysphoria
  ⋄ synesthesia
+ tachycardia
+ hypertension

+ tachypnea
+ hyperthermia
+ mydriasis
+ emesis
+ horizontal and vertical nystagmus
+ muscle tremors or contractions

Treatment and Management

+ Place patient in calm, quiet environment.
+ Supportive care for symptoms can include:
  ⋄ benzodiazepines for severe agitation
  ⋄ cooling measures for hyperthermia
+ Gastrointestinal decontamination (activated charcoal) should be used only when large quantities of hallucinogens have been ingested < 1 hour earlier.

SYMPATHOMIMETIC

Sympathomimetic agents mimic endogenous sympathetic nervous system agonists (e.g., epinephrine, dopamine), causing direct stimulation of the alpha- and beta-adrenergic receptors.

Most common causes:

+ cocaine
+ amphetamines
+ methamphetamines
+ hallucinogenic amphetamines (MDMA, MDA)

+ khat and related substances (methcathinone, "bath salts")
+ cold medications
+ diet supplements containing ephedrine

Signs and Symptoms

+ sinus tachycardia
+ hypertension
+ tachypnea
+ hyperthermia
+ mydriasis
+ diaphoresis
+ flushing

+ rhabdomyolysis
+ hyperkalemia
+ metabolic acidosis
+ agitation or anxiety
+ hallucinations
+ seizures

Treatment and Management

+ Cardiac monitoring may be necessary.
+ Administer IV fluids.
+ Perform gastric decontamination to limit further absorption.
    ⋄ activated charcoal
    ⋄ whole bowel irrigation

+ Supportive care for symptoms can include:
    ⋄ benzodiazepines for chest pain, hypertension, agitation, or seizures
    ⋄ nitroglycerin for chest pain and hypertension
    ⋄ cooling measures for hyperthermia

SEDATIVE-HYPNOTIC

Most **sedative-hypnotics** cause an increase in the effects of gamma-aminobutyric acid (GABA) at specific receptors. This state inhibits cellular excitation.

Most common causes:

+ benzodiazepines
+ barbiturates
+ antipsychotics

+ zolpidem (Ambien)
+ clonidine
+ GHB

Signs and Symptoms

+ bradycardia
+ hypotension
+ bradypnea
+ hypothermia
+ ataxia
+ mydriasis

+ blurred vision
+ slurred speech
+ dry mouth
+ lethargy
+ hallucinations
+ confusion

Treatment and Management

+ Manage airway and breathing.
    ⋄ EtCO$_2$ monitoring for patients with hypoventilation
+ Cardiac monitoring may be necessary.
+ Provide supportive care for symptoms.
+ Naloxone (Narcan) may be required for patients with decreased LOC.

+ Flumazenil (Romazicon) may be administered in case of benzodiazepine overdose.
    ⋄ Flumazenil (Romazicon) may be administered in case of benzodiazepine overdose.

Acids and Alkalis

Pathophysiology

Acids are compounds that release hydrogen ions and taste sour; **alkalis** are compounds that accept hydrogen ions and are slippery or soapy. On the pH scale (1 to 14), acids have a value lower than 7, alkalis have a value greater than 7, and 7 is neutral.

Common household acids:

+ swimming pool and toilet cleaners
+ anti-rust cleaners
+ battery acid

Common household alkalis:

+ common bleach
+ drain cleaner

Ingestion of acids and alkalis is most common in young children. Ingestion in adults is usually linked to severe mental illness or suicidal behaviors. Ingestion of acids usually causes injuries to the upper respiratory tract as the pain and sour taste prompt gagging or spitting, which may lead to aspiration. The acid may also cause coagulative necrosis in the stomach. Alkali ingestion will cause liquefactive necrosis in the esophagus and will continue to cause damage until it has been neutralized.

Signs and Symptoms

+ drooling
+ dysphagia
+ excessive thirst
+ visible oral burns
+ GI pain
+ emesis (can appear brown)
+ bleeding in mouth, throat, or stomach

+ esophageal perforation:
  ⋄ chest pain
  ⋄ tachycardia
  ⋄ tachypnea
  ⋄ fever
  ⋄ shock
+ airway injury:
  ⋄ stridor
  ⋄ dyspnea

Treatment and Management

+ Absence of symptoms in the mouth and throat does not mean that there is not damage further along the GI tract. An endoscopy needs to be performed even in the absence of symptoms.
+ Maintain airway and breathing.
  ⋄ Intubation is required for patients with severe oropharyngeal edema or necrosis.
+ Dilute with water or milk (only during first few minutes after ingestion).
+ Treatments that are contraindicated include:
  ⋄ gastric emptying by emesis
  ⋄ activated charcoal
  ⋄ neutralizing agents
  ⋄ gastric lavage
  ⋄ nasogastric tube
+ Supportive care for symptoms includes:
  ⋄ pain management
  ⋄ liquid diet
+ Perforation or necrosis in the esophagus or stomach requires immediate surgery.

QUICK REVIEW QUESTION

1. A 15-year-old patient is brought to the ED by her mother, who states that the patient mistook a bottle of ammonia for lemonade and drank it. The mother is very upset that the emergency room staff is not trying to make the patient throw it back up to get it out of her system. How do you explain this action to the patient's mother?

Acute Substance Withdrawal

ALCOHOL WITHDRAWAL

Pathophysiology

Alcohol is a central nervous system depressant that directly binds to gamma-aminobutyric acid (GABA) receptors and inhibits glutamate-induced excitation. Chronic alcohol use alters the sensitivity of these receptors; when alcohol use is stopped, the result is hyperactivity in the central nervous system. Alcohol withdrawal can be fatal.

Chronic alcohol use inhibits the absorption of nutrients, including thiamine and folic acid. Consequently, patients admitted with symptoms of alcohol withdrawal are also at risk for disorders related to vitamin deficiency, including Wernicke's encephalopathy and megaloblastic anemia.

Signs and Symptoms

+ mild (6 – 24 hours after last drink):
    ⋄ sinus tachycardia
    ⋄ systolic hypertension
    ⋄ agitation
    ⋄ restlessness
    ⋄ tremor
    ⋄ insomnia
    ⋄ hyperactive reflexes
    ⋄ diaphoresis
    ⋄ headache
    ⋄ nausea and emesis

+ severe:
    ⋄ hallucinations (12 – 48 hours after last drink)
    ⋄ tonic-clonic seizures (6 – 48 hours after last drink)
    ⋄ delirium tremens (DTs) (72 – 96 hours after last drink):
        • anxiety
        • tachycardia
        • hypertension
        • ataxia
        • diaphoresis

Assessment

+ The **Clinical Institute Withdrawal Assessment (CIWA)** is a ten-item scale used to objectively assess withdrawal symptoms and ensure withdrawing patients are given the correct amount of medication.

+ Patients are given a score of 0 to 7 for each symptom, based on its severity, except orientation, which is scored from 0 to 4.
    ⋄ nausea and emesis
    ⋄ paroxysmal sweats
    ⋄ level of anxiety
    ⋄ level of agitation
    ⋄ tremors
    ⋄ headache symptoms
    ⋄ auditory disturbances
    ⋄ visual disturbances
    ⋄ tactile disturbances
    ⋄ orientation

+ The numerical values for the sections are totaled and the number is used to guide the use of withdrawal medication.
    ⋄ For a CIWA score below 8, no medication is needed.
    ⋄ A score of 8 – 14 calls for 5 – 10 mg diazepam (Valium) or equivalent lorazepam (Ativan) (0.5 – 1 mg).

- A score of 15 – 19 calls for 10 – 15 mg diazepam or equivalent.
- A score of 20 – 25 calls for 20 mg diazepam or equivalent.
- A score of 25 – 30 calls for 25 – 30 mg diazepam or equivalent.

Treatment and Management

- Administer IV fluids.
- Monitor for electrolyte imbalances.
- Treat for vitamin deficiencies and malnutrition by administering:
  - glucose
  - thiamine
  - folate
  - parenteral multivitamins
- Administer benzodiazepines for agitation.
- Administer lorazepam for seizures.
- For severe drug-resistant DTs:
  - drug "cocktail" that includes lorazepam, diazepam, and midazolam (Versed) or propofol
  - mechanical ventilation if needed
  - mechanical restraints if needed

QUICK REVIEW QUESTION

2. A 45-year-old man is admitted to the ED with vomiting, profuse sweating, and complaint of a headache. Assessment shows a HR of 130 bpm and blood pressure of 130/102 mm Hg. The nurse checks the patient's chart and notes that the patient has a history of alcohol abuse. What should the nurse prepare to do next?

OPIOID WITHDRAWAL
Pathophysiology

Opioids are synthetically and naturally occurring substances that bind to opioid receptors in the brain, depressing the central nervous system. (The term "opiate" is sometimes used to refer only to naturally occurring opioids.) Chronic use of opioids increases excitability of noradrenergic neurons, and withdrawal leads to hypersensitivity of the central nervous system. Opioid withdrawal is rarely fatal, but death can occur, usually as a result of hemodynamic instability or electrolyte imbalances.

Opioids include:

- codeine
- fentanyl
- heroin
- hydrocodone
- hydromorphone
- meperidine
- methadone
- morphine
- oxycodone

Signs and Symptoms

- drug craving
- nausea and emesis
- diarrhea
- abdominal cramping
- dysphoria
- anxiety
- yawning
- rhinorrhea
- lacrimation
- mydriasis

- ✦ piloerection
- ✦ sweating
- ✦ muscle pain and twitching
- ✦ tachycardia
- ✦ tachypnea
- ✦ hypertension

Assessment

- ✦ The **Clinical Opiate Withdrawal Scale (COWS)** is an 11-item scale to help objectively assess withdrawal symptoms and ensure that patients are given the correct amount of medication.
- ✦ Patients are given a score based on the severity of each symptom.
    - ✧ resting heart rate
    - ✧ sweating
    - ✧ restlessness
    - ✧ pupil size
    - ✧ bone or joint aches
    - ✧ rhinorrhea or lacrimation
    - ✧ GI upset
    - ✧ tremor
    - ✧ yawning
    - ✧ anxiety or irritability
    - ✧ piloerection
- ✦ The numerical values for the sections are totaled and the amount is used to guide the use of withdrawal medication.
    - ✧ 5 – 12: mild withdrawal
    - ✧ 13 – 24: moderate withdrawal
    - ✧ 25 – 36: moderate to severe withdrawal
    - ✧ 36: severe withdrawal

Treatment and Management

- ✦ Supportive care for symptoms can include:
    - ✧ benzodiazepines for anxiety, tachycardia, and hypertension
    - ✧ antiemetics
    - ✧ clonidine for tachycardia and hypertension
    - ✧ antidiarrheals
- ✦ Possible treatments for opioid withdrawal:
    - ✧ Immediately cease taking opiates.
    - ✧ Opioid antagonists: naltrexone and naloxone block the effects of opioids.
    - ✧ Opioid replacement therapy: methadone or buprenorphine relieve symptoms without producing intoxication.

QUICK REVIEW QUESTION

3. The nurse takes the vitals of a patient in the ED who was admitted for opioid withdrawal. The patient's HR is 102 bpm and her blood pressure is 110/105 mm Hg. What should the nurse anticipate will be ordered for this patient?

Carbon Monoxide

Pathophysiology

Carbon monoxide (CO) displaces oxygen from hemoglobin, which prevents the transport and utilization of oxygen throughout the body. Mild **CO poisoning** can be resolved in the ED; severe CO poisoning can lead to myocardial ischemia, dysrhythmias, pulmonary edema, and coma. Sources of CO include smoke from fires, malfunctioning heaters and generators, and motor vehicle exhaust. CO poisoning and cyanide poisoning often occur together.

Signs and Symptoms

+ mild:
  - headache
  - altered LOC
  - dizziness
  - confusion
  - visual disturbances
  - dyspnea on exertion
  - emesis
  - muscle weakness and cramps

+ severe:
  - syncope
  - seizures
  - signs and symptoms of cardiopulmonary complications
  - coma

Treatment and Management

+ Administer 100% oxygen through non-rebreather.
+ Hyperbaric oxygen may be used to treat patients with:
  - carboxyhemoglobin level greater than 25%
  - cardiopulmonary complications
  - loss of consciousness
  - severe metabolic acidosis

QUICK REVIEW QUESTION

4. A patient in the ED is diagnosed with carbon monoxide (CO) poisoning. The patient states that she had carbon monoxide monitors installed with the smoke detectors throughout her house, so this diagnosis can't be right. What education can the nurse provide to the patient regarding proper carbon monoxide detector placement?

Cyanide

Pathophysiology

Cyanide interferes with the production of ATP in mitochondria. **Cyanide poisoning** is rare but usually fatal without medical intervention. Sources of cyanide include smoke from fires, medications (e.g., sodium nitroprusside), and pits/seeds from the family Rosaceae (which includes bitter almonds, apricots, peaches, and apples).

Signs and Symptoms

+ bitter almond smell on breath
+ anxiety
+ agitation
+ headache

+ confusion
+ bloody emesis
+ diarrhea
+ flushed, red skin

- tachycardia
- tachypnea
- hypertension

- seizure
- hypovolemic shock
- coma

Treatment and Management

- Decontaminate patient.
- Administer 100% oxygen through a non-rebreather.
- Intubation is usually required.
- Administer IV fluids.
- Use activated charcoal if airway is not compromised.

- Cyanide antidotes include:
  - hydroxocobalamin
  - amyl nitrite
  - sodium nitrite
  - sodium thiosulfate

QUICK REVIEW QUESTION

5. Which situations in a patient's history should alert the ED nurse to the possibility of cyanide poisoning?

Overdose

Table 14.2 provides information about overdose for various substances.

Table 14.2. Managing Overdose: Various Substances

Substance	Signs and Symptoms	Treatment and Management	Nursing Considerations
Opioid	respiratory depression, shallow breathing, pinpoint pupils, cyanosis, bradycardia, emesis or gurgling, inability to be aroused	naltrexone, ET tube, mechanical ventilation	Observe respiration rate.
Acetaminophen	gastroenteritis, renal failure, pancreatitis, hepatotoxicity leading to multiple organ failure	N-acetylcysteine, activated charcoal	Rumack-Matthew nomogram needed for serum level lab work.
Benzodiazepine	nystagmus, miosis, altered LOC, respiratory depression	flumazenil, intubation, mechanical ventilation	Observe respiration rate; check gag reflex.
Salicylate	nausea and emesis; tinnitus; fever; confusion; seizures; rhabdomyolysis; acute renal failure; hyperventilation and respiratory alkalosis (early), hypoventilation and respiratory acidosis (late), respiratory failure; hyperactivity that can turn into lethargy	activated charcoal, alkaline diuresis with extra KCl, ET tube, mechanical ventilation	Expect to draw salicylate level and ABGs.
Calcium channel blockers	hyperglycemia, hypotension, bradycardia, reflexive tachycardia, peripheral edema, heart block	high-dose insulin, vasopressors, inotrope	Expect to run ECG, check blood pressure every 15 minutes, and monitor blood glucose.

Table 14.2. Managing Overdose: Various Substances (continued)

Substance	Signs and Symptoms	Treatment and Management	Nursing Considerations
Beta blockers	cardiac: bradycardia, hypotension, bronchospasms, prolonged Q–T interval, prolonged QRS complex, ventricular dysrhythmias, AV block GI: esophageal spasms, hyperkalemia, hypoglycemia	glucagon, dopamine, norepinephrine, ipratropium for patients with esophageal spasms	Run ECG and monitor blood glucose, blood pressure, and heart rate.
Digitalis	nausea, emesis, abdominal pain, headache, dizziness, confusion, delirium, blurred vision, halo vision, bradycardia, tachydysrythmias (paroxysmal atrial tachycardia with block most common)	digoxin immune fab, potassium supplementation, atropine in case of AV block or severe bradycardia, lidocaine or phenytoin to prevent cardioversion	ECG should be left on through treatment as hyperkalemia could lead to AV block.
Heavy metals	altered LOC, fatigue, muscle and joint pain, hypertension, constipation, nausea and emesis, renal failure, numbness and pain in extremities, anemia, dark eye circles, jaundice, rash, itching, hearing loss, insomnia, depression, mood swings Severe lead toxicity will lead to wrist drop, encephalopathy, colic, and Burton's line (blue-black line on the gums). Mercury poisoning can lead to "mad hatters disease," with signs and symptoms including slurred speech, irritability, and depression.	chelation therapy, dialysis	Most common are arsenic, cadmium, lead, and mercury. Mees' lines can be seen in heavy metal poisoning but can be indicative of many other conditions.
Iron	stage 1: GI upset, nausea, emesis, pain stage 2 (latent phase): milder GI upset stage 3: shock and metabolic acidosis, dehydration, lactic acid stage 4: hepatotoxicity, necrosis stage 5: bowel obstruction from GI healing leading to scarring	deferoxamine mesylate (DFO) for acute iron toxicity, intermittent phlebotomy for chronic iron toxicity from hemochromatosis	This is especially toxic in small children, usually after consumption of multiple iron tablets, and can be seen in patients who have had repeated blood transfusions.

Substance	Signs and Symptoms	Treatment and Management	Nursing Considerations
Oral hypoglycemic	mild: dizziness, lightheadedness, nausea severe: altered LOC, CNS depression, seizures, coma, hypokalemia, hypomagnesemia	sulfonylurea supplemented with octreotide if needed for GI symptoms, IV dextrose bolus followed by dextrose 10% continuous infusion	Check blood sugars before administering oral hypoglycemic medications to patients. Do not administer to patients with low blood sugar levels.
Warfarin	bloody, red, or black tarry stool; pink, red, or dark urine; spitting or coughing up blood; "coffee ground" emesis; hemorrhage	vitamin K	Monitor PT/INR.
Tricyclic antidepressants	blurred vision, dilated pupils, lethargy, change in LOC, hallucinations, hyperthermia, seizures, respiratory distress, hypotension, tachycardia, cardiac arrest	sodium bicarbonate, metoprolol as needed to correct cardiac dysrhythmias, benzodiazepines to treat or prevent seizures	Monitor cardiac rhythms and respiratory status.

QUICK REVIEW QUESTION

6. A patient presents in the ED with constricted pupils, slow and shallow breathing, confusion, and blue-toned skin. Based on the scene, EMS suspects an opioid overdose. What is the nursing priority for this patient?

ANSWER KEY

1. Inducing vomiting is contraindicated when a patient ingests a caustic agent. Causing regurgitation will re-expose the upper GI tract to the caustic agent.

2. The nurse should anticipate assessing the patient using the CIWA scale and administering medications per the ED's protocol.

3. The nurse should anticipate administering clonidine to the patient for hypertension and tachycardia.

4. Unlike smoke from fire, which is lighter than air and rises, carbon monoxide mixes with air. Due to this property, the best placement for a carbon monoxide meter is 5 feet off the ground. By the time there is enough carbon monoxide in a room to trigger an alarm placed on the ceiling, there are lethal levels of carbon monoxide in the room.

5. Nurses should consider cyanide toxicity when patients present to the ED after being around a fire: inhaled fumes from burning polymer products such as vinyl and polyurethane will produce cyanide poisoning. Cyanide toxicity can also be caused by a nitroprusside IV infusion.

6. Opioid overdose can quickly lead to respiratory distress. Administer oxygen and intubate and provide mechanical ventilation if needed.

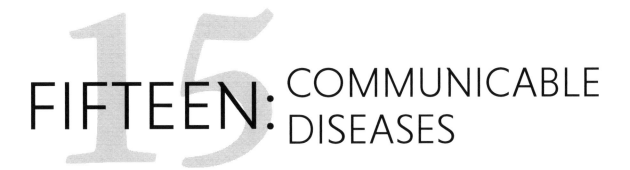

FIFTEEN: COMMUNICABLE DISEASES

Isolation Precautions

Purpose

Isolation precautions are used to prevent the spread of infection. The precautions are guidelines set by organizations like the World Health Organization (WHO) and the Centers for Disease Control (CDC) to prevent the transmission of microorganisms that are responsible for causing infection. There are two tiers of isolation precautions: the first tier is standard precautions, and the second tier consists of three transmission precautions (airborne, droplet, and contact).

Standard Precautions

+ Assume that all patients are carrying a microorganism.
+ Use **personal protective equipment (PPE)**.
    ✧ gloves
    ✧ mask
    ✧ gown
    ✧ protective eye wear
+ Practice hand hygiene.
    ✧ Use soap and water when hands are visibly soiled.
    ✧ Antimicrobial foam or gel may be used if hands are not visibly soiled.
+ Wear gloves.
    ✧ Gloves must be discarded between each patient.
    ✧ Gloves may need to be discarded when soiled and a new pair applied.
    ✧ Practice hand hygiene after removing gloves.
+ Prevent needle sticks.
    ✧ Immediately place used needles in puncture-resistant containers.
    ✧ Recap using mechanical device or one-handed technique.
+ Avoid splash and spray.
    ✧ Wear appropriate PPE if there is a possibility of body fluids splashing or spraying.

Airborne Precautions

+ Patient should be placed in a private room with a negative-pressure air system and the door kept closed.

+ Wear N95 respirator mask; place on before entering the room and keep on until after leaving the room.

+ Place N95 or surgical mask on patient during transport.

Droplet Precautions

+ Place patient in a private room; the door may remain open.

+ Wear appropriate PPE within 3 feet of patient.

+ Wash hands with antimicrobial soap after removing gloves and mask, before leaving the patient's room.

+ Place surgical mask on patient during transport.

Contact Precautions

+ Place the patient in a private room; the door may remain open.

+ Wear gloves.
    ⋄ Change gloves after touching infected materials.
    ⋄ Remove gloves before leaving patient's room.

+ Wear gown; remove before leaving patient's room.

+ Practice hand hygiene.
    ⋄ Use soap and water when hands are visibly soiled.
    ⋄ Antimicrobial foam or gel may be used if hands are not visibly soiled.

+ Use patient-dedicated equipment if possible; community equipment is to be used clean and disinfected between patients.

+ During transport keep precautions in place and notify different areas as needed.

C. Difficile

Pathophysiology

Clostridium difficile (commonly called **C. diff**) is an acute bacterial infection in the intestine most commonly seen after antibiotic use. The antibiotics disrupt the normal intestinal flora, allowing the antibiotic-resistant C. *diff* spores to proliferate in the intestines. The bacterium releases a toxin that causes the intestine to produce yellow-white plaques on the intestinal lining.

The C. *diff* infection can produce inflammation in the intestines, resulting in toxic colitis (toxic megacolon) or pseudomembranous colitis, and may also lead to perforation and sepsis.

Transmission

+ fecal to oral
  - touching feces
  - touching surfaces soiled with feces

Precautions

+ Use contact precautions.
+ Practice hand hygiene.
  - Wash hands using soap and warm water.
  - Do not use foams and gels (they will not kill the spores).
+ CDC recommends an environmental cleanse of a 1:10 bleach-to-water solution.
+ Proton inhibitors and H2 blockers have both been shown to be risk factors for *C. diff* infection.

Signs and Symptoms

+ diarrhea:
  - 5 – 10 days after start of antibiotic
  - foul smelling
  - sometimes bloody
+ abdominal pain

+ in patients who develop toxic colitis:
  - tachycardia
  - abdominal distension and tenderness
+ peritoneal signs and symptoms if perforation of the bowel occurs

Diagnostic Tests and Findings

+ Collect a stool specimen.
+ Enzyme immunoassay (EIA) is the most commonly run diagnostic test.
  - results in 3 hours
+ Polymerase chain reaction (PCR) test can be run on the stool specimen.
  - most sensitive and specific diagnostic test
  - results in 1 hour

Treatment and Management

+ For antibiotic-induced *C. diff*, stop current use of antibiotics if possible.
+ May need to be treated with antibiotics.
  - oral antibiotics
  - IV if oral antibiotics cannot be tolerated
  - metronidazole (Flagyl)
  - vancomycin (Vancocin)
  - fidaxomicin (Dificid)

+ Probiotics may be prescribed.
+ In refractory or severe cases:
  - fecal transplant
  - colectomy

QUICK REVIEW QUESTION

1.   A patient is admitted to the ED with a suspected *C. difficile* infection. What PPE should the nurse use?

Childhood Diseases

MEASLES

Pathophysiology

Measles is an acute infection caused by a paramyxovirus. The virus enters through the upper respiratory tract or conjunctiva and spreads systemically through the lymph nodes, triggering a systemic inflammatory response.

Transmission

+ person to person through respiratory droplets:
    ⋄ coughing
    ⋄ sneezing
+ can live in the air or on hard surfaces for up to 2 hours

Precautions

+ airborne precautions
+ droplet precautions
+ contact precautions

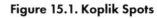

Figure 15.1. Koplik Spots

Signs and Symptoms

+ fever
+ cough
+ runny nose
+ conjunctivitis
+ sore throat
+ Koplik spots
+ rash:
    ⋄ cephalocaudal; usually starts behind the ears
    ⋄ irregular macules
    ⋄ causes itching
+ photophobia
+ in immunocompromised patients:
    ⋄ no rash
    ⋄ severe, progressive giant-cell pneumonia
+ complications:
    ⋄ subacute sclerosing panencephalitis
    ⋄ encephalitis
    ⋄ acute thrombocytopenic purpura
    ⋄ bacterial superinfection
    ⋄ transient hepatitis

Diagnostic Tests and Findings

+ swab of cheek saliva, saliva sample, or blood sample:
    ⋄ swab, saliva, or blood samples tested for measles-specific immunoglobulin M (IgM)
    ⋄ IgM present in the blood for up to 6 weeks after onset of disease

- test blood sample for IgM antibodies using ELISA or EIA
- test urine sample for the virus or IgM

Treatment and Management

- Provide supportive care for symptoms.
- Administer vitamin A.

QUICK REVIEW QUESTION

2. The nurse is assigned to a patient who has a positive diagnosis of measles. What PPE should the nurse wear?

MUMPS

Pathophysiology

Mumps is an acute infection caused by a paramyxovirus. The virus enters the nose or mouth and replicates in the respiratory tract, GI tract, or eyes. The viral replication causes an inflammatory response that results in swelling of the salivary glands (usually the parotid glands).

Transmission

- person to person through respiratory droplets in close proximity:
  - coughing
  - sneezing

Precautions

- droplet precautions

Signs and Symptoms

- after incubation period (12 – 24 days):
  - headache
  - low-grade fever
  - anorexia
  - fatigue
- 12 – 24 hours after symptoms begin:
  - salivary gland edema
  - fever for 24 – 48 hours
  - parotitis
  - pain when chewing or swallowing, especially acidic beverages or food
  - submandibular glands may swell, causing edema below the jawline
  - tongue may swell

- complications in prepubescent patients:
  - orchitis or oophoritis
  - meningitis or encephalitis
  - pancreatitis

Diagnostic Tests and Findings

+ serological assay (EIA) on blood sample to detect IgM

+ RT–PCR (real-time–polymerase chain reaction) on the blood sample to detect viral mumps RNA

Treatment and Management

+ Supportive care includes:
  ⋄ soft diet
  ⋄ avoidance of acidic substances

+ Isolate until glandular swelling is gone.

QUICK REVIEW QUESTION

3. A nurse is assessing a patient and notes a temperature of 102°F (38.9°C) and swelling in the patient's neck under the jawline. The patient also reports that their throat burned this morning when they drank their orange juice. Which diagnostic test should the nurse anticipate will be ordered?

PERTUSSIS

Pathophysiology

Pertussis, also known as whooping cough, is an infection caused by the bacterium *Bordetella pertussis*. The infection causes a mucopurulent sanguineous exudate that can compromise the respiratory tract. The bacterium infects the respiratory system, initially producing nonspecific upper respiratory infection symptoms. The infection then progresses to a hallmark paroxysmal or spasmodic cough, known as the "whoop," that ends in a prolonged, high-pitched inspiration.

Transmission

+ person-to-person in close proximity through respiratory droplets:
  ⋄ talking or singing
  ⋄ sneezing
  ⋄ coughing

Precautions

+ droplet precautions

Signs and Symptoms

+ catarrhal stage:
  ⋄ sneezing
  ⋄ watery eyes
+ paroxysmal stage (after 10 – 14 days):
  ⋄ cough increases in severity and occurrence
  ⋄ increase in mucus
  ⋄ nausea and vomiting

  ⋄ nocturnal cough
  ⋄ hoarseness

  ⋄ rapid bouts of coughing followed by hallmark "whoop"
  ⋄ choking spells in infants

- convalescent stage (4 weeks following onset):
  - paroxysmal cough
  - sensitive respiratory tract

Diagnostic Tests and Findings

- nose or throat swab tested for the presence of pertussis bacterium:
  - most commonly used
- PCR test run on the swab:
  - preferred as it is the most sensitive

Treatment and Management

- Administer antibiotics:
  - erythromycin
  - azithromycin (Zithromax)
- Supportive care includes:
  - suctioning in infants
  - tracheostomy or nasotracheal intubation needed in emergent severe cases

QUICK REVIEW QUESTION

4. A mother brings her 2-year-old into the ED with complaints of a persistent cough and hoarseness. What tests should the nurse anticipate to determine if the child has pertussis?

CHICKEN POX

Pathophysiology

The **varicella zoster virus**, also known as **chicken pox**, is highly contagious. Inhaled contaminated droplets infect the conjunctiva or the mucous membranes of the upper respiratory tract. The viral infection then spreads, causing the hallmark rash of small, itchy, fluid-filled blisters all over the body.

Transmission

- person-to-person through direct contact
- person-to-person through airborne droplets

Precautions

- airborne precautions
- droplet precautions
- contact precautions

Signs and Symptoms

- rash:
  - itchy rash that forms small fluid-filled blisters that eventually scab
  - first appears on face and trunk and then can spread to the rest of the body

+ mild headache

+ moderate fever

+ fatigue

+ more severe complications in immunocompromised patients:
    ⋄ secondary bacterial infection, including cellulitis, necrosis, and streptococcal toxic shock
    ⋄ pneumonia
    ⋄ myocarditis
    ⋄ hepatitis
    ⋄ cerebellar ataxia
    ⋄ transverse myelitis
    ⋄ encephalitis

Diagnostic Tests and Findings

+ varicella titer test on a blood sample

+ Tzanck test performed on a swab sample of the lesion area
    ⋄ positive for chicken pox or herpes zoster

Treatment and Management

+ In mild cases:
    ⋄ symptomatic treatment aimed at stopping itching
    ⋄ systemic antihistamines
    ⋄ colloidal oatmeal baths
    ⋄ no aspirin for pediatric patients

+ In immunocompromised patients or more severe cases:
    ⋄ antivirals:
        + valacyclovir (Valtrex)
        + famciclovir (Famvir)
        + acyclovir (Zovirax)
        + IV for immunocompromised patients
        + oral for more severe cases

QUICK REVIEW QUESTION

5. The nurse is preparing to discharge a 2-year-old patient diagnosed with chicken pox. What information about OTC medications should the nurse include in his teaching?

DIPHTHERIA

Pathophysiology

Diphtheria is an infection caused by the bacterium *Corynebacterium diphtheriae*. The bacterium gains entry through the pharynx or the skin and releases a toxin that causes inflammation and necrosis of the infected area. In the pharynx it initially causes a white, glossy exudate that progresses to tough fibers that adhere themselves to the epithelial lining of the pharynx. Removal of the fibers will cause bleeding. Infection in the skin causes a variety of appearances that are often hard to distinguish from other chronic skin conditions.

Transmission

+ person-to-person through respiratory droplets for pharyngeal infection:
    - coughing
    - sneezing
+ person-to-person skin contact for skin infection

Precautions

+ droplet precautions
+ contact precautions

Signs and Symptoms

+ pharyngeal infection:
    - white or gray glossy exudate in the back of the throat
    - mild sore throat
    - serosanguinous or purulent discharge
    - difficulty swallowing or getting food stuck in throat
    - hoarseness
    - edema, visibly swollen neck (bull neck)
    - stridor
    - low-grade fever
    - tachycardia
    - nausea and vomiting
    - chills
    - headache
+ skin infection:
    - often indistinguishable from symptoms that look like a variety of chronic skin diseases
    - pain and tenderness
    - numbness possible when high amounts of toxins are present
+ more serious symptoms with high amounts of toxins:
    - severe prostration
    - pallor
    - tachycardia
    - acute renal failure
    - stupor
    - coma
+ main critical symptoms that can develop:
    - myocarditis:
        + complete heart block
        + ventricular arrhythmias
        + atrioventricular dissociation
        + heart failure
    - nervous system toxicity:
        + demyelinating polyneuropathy affecting cranial and peripheral nerves
        + loss of ocular accommodation
        + bulbar palsy
        + diaphragm paralysis

Diagnostic Tests and Findings

+ pharyngeal infection:
    - swab of the pharyngeal area:
        + a metachromatic (beaded) gram stain of specimen from the swab
        + gram-positive bacilli found in patients with diphtheria

- skin infection:
  - swab or biopsy of skin from rash area
    - a metachromatic (beaded) gram stain of swab
    - gram-positive bacilli found in patients with diphtheria

Treatment and Management

- For pharyngeal infection:
  - Administer diphtheria antitoxin (IM or IV).
  - Administer antibiotics:
    - penicillin
    - erythromycin
    - IM or IV until oral can be tolerated
- For skin infection:
  - Clean area with soap and water.
  - Administer antibiotics.
    - penicillin
    - erythromycin

- Serial ECGs are performed if myocarditis is suspected.
- Diphtheria vaccination is given after recovery.
- Close contacts should receive antibiotics.
- Close contacts should receive vaccinations if not previously vaccinated.

QUICK REVIEW QUESTION

6. The nurse is discharging a 4-year-old patient diagnosed with diphtheria. What instructions should she provide to the parents about vaccinations?

Herpes Zoster

Pathophysiology

Herpes zoster, more commonly known as **shingles**, is an acute viral infection that is the result of the varicella zoster virus reactivating in a posterior dorsal root ganglion. The varicella zoster virus initially infects most patients as children during an episode of chicken pox. In adulthood, the virus comes out of latency and inflames the sensory root ganglion, the dermatome, and the skin associated with the dermatome.

Transmission

- contact with fluid from blisters caused by rash
- having had chicken pox

Precautions

- before blisters appear and after blisters are completely dry and crusted:
  - Take standard precautions.
  - Completely cover lesions.

+ before blisters are completely dry and crusted:
    ◇ Take contact precautions.
    ◇ Take airborne precautions.

Signs and Symptoms

+ redness and rash of blisters:
    ◇ usually occur in a linear fashion on one side of the body
    ◇ usually appear in the truncal area
    ◇ typically scab over in 7 – 10 days (blisters)
    ◇ clears in 2 – 4 weeks (rash)

+ pain:
    ◇ sharp, burning sensation
    ◇ tingling
+ itching

Diagnostic Tests and Findings

+ Diagnosis is based on symptoms of characteristic painful rash that follows a dermatomal distribution.
+ Tzanck test can be performed on a swab sample of the lesion area.
    ◇ positive for chicken pox or herpes zoster
+ Blood sample can tested through PCR.

Treatment and Management

+ Administer oral or IV antivirals.
    ◇ acyclovir (Zovirax)
    ◇ famciclovir (Famvir)
    ◇ valacyclovir (Valtrex)
+ Blister areas can be treated with a wet compress.
+ Patient should see an ophthalmologist immediately if the virus is suspected in the eye.

+ Pain can be treated:
    ◇ systemically with gabapentin (Neurontin) or cyclic antidepressants
    ◇ locally with topical capsaicin or xylocaine (Lidocaine) ointment

QUICK REVIEW QUESTION

7. A topical analgesic has been applied to a patient with shingles, but the patient still complains of pain. What medication should the nurse expect to administer to the patient?

Mononucleosis

Pathophysiology

Mononucleosis, commonly known as mono, is an infection caused by the Epstein-Barr virus. The virus replicates in the epithelial cells of the pharynx and in B lymphocytes, triggering a response from the body's immune system. Mono is common in children and presents with mild symptoms. Symptoms can be more severe in young and older adults.

Transmission

+ body secretions
+ most commonly transmitted through saliva during kissing
+ transfusion of blood products

Precautions

+ contact precautions

Signs and Symptoms

+ fatigue lasting from a few weeks to months
+ fever
+ pharyngitis
+ palatal petechiae
+ lymphadenopathy
+ airway obstruction
+ adenopathy
  ✧ posterior cervical
  ✧ auricular
  ✧ inguinal
+ splenic rupture

Diagnostic Tests and Findings

+ Collect blood sample for mononuclear spot test (usually Monospot).
+ Due to risk of splenic rupture, avoid deep pressure palpation of the abdomen.

Treatment and Management

+ Provide supportive care.
+ Administer corticosteroids for severe symptoms, such as airway obstruction.
+ Teach patient at discharge:
  ✧ Rest.
  ✧ Avoid heavy lifting and contact sports for 1 month or until splenomegaly resolves.

QUICK REVIEW QUESTION

8. A patient arrives at the ED with symptoms of mononucleosis. What should the nurse avoid while assessing the patient?

Multi-Drug-Resistant Organisms

MRSA

Pathophysiology

Methicillin-resistant *Staphylococcus aureus* (MRSA) is a bacterial infection caused by a strain of *Staphylococcus* ("staph") that is resistant to many of the antibiotics normally used to treat staph infections, beta-lactam agents including ampicillin, amoxicillin, methicillin, penicillin, and cephalosporin. MRSA can be hospital acquired (HA-MRSA) or community acquired (CA-MRSA). MRSA can spread to the lungs, heart, bloodstream, and joints.

Transmission

+ hospital acquired:
    ✧ invasive procedures or devices
    ✧ IV insertion
    ✧ IV tubing
    ✧ surgery
    ✧ artificial joints

+ community acquired:
    ✧ cuts
    ✧ abrasion
    ✧ skin-to-skin contact

Precautions

+ contact precautions

Signs and Symptoms

+ red area on the skin
+ swelling
+ pain

+ warm to the touch
+ pus or drainage from bumps on skin
+ fever

Diagnostic Tests and Findings

+ tissue sample of area suspected of MRSA or nasal swab:
    ✧ Swab is cultured and tested for the presence of the MRSA bacterium.

Treatment and Management

+ Administer antibiotics:
    ✧ oral for skin infections
    ✧ IV therapy if infection advances
    ✧ trimethoprim (Primsol)

    ✧ sulfamethoxazole (Bactrim)
    ✧ clindamycin (Cleocin)
    ✧ linezolid (Zyvox)

QUICK REVIEW QUESTION

9. Which antibiotics should NOT be used to treat patients with methicillin-resistant *Staphylococcus aureus* (MRSA)?

VRE

Pathophysiology

Vancomycin-resistant enterococci (VRE) is a bacterial infection caused by strains of enterococci bacteria that are resistant to vancomycin. Enterococci are normal flora in the intestinal tract that are commonly associated with skin infections or cellulitis, UTIs, sepsis, endocarditis, meningitis, intra-abdominal infections, pelvic infections, and infections in wounds.

Transmission

+ person-to-person physical contact

+ touching contaminated objects

Precautions

+ contact precautions

Signs and Symptoms

+ varied symptoms depending on location of infection
+ infected wounds:
  - red
  - warm to touch
  - painful
  - swollen
  - may have pus or drainage
+ pneumonia:
  - fever
  - cough
  - dyspnea
+ UTI:
  - increased urination
  - burning on urination
  - back pain
  - fever

+ meningitis:
  - headache
  - confusion
  - stiff neck
  - fever
+ sepsis:
  - fever
  - tachycardia
  - nausea and vomiting
  - diarrhea

Diagnostic Tests and Findings

+ peri-rectal or anal swabs, stool sample, or swab of infected area:
  - Sample is swabbed on auger in a petri dish containing vancomycin.
  - Growth of black bacteria on the plate indicates positive result.

Treatment and Management

+ Send samples to lab for culture and sensitivity.
  - Lab identifies which antibiotics the VRE may be sensitive to.
+ Administer antibiotics.
  - amoxicillin
  - ampicillin
  - gentamicin
  - penicillin
  - piperacillin
  - streptomycin
+ Treat skin infections with:
  - daptomycin (Cubicin)
  - linezolid
  - tedizolid (Sivextro)
  - tigecycline (Tygacil)
+ Treat intra-abdominal infections with:
  - piperacillin-tazobactam (Zosyn)
  - imipenem (Primaxin)
  - meropenem (Merrem)

> ## QUICK REVIEW QUESTION
>
> **10.** Why is it not advised to use alcohol-based wipes on equipment and hard surfaces in the room of a patient with VRE?

Tuberculosis

Pathophysiology

Tuberculosis (TB) is a chronic, progressive bacterial infection of the lungs. There is an initial asymptomatic infection followed by a period of latency that may develop into active disease. Active TB produces granulomatous necrosis, more commonly known as lesions. The rupturing of the lesions in the pleural space can cause empyema, bronchopleural fistulas, or a pneumothorax.

Transmission

+ person-to-person through respiratory droplets:
  - coughing
  - sneezing
+ induction of sputum by medical staff

Precautions

+ airborne precautions

Signs and Symptoms

+ prolonged productive cough
+ fever
+ anorexia or weight loss
+ fatigue
+ night sweats
+ hemoptysis
+ dyspnea

Diagnostic Tests and Findings

+ TB skin test (Mantoux skin test):
    ✧ Positive results indicate patient is infected.
    ✧ Tests do not distinguish latent TB infection from active TB disease.
+ chest X-ray showing multinodular infiltrate near the clavicle
+ sputum sample:
    ✧ Sample is placed on slide and checked for acid-fast bacilli.
    ✧ Sample can also be cultured to isolate TB bacterium.

Treatment and Management

+ Begin with 2 months of treatment with:
    ✧ isoniazid (INH)
    ✧ rifampin (RIF)
    ✧ pyrazinamide (PZA)
    ✧ ethambutol (EMB)
+ After 2 months of treatment, PZA and EMB are discontinued. INH and RIF are continued for another 4 – 7 months or longer, depending on clinical findings and symptoms.

QUICK REVIEW QUESTION

11. A patient in the ED complains of a cough that has lasted for several weeks and also states that they have been waking up at night covered in sweat. Which diagnostic test should the nurse prepare for?

ANSWER KEY

1. *C. difficile* requires contact protections, so the nurse should use gloves and an isolation gown.

2. The nurse should use an N95 respirator in addition to gloves.

3. The nurse should anticipate drawing a blood sample for lab testing to confirm mumps.

4. The diagnostic tests for pertussis include nasopharyngeal culture and PCR testing. The PCR test is preferred because it is the most sensitive.

5. The nurse should tell the parents not to give aspirin to a child with chicken pox. Aspirin increases these children's risk of developing Reye's syndrome, a life-threatening encephalopathy linked to viral infections and aspirin use.

6. The patient will need to be given the diphtheria vaccine once he has recovered. The parents should make sure that anyone who comes in close contact with the child also has an up-to-date diphtheria vaccine.

7. The nurse should expect to administer gabapentin, which treats neuropathic pain.

8. The nurse should avoid deep abdominal palpation due to the risk of splenic rupture in patients with mononucleosis.

9. MRSA is resistant to beta-lactam agents, including ampicillin, amoxicillin, methicillin, penicillin, and cephalosporin.

10. Alcohol-based wipes are not sufficient to kill the bacteria that cause VRE on equipment and hard surfaces. Germicidal wipes should be used instead.

11. The nurse should prepare the patient for a chest X-ray to confirm tuberculosis.

SIXTEEN: PROFESSIONAL ISSUES

Nurse

CRITICAL INCIDENT STRESS MANAGEMENT

+ **Critical incidents** are sudden and unexpected events that can impact an individual or group in such a way that it overwhelms the ability of the individual or group to cope, resulting in significant psychological distress.

+ **Critical incident stress management (CISM)** programs are comprehensive, with the goal of helping personnel return to a baseline state of emotional health. There are several components to a CISM system:

  - precrisis preparation
  - demobilization and consultation
  - defusing
  - critical incident stress debriefing

  - crisis intervention
  - family CISM
  - follow-up

+ Debriefing is a key element to CISM, and can occur immediately after the event, or as soon as it is possible to assemble all key players (up to 14 days later).

  - provides perspective and closure for staff involved
  - prevents personal feelings of blame or responsibility

  - opens discussion for improvement for future events

QUICK REVIEW QUESTION

1. A charge nurse in the ED notices that a new nurse in the department is withdrawn, quiet, and struggling to keep up with tasks in her assignment. The charge knows this nurse experienced her first pediatric resuscitation on the previous shift, and there was a poor outcome. What can the charge do to help this nurse?

ETHICAL DILEMMAS

+ **Ethical dilemmas** are situations that require healthcare providers to balance competing ethical principles; such situations are present in all areas of healthcare. Ethical dilemmas that occur in the emergency department include decisional capacity determination, medical futility considerations, and refusals of care.

+ **Decisional capacity** relates to the expectation that patients have a responsibility to participate in their own care, whenever able. Decisional capacity is fluid and can change based on the patient's presentation and status throughout emergency care. In some cases, decreased decisional capacity can be reversed.

  ❖ **Diminished decisional capacity** can be due to several factors:

  + alcohol intoxication
  + trauma
  + sedation
  + extreme stress
  + hypoxia
  + developmental delay

  ❖ Assessment of decisional capacity is based on the patient's:

  + ability to provide an accurate and detailed medical history
  + cooperation with the physical evaluation
  + understanding of the recommended treatments

  ❖ If decisional capacity is determined to be diminished, a surrogate or medical power of attorney may be used.

  ❖ In cases of acute emergency, when there is no time to obtain consent from the patient, implied consent is understood. Implied consent is the assumption that a rational human being wants to live as long as possible.

+ **Medical futility** refers to medical interventions in emergency situations that are not likely to result in significant positive outcomes for the patient. Interventions that are futile are characterized as ones that maintain permanent states of unconsciousness.

  ❖ In the ED setting, there are some interventions that are carried out automatically, even in the absence of a medical history.

  + CPR
  + fluid resuscitation (blood products in the presence of hemorrhagic shock)
  + intubation and ventilation in respiratory distress or arrest

  ❖ If a case of futility is questioned, the ED healthcare team should act in line with the standard ethical principles for medical and nursing practice. If there is time, an ethics committee can be convened to assist with decision-making in cases such as these.

+ Patients who are deemed to have intact decisional capacity have the **right to refuse any and all care.** The responsibility of the ED nurse is to provide the patient with as much information as they can to allow the patient to make an informed decision to refuse care. This applies to surrogates or family members responsible for making care decisions as well.

  ❖ **Leaving against medical advice (AMA)** is when a patient requests to leave the care of the emergency physician and depart the ED. If the patient chooses to do so, the physician will counsel the patient on the risks of such a departure, and then ask the patient to provide a signature acknowledging these risks.

  ❖ **Involuntary commitment** is a legal process under which a physician determines that a patient is unsafe to themselves or others and requires close observation under medical care for the sake of safety. State laws govern involuntary commitment and should be reviewed prior to involuntarily committing a patient to care.

+ Decisions in these cases are made based on the ethical principles of autonomy, beneficence, non-maleficence, justice, and veracity.

- **Autonomy**: Recognition that a patient is a unique individual with the right to have their own opinions, values, beliefs, and perspectives. Nurses advocate for patients without judgment, coercion, or assertion of the nurse's own beliefs or values.
- **Beneficence**: Acting with the intent of doing good or the right thing. This principle addresses the obligation to act in the best interest of the patient when there may be other competing interests.
- **Non-maleficence**: "Do no harm." This principle relates to the nurse's responsibility to protect the public and the patient from harm in the context of the care setting.
- **Justice**: Provision of equitable access to care. This principle covers providing care to all patients regardless of socioeconomic status, insurance coverage, or any other demographic category.
- **Veracity**: The practice of complete truthfulness with patients and families.

QUICK REVIEW QUESTION

2. An adult patient arrives at the ED with evidence of polytrauma, and CPR is in progress. The emergency physician and trauma surgeon disagree on the futility of further intervention. How can the charge nurse help address the situation?

EVIDENCE-BASED PRACTICE

+ **Evidence-based practice (EBP)** is the use of high-quality research outcomes to inform clinical practice. EBP is typically implemented through the establishment of a **clinical practice guideline (CPG)**, either at the local organization or professional association (such as the Emergency Nurses Association) level.
  - EBP is developed based on a combination of research data and evidence and clinical experience meeting the needs of a specific organization.
  - Nurses have a responsibility to practice with the most up-to-date evidence guiding them. However, implementation of such practice is not done on an individual basis and should be a collaborative effort within the disciplines of healthcare.
+ There are many types of research. The following types are listed in order of the value of the evidence that comes from them. The first listed are generally recognized as providing the highest level of evidence and are therefore the most useful in the EBP implementation process.
  - Systematic reviews and meta-analysis (quantitative) are the most reliable sources of evidence, and practice policies or guidelines can be based on them.
  - Randomized controlled trials (quantitative) are used in medical research more often than in nursing research, but they are the standard method when studying very specific interventions, such as in pharmacological research.
  - Cohort studies (quantitative) compare two groups of subjects, one with and one without a certain characteristic, over time. Comparisons are made in order to predict the outcomes based on demographic and other variables.
  - Qualitative studies collect the thoughts, feelings, and perspectives of patients concerning a topic; the results are then used to inform practice.
  - Case studies are presentations of interesting patient cases, typically written by providers.
+ There are steps to implementing research into EBP. Two models used for such implementation are the Iowa and Stetler models.

- The **Iowa Model** is a seven-step process: identifying a problem, forming a team, collecting evidence, grading the evidence, creating a CPG, implementing it, and evaluating it.
- The **Stetler Model** is a five-step process: preparation, validation, comparative evaluation, translation, and evaluation.

QUICK REVIEW QUESTION

3. An ED nurse is noted to have tried new nursing interventions that are not in the current local CPG. When approached, the nurse says, "I read an article that said this improves patient outcomes." Why were these actions inappropriate?

RESEARCH

- Emergency nurses who choose to read research studies to inform their personal practice must know how to identify reliable sources of evidence. An assessment should be done on each article read to determine if it is valid and reliable. Consider the following questions:
  - Is the evidence recent, published within the last 5 – 7 years?
  - Was it carried out in an ethical, legal manner?
  - Was the design appropriate for the research question?
  - Was the population chosen appropriate to the research question?
  - Was the sample size adequate?
  - Was a literature review performed?
  - If instruments were used, were they validated?
  - Do the findings address the current clinical problem?

- Nursing research conducted in EDs must follow all ethical and legal regulations in order to be done reliably and correctly. Emergency nurses interested in performing research typically follow a continuum of nursing research.
  - understand research concepts
  - critique research for use in practice
  - systematically review the literature on a topic
  - participate in clinical-practice change projects
  - participate in a research study
  - act as primary investigator in a nursing research study

QUICK REVIEW QUESTION

4. How can emergency nurses demonstrate interest in the research process and join a research protocol in the agency?

LIFELONG LEARNING

- Emergency nursing is a specialty practice that must be promoted within the overall profession of nursing. Professional nursing associations advance their mission and vision statements and establish standards of professional practice.

- **Certification** in the specialty demonstrates a commitment to the profession and to lifelong learning and growth within the discipline.

- Earning **continuing education** credits demonstrates current practice knowledge and is often required for licensure and recertification in the specialty. Examples of continuing education activity include:
  - conference attendance
  - webinar participation
  - lunch-and-learn participation
  - grand rounds presentations
  - higher-level nursing education (BSN, MSN, DNP, PhD)

QUICK REVIEW QUESTION

5. How can an emergency nurse demonstrate continuing education to licensing bodies and to prospective employers?

Patient

DISCHARGE PLANNING AND TRANSITIONS OF CARE

- **Discharge planning** in the setting of the ED generally consists of arranging for follow-up care either with primary care services or specialty care consultations. Patients discharged from the ED are considered stable and should not require extensive discharge planning services.
  - Emergency nurses can offer community resources to patients who are homeless or otherwise require community or state assistance, but this should not prevent discharge from the ED of an otherwise healthy patient.
  - Resources may be available through social work or case management within the hospital or agency.
- **Transition of care** is the process of moving patients from one care setting to another.
  - Key considerations for transitions of care include:
    - accessibility of services
    - information sharing and communication
    - community partnerships
    - care coordination
    - health care utilization and costs
    - safety
  - The flow of information from emergency care back to primary and follow-up care must be considered.
  - **Care coordination**—the organization of patient care activities between two medical entities (ED and primary care, community care, etc.)—is ideal.
- As EDs continue to act as the safety net of the US healthcare system, patients seeking care for issues better served in primary care will continue to present to departments. Well-executed care coordination will, over time, decrease over-reliance on ED and urgent care settings, and support the shift toward preventative medicine.

QUICK REVIEW QUESTION

6. What is the role of the emergency nurse in the transition of care for patients seen in the ED?

+ **Organ and tissue donation** is an important step in end-of-life care in the ED. When a patient dies, there is only a short window of time in which to arrange for donation; certain steps are required to do so successfully.

+ Typically, the organ and tissue procurement agency is called for every death in the ED to determine if the patient is eligible for procurement.

+ This should be done no matter what the known preference of the patient is. Often, the agency will speak with family members to discuss if they are willing to consider donating their loved one's tissue.

+ The steps to successful procurement are as follows:

  ◇ **Determination of death**, followed by **declaration of death**. Brain death is generally declared if there are fixed pupils, an absence of reflexes in the brain stem, or no respiratory effort, or if tests have confirmed the absence of perfusion or electrical activity in the brain tissue.

  ◇ **Medical examiner review and approval.** Depending on the mechanism of the patient's death, the medical examiner may need to grant approval for organ procurement. (This requirement is governed by state laws and may vary.) Examples of such situations include:

    + suicide
    + homicide
    + accidental death
    + pediatric death
    + death after admission to hospital or long-term care facility

  ◇ **Notification of local organ procurement organization.** The procurement organization should be called in every event.

  ◇ **Review of patient consent or wishes.** There are circumstances in which the patient's wishes are clear, such as in advance directives, a will, or indication on the driver's license. In these cases, no further consent is needed. If the patient's preference is unclear, the legal next of kin must provide consent.

+ The process of organ procurement can be a long one due to these steps and other factors.

  ◇ Care of the patient awaiting procurement must consider the preservation of tissues. The following parameters are preferred (in the case of patients in a vegetative state but still functionally alive).

    + Maintain intravascular volume when possible.
    + Maintain vital signs within normal limits to include temperature.
    + Promote diuresis if possible.
    + Manage tissue oxygenation and acid-base balance.

  ◇ If the patient is not in a vegetative state, but tissue is still eligible for donation (eye donors) follow these parameters:

    + Maintain the head of the bed at 20 degrees.
    + Instill artificial tears or saline to preserve tissue.
    + Tape eyes closed using paper tape, and place compresses over eyes to deter swelling.

QUICK REVIEW QUESTION

7. A patient has been declared brain dead in the ED, but is still hemodynamically stable via mechanical ventilation. What steps should the nurse take following the declaration of brain death?

ADVANCE DIRECTIVES

+ **Advance directives** are written statements of individuals' wishes with regard to medical treatment decisions such as resuscitation, intubation, and other interventions. They are made to ensure the wishes of the individual are carried out in the event the person is unable to express those wishes at the time of care.

+ They are used to provide answers to difficult questions or decisions needing to be made in the context of end-of-life care. States and organizations may have policies that guide the establishment and use of advance directives.

+ Advance directives must be valid, up to date, and documented before they can be honored in the ED. In order to honor an advance directive, the physician must see the paperwork, validate the paperwork, and place an order that indicates the advance directive status of the patient.

+ Advance directives generally dictate the level of life-saving measures taken in certain circumstances.
    + **Do not resuscitate (DNR)** typically indicates that no heroic measures should be taken to sustain the patient's life.
    + **Do not intubate (DNI)** indicates that the patient does not wish to be intubated if the need presents.
    + **Allow natural death (AND)** indicates the patient does not want any intervention that may sustain life or prevent a natural progression to death.

+ Any combination of DNR, DNI, and AND may be requested, and other requests may be present in the documentation if applicable to the patient's circumstance.

+ DNR, DNI, and AND all allow for palliative care and comfort measures.

+ **Living wills** are also used in situations where a patient may have a terminal illness or is acutely in a vegetative state.
    + Living wills allow an individual to state which treatments they would like in the event they are unable to express such at the time of illness.
    + The document must be present and valid in order to be applied to care in the ED.

+ **Durable powers of attorney** or **medical powers of attorney** may also be used in situations at the end of life.
    + A power of attorney designates an individual to make decisions in place of the patient when the patient does not have the capacity to do so. It may be general or very specific in the range of decisions this surrogate can make.
    + It must be present and valid in order to be used for decisions in care.

+ Decisions to withhold, withdraw, or transition to palliative care are typically made before or after an ED visit. The ED is not the ideal place to make decisions of this nature.

+ If circumstances present that necessitate such decisions, conformity to living wills, advance directives, and powers of attorney must occur.

+ In the absence of legal documentation to guide such decisions, a multidisciplinary approach should be taken to inform patients and families of options for these decisions. Teams that should be involved in the decision include:
    + emergency physicians
    + social workers
    + chaplains
    + ethics committee
    + legal advisors
    + intensivist/critical care physician
    + specialty consultation if appropriate

FAMILY PRESENCE

+ Family presence in the ED, particularly during procedures or resuscitation, is a complex and controversial topic.

+ Generally, family presence, even during invasive procedure and resuscitation, is recommended. Evidence shows that family members assert that it is their preference and right to be present for these efforts, especially in the case of pediatric care.

+ Family members may find the experience difficult, and a staff member should be assigned to be available to discuss the events occurring.

   ⬦ If family members elect to be present, consider calling chaplain support if it is in line with the family's wishes.

   ⬦ Consider CISM resources if available to patients and families.

+ Family member presence should be offered if appropriate and should be governed by local policy and guidelines for consistency and provision of boundaries.

+ If a family member is behaving inappropriately or interfering with care, they should not be present.

FORENSIC EVIDENCE COLLECTION

+ Forensic evidence collection occurs in the emergency setting when a crime is known or suspected to have been committed, and collection of evidence is vital to the care of the patient and potential victims. Situations in which forensic evidence may be collected include:

   ⬦ GSWs
   ⬦ trauma
   ⬦ sexual assault
   ⬦ domestic abuse
   ⬦ child abuse

+ Evidence collection should be systematic and done with high accountability for detail and inventory. The ED nurse must have a solid understanding of collection techniques as well as chain-of-custody considerations.

+ Remove clothing.

   ⬦ Place clean sheets or other clean barrier on the floor or a large table.

   ⬦ Remove clothing by cutting, being careful to avoid any tears, bullet holes, or obviously soiled areas to prevent deterioration of evidence on the clothing.

   ⬦ Remove clothing one article at a time, being careful not to make a pile with the removed clothing.

   ⬦ Paper bags must be used for packaging. Package each item or article separately. Avoid excessive handling of evidence.

- To close the bag, fold the top over at least two times, and apply tape from one end of the fold to the other. Do not staple the bag. Sign or initial across the seal to deter tampering.
- Place sheet or barrier used in separate bag to submit to evidence as well.
+ Retrieve non-clothing evidence.
    - Place evidence on a clean white sheet of paper using sterile or clean gloves.
    - Fold the paper into thirds, turn the paper 90 degrees and fold into thirds again, keeping the evidence in the center of the page.
    - Tuck the ends into one another, place in an envelope, tape shut, and sign across seal to deter tampering.
+ Collect evidence from gunshot wounds.
    - Cover victim's hands, if possible, to preserve gunpowder residue if it is present.
    - If the bullet is retained, or found in the clothing, handle it as little as possible, wrap it in gauze, and place in a sterile collection cup with a lid that twists on. Tape the lid and label with signature or initials to deter tampering.
    - If a wound is found to have gunpowder around it, make every attempt to photograph the area and collect residue before cleaning the area.
+ Collect other evidence from the body.
    - Collect evidence from under fingernails by scraping the contents under the nail onto a white sheet of paper to be folded and placed in an envelope as described above.
    - Evidence of suspected or reported bodily fluids should be removed with a cotton-tipped applicator. Allow the swab tip to dry, and place in a signed, sealed envelope.
+ Document chain of custody.
    - If possible, limit the number of people in the chain of custody to preserve the integrity of the evidence.
    - When the evidence is given to law enforcement, the following information should be documented in the medical record:
        - inventory of the items released as evidence to law enforcement
        - name, badge number, and department of law enforcement officer
    - Label the evidence (every item) with the following information (many law enforcement agencies and hospitals have an official form to document all the listed information):
        - patient name
        - description of item in bag or envelope
        - name of agency taking item
        - name of people sealing, releasing, and accepting the item, each with a date and time
+ Examination by a sexual assault forensic nurse.
    - Sexual assault nurse examiners (SANE nurses) are registered nurses who have completed specialized certification and training for clinical practice in medical forensic care of victims and alleged perpetrators.
    - SANE nurses should be used whenever possible to collect evidence for a rape kit. It is best practice to use this resource due to the sensitivity and obligation to collect the evidence in a careful manner. Evidence collected incorrectly will not be admissible if ever seen in court proceedings.

10. The nurse is supervising a technician as he cuts away clothing on a trauma patient. She notes that the technician is cutting the clothing with no regard for evidence that may be retained on the garments. How should the nurse approach this issue?

PAIN MANAGEMENT AND PROCEDURAL SEDATION

+ **Pain management** in the ED is a complex and controversial issue in the context of the current opioid crisis facing the United States.

+ Responsible administration and prescription of opioid medications in the ED is required.

+ Both non-pharmacological and pharmacological approaches to pain should be considered.

+ Nursing considerations for the care of patients in pain:

  ⋄ Pain assessment is a numerical score as well as a subjective description of the nature of pain from a patient's perspective.

  ⋄ Measurement of pain should occur as frequently as every measurement of vital signs, or more frequently if indicated.

  ⋄ Nurses are charged with managing expectations for pain relief with patients. Patients may have unrealistic expectations of pain management and will need education on the subject. Establishing a goal for pain with the patient may help mitigate this issue.

+ **Procedural sedation** in the ED is performed with a sedation-certified registered nurse, the emergency physician, and occasionally a consult such as cardiology, orthopedics, or general surgery. It is indicated for anxiolysis, analgesia, and amnesia for uncomfortable procedures that do not require general anesthesia or admission to the operating room.

+ Procedures commonly done under sedation include:

  ⋄ synchronized cardioversion
  ⋄ reduction of fractures
  ⋄ suturing of lacerations
  ⋄ incision and drainage

+ Procedural sedation requires informed consent to be collected for both the procedure to be performed and the moderate sedation.

+ The ED nurse's role in procedural sedation is to assist during the procedure and help the patient recover from the moderate sedation. Nurses should confirm that all consents are in place before beginning and participate in the time-out and debriefing before and after the procedure.

11. A pediatric patient's mother asks about the procedural sedation process for her son who was climbing a fence, fell, and broke his arm. She is concerned that the procedure should be performed in the operating room, and does not feel comfortable with it happening in the ED. How can the nurse respond to this mother?

PATIENT SAFETY AND RISK MANAGEMENT

+ Potential **patient safety** issues in the ED include patient falls, medication errors, and the safety of moderately ill patients in waiting rooms.

  ⋄ **Preventing falls** in the ED is a difficult endeavor due to the chaotic and fast-paced nature of the work. Communication with the patient, provision of call lights, and hourly rounding are good ways to mitigate the risk of patient falls.

- **Medication errors** in emergency situations or resuscitation efforts are at a greater risk of occurring in the ED. Drills and practice in these situations allow the nurse to be confident and efficient in administering emergency drugs.
  - ED **overcrowding** can lead to poor patient outcomes in the waiting room before a patient can be seen. Hourly rounding and reassessment of patients can prevent deterioration or waiting room deaths.

- **Risk managers** typically assess risk in the hospital system or agency overall. However, they will also assess certain events occurring in the ED: adverse or sentinel events, or any patient complaint or concern that might lead to litigation.

- Risk managers get case referrals from many sources:
  - medical or nursing quality councils
  - internal patient safety reporting systems
  - nursing or provider referral
  - adverse or sentinel event reporting
  - patient referral through patient relations avenues

- Risk managers then perform formal root-cause analysis of these cases to identify what led to the poor outcome.

- Root-cause analysis is a stepwise process.
  - examines policy compliance or presence of standard operating procedures to govern processes
  - considers decision-making leading up to the event
  - establishes a sequence of events or a timeline leading to the event
  - considers individuals or groups of individuals involved
  - often done in focus group setting with multidisciplinary participation
  - may take several months to complete the investigation

- After root causes are identified, the risk manager recommends changes to be made to the department and follows up on them.

QUICK REVIEW QUESTION

12. An ED nurse identifies a near-miss event that could have resulted in a sentinel event for a patient. He asks his nurse manager how to properly report the incident to prevent it from happening again. What is the best response by the nurse manager?

PATIENT SATISFACTION

- **Patient satisfaction** is measured to determine if and what areas of the overall patient care experience need improvement.

- Different regulatory bodies may be concerned with patient satisfaction rates, and they use different tools and processes to measure patient satisfaction.

- One common patient satisfaction survey is the **Hospital Consumer Assessment of Healthcare Providers and Systems (HCAHPS)** survey.
  - The HCAHPS survey addresses over 20 patient perspectives on care and allows the patient to rate their experiences.
  - HCAHPS scores can be used in the context of quality assurance and performance appraisal and measurement, and as a means to improve on the departmental or unit level.

- Patient satisfaction is driven by many variables, some of which are under the control of the department and many of which are not.
    - care outcomes
    - facility services
    - customer service practices
    - overall appearance of facility
    - attitude/knowledge of staff
    - availability of equipment or supplies
    - pain management

QUICK REVIEW QUESTION

13. Why are patient satisfaction scores important to nursing in the ED?

TRANSFER AND STABILIZATION

- Transfer and stabilization of patients in the ED is governed by federal regulations in the **Consolidated Omnibus Budget Reconciliation Act (COBRA)**, which includes the **Emergency Medical Treatment and Active Labor Act (EMTALA)**.
- According to EMTALA, any patient presenting to an ED requesting care must at a minimum receive the following:
    - Medical screening exam performed by a qualified medical provider. Triage by a registered nurse does not qualify.
    - If the exam reveals a condition requiring immediate or near-immediate care, the following must occur:
        - The patient receives care and is discharged to home if stable.
        - The patient is admitted to the facility if the appropriate resources are available.
        - The patient is transferred to another facility with the appropriate level of care.
- Transfers of patients to higher levels of care require the following:
    - The patient must be stable for transport.
    - There must be an accepting physician at a receiving hospital that has the right services for the care of the patient.
    - The risks and benefits of transfer must be disclosed to the patient, and written, informed consent must be signed and sent with the patient.
    - Medical records must be sent from the transporting hospital to the destination, and a report must be sent or called in before patient arrives.
    - The method of transfer must be appropriate to the scale of the patient's condition.
- Transport methods must be appropriate to the patient's needs; excessive cost or use of resources that may be needed elsewhere should be avoided.
    - **Surface transport** is typically the lowest-cost option; however, it takes the most time. It can accommodate large patients or large equipment and is less affected by weather conditions.
    - **Rotor-wing transport** (helicopters) provides rapid transport from two points, either hospital to hospital or point of injury to hospital. It can be limited by weather conditions and distance between points due to fuel concerns and by weight of crew, patient, and equipment, and it is moderately expensive. It does not require an airport or landing strip.
    - **Fixed-wing transport** (airplanes) is the most expensive and is used when other modes are not available. It can cover long distances, has a pressurized cabin, and can accommodate gear and people. It requires a landing strip.

- Nursing considerations for the care of a patient needing transport:
  - Ensure peripheral or central line access is patent. If peripheral, establish two access sites.
  - Decompress gastric gases if patient is transporting via rotor-wing transport.
  - Insert urinary catheter.
  - Determine if blood products need to be packed and sent with patient or if the crew has their own.
  - Consider the impact of higher elevation on equipment and hollow organs. Consider chest tube placement if appropriate for the patient's condition.

QUICK REVIEW QUESTION

14. What is the nurse's role and responsibility in preparing a patient for transfer?

CULTURAL CONSIDERATIONS

Cultural considerations in the context of emergency nursing include respecting cultural practices that inform patients' decisions to accept certain treatments, and demonstrating cultural competence in care.

- Areas of diversity to consider are the following:
  - age
  - gender and gender identity
  - culture
  - ethnicity
  - sexual orientation
  - nationality
  - race
  - religion
  - marginalization (those considered by some to be unworthy of care based on actions, like using drugs or having committed a criminal offense)

- Each area of diversity influences patient and family responses to medical care, medical decision-making, compliance with care, response to serious illness, etc.

- Delivery of competent nursing care requires cultural competence. Quality care can be achieved when diversity is approached in a nonjudgmental, positive, and sensitive manner.

QUICK REVIEW QUESTION

15. An emergency nurse encounters a patient with religious beliefs that he is not familiar with. What is the best way to respect the patient's beliefs during the course of care?

System

DELEGATION OF TASKS

- Delegation of tasks is governed by local organizational policies, state nurse practice acts, and professional association practice guidelines.

- State nurse practice acts outline specific scopes of practice for all licensed personnel working in healthcare settings. Registered nurses in the ED may delegate tasks to the following licensed personnel:
  - paramedics working in the ED
  - EMTs working in the ED
  - LPNs/LVNs
  - medical assistants
  - nursing assistants
  - technicians

+ Tasks must be delegated with the following understandings:

  ✧ Delegation does not take away the nurse's responsibility for the completion of the task and its outcome.

  ✧ Delegation should take into account the scope of practice and, to the extent possible, the skills and abilities of the individual to whom the task is delegated.

QUICK REVIEW QUESTION

16 If an ED nurse is unsure what tasks are appropriate to delegate to technicians, where can this information be found?

DISASTER MANAGEMENT

Disaster management in the context of emergency nursing includes considerations for mass casualty incidents; natural disasters; pandemic, endemic, or epidemic illness; and decontamination of patients.

+ **Mass casualty incidents (MCIs)** are characterized by a rapid influx of patients that overwhelms the resources available in the ED, resulting in the activation of a contingency plan to bring more resources (staff, supplies, etc.) where they are needed. MCIs include:

  ✧ mass shootings

  ✧ sudden onset of contagious disease (a particularly bad flu season, for example)

  ✧ MVCs involving buses or a large number of vehicles

  ✧ train and airplane accidents

  ✧ biological or chemical accidents or attacks

+ Triage of patients is done differently during MCIs.

  ✧ Disaster triage is defined as doing the most good for as many people as possible.

  ✧ One method of disaster triage is known as **START triage** (simple triage and rapid treatment). Four triage categories are used:

    + Expectant: Black color. The victim is unlikely to survive injuries despite efforts to resuscitate. Palliative care measures only.

    + Immediate: Red color. Victims require immediate intervention with reasonable expectation of preserving life.

    + Delayed: Yellow color. Victim's transport and care can be delayed. May include serious, potentially life-threatening injuries, but deterioration is not imminent.

    + Minor: Green color. "The walking wounded." Immediate care is not needed; these victims have relatively minor injuries and can wait for treatment.

+ **Natural disasters** often result in widespread power outages, necessitating the evacuation of large hospital systems and care of patient populations long after the disaster has occurred. EDs, within the hospital system overall, must have a contingency plan for evacuation and support of patients requiring care following a large natural disaster.

+ There are three categories of widespread illness that may require the activation of disaster management processes.

  ✧ **pandemic:** an infectious disease that is prevalent on a global scale

  ✧ **endemic:** an infectious disease found among a group of people or restricted to a certain area

  ✧ **epidemic:** an infectious disease that occurs in a community at a particular time, such as influenza

- **Decontamination** must be performed by trained or certified individuals with a strong working knowledge of contaminants. Decontamination areas must be set up a good distance from any entrance into a hospital to avoid cross contamination of the area and building.
  - The **hot zone** of care is the point of entry to the decontamination process following an incident. Patients triaged as immediate, delayed, or nonambulatory will be decontaminated first. They are triaged in the hot zone and have their clothes removed as they approach the warm zone.
  - The **warm zone** is where active decontamination occurs. Decontamination usually includes the use of water, but this will depend on the chemical, biological, or radioactive agent the patient is exposed to.
  - The **cold zone** is the point of exit from the decontamination area. The patient enters the cold zone and may be treated onsite or transported to an appropriate level of care.
- **Disaster preparedness** is usually managed in the form of large-scale drills or tabletop exercises to determine how to mitigate weaknesses and identify needs in disaster management plans.
- Many organizations use the **incident command system (ICS)** promoted by FEMA to manage disaster situations.
- The following are four steps to disaster management and preparedness.
  - Mitigation: Identify vulnerabilities to threats or weaknesses in current plans.
  - Preparedness: Develop mutual aid agreements, create disaster management plans, determine supply thresholds and needs, consider stockpiles, and establish a command and control structure.
  - Response: Warn (notify), isolate (during the disaster), and rescue (following the disaster).
  - Recovery: Inventory supplies and resources, relieve staff members present during the isolation phase, incorporate records into the EMR, implement CISM program if needed, and activate employee assistance programs if needed.
- The ICS uses the following hierarchy:
  - incident commander
    - command staff (public information officer, security officer, liaison officer)
    - general staff (operations, planning, logistics, finance/administration)
- Each role in the ICS is preassigned and drilled in preparation for disaster events. Organizations may customize the hierarchy below the general staff to fit the needs of their own system.

QUICK REVIEW QUESTION

17. What role does a nurse play in disaster management?

THE HEALTH INSURANCE PORTABILITY AND ACCOUNTABILITY ACT (HIPAA)

- The **Health Insurance Portability and Accountability Act (HIPAA)** requires that individual healthcare providers and healthcare organizations make every attempt to safeguard the **protected health information (PHI)** of the patient.
- PHI is defined as any information that concerns the past, present, or future mental or physical health of the patient, along with the treatments of such health conditions and the methods of payment for health services rendered.
- Organizations are required to take measures to protect all PHI on electronic platforms or in electronic formats.

- HIPAA is based on the **minimum necessary requirement**; i.e., the minimum amount of PHI needed to accomplish a task should be shared.

- Sharing of PHI with patient's family, friends, or others is only possible with the patient's consent.

- Sharing of PHI is permissible under HIPAA in the following contexts:
  - activities involving reimbursement or payment for care premiums, determining coverage or provision of benefits, etc.
  - health care operations such as quality improvement activities
  - competency assurance
  - audits of medical records for legal or competency reviews
  - insurance use
  - business planning, development, or management

- PHI may also be released for the following reasons:
  - public health reporting
  - fraud reporting
  - abuse and neglect reporting
  - organ and tissue donation
  - law enforcement proceedings
  - crime reporting
  - military and veterans' health and national security

- Many organizations employ HIPAA compliance officers in order to support both patients and the organization with compliance issues and training.

- If a patient believes their PHI was not protected appropriately, they should be referred to the compliance officer or the United States Department of Health and Human Services.

- Patient's rights under HIPAA include:
  - the right to receive information regarding how their PHI is used and protected
  - access to personal medical records (with some exceptions)
  - access to lists of nonroutine disclosures of their PHI
  - the right to dictate authorization to use their PHI and to restrict certain uses

QUICK REVIEW QUESTION

18. What should a nurse do when made aware of a possible HIPAA breach or violation?

PATIENT CONSENT FOR TREATMENT

- Patient **consent for treatment** is a complex and nebulous issue in the ED. Considerations include capacity for consent, age of consent, and state and federal laws governing when these considerations may be waived.

- In general, there are four types of consent.
  - **Informed consent** is used in situations where moderately invasive or high-risk procedures are going to be performed. The provider must cover key elements for informed consent to be valid.
    - description of the procedure
    - risks and benefits of the procedure
    - alternative options available to the patient
  - **Implied consent** is given in situations where patients are at risk to lose life or limb, and they are unable to provide informed consent. This type of consent is only applicable during resuscitation and is no longer implied if the patient is able to give and/or express informed consent.

- ✧ **Express consent** is characterized by the assumption of consent to perform noninvasive to minimally invasive procedures in the ED. Some departments require a signature for express consent; others take verbal consent based on words or actions of patients.
  - ✧ **Involuntary consent** is given when a patient is deemed not to have decisional capacity due to reasons such as altered mental status or mental health issues. Physicians, law enforcement officers, and psychiatrists typically enact this type of consent.
- ✦ **Pediatric consent** is another complex issue. If a pediatric patient presents for care without the presence of a legally responsible adult, the emergency nurse must get consent for care from the legal custodian of the patient. There are some exceptions to this rule:
  - ✧ Treatment can be provided if there is immediate danger to life or limb.
  - ✧ Some states allow pediatric patients to come to the ED for care STIs or similar issues in the absence of the legal custodian.
  - ✧ Treatment can be provided when there is high suspicion of non-accidental trauma or domestic abuse. Consent for treatment is implied until the local child services system can determine temporary legal guardianship terms.

QUICK REVIEW QUESTION

19. A 15-year-old male patient arrives at the ED requesting an evaluation for a possible STI. What kind of consent for treatment should be established?

PROCESS IMPROVEMENT

- ✦ There are many opportunities to apply process improvement initiatives in the ED.
- ✦ The greatest opportunity for process improvement is in throughput and patient flow through the department, a task that nurses are largely responsible for managing.
- ✦ Measurement of metrics such as arrival to triage times, arrival to provider times, arrival to bed times, and arrival to disposition times can give excellent insight into process issues that can be addressed.
- ✦ Process improvement projects normally follow structured programs such as Lean Six Sigma or 4DX in order to provide a framework to carry out the project.
- ✦ Generally, steps in process improvement include:
  - ✧ identifying the problem
  - ✧ measuring relevant variables for baseline metrics
  - ✧ identifying, developing, and implementing a solution or change
  - ✧ measuring the impact of the change

QUICK REVIEW QUESTION

20. The ED manager has noticed a steady increase in the percentage of patients leaving without being seen or leaving before being triaged. How should she investigate this problem?

SYMPTOM SURVEILLANCE

- ✦ In general, the emergency nurse is not required to recognize **symptom clusters** through sophisticated statistical methods such as spatial analysis. However, there is an obligation to report a concern of an acute influx of like symptoms within a community or population.

- Sources of infectious disease clustering may include places where large numbers of people gather at a given time, such as schools, churches, large events, movie theaters, etc.
  - Infectious disease can be spread through pediatric populations at schools or day cares.
  - Foodborne illness can be spread through the distribution of food at grocery stores, restaurants, festivals, local farming co-ops, etc.
- Screening for infectious disease exposure typically occurs at triage through a series of questions about travel, recent social activities, or attendance at schools or churches.
- Disease surveillance is achieved through the systematic collection of data on certain **mandatorily reported diseases**. These diseases include:
  - anthrax
  - STIs
  - viral diseases spread by mosquitos or other insect vectors
  - botulism
  - chicken pox
  - cholera
  - all vaccine-preventable diseases
  - SARS
- There are many more diseases that are mandatory to report. Hospital systems have mechanisms to prompt reporting through ICD-10 coding, and generally do not require that individual practitioners submit such reports.

QUICK REVIEW QUESTION

21. An emergency nurse is on his third scheduled shift in a row, and he has noticed several pediatric patients presenting to the department with similar but vague symptoms. What should he do with this information?

Triage

- **Triage** in the ED is defined as the method of sorting patients based on chief complaint, physical presentation, anticipated needed resources, and vital signs.
- There is not a universal triage system used in the United States.
- Some departments use the three-level triage system, categorizing patients as emergent, urgent, and nonurgent.
  - **Emergent patients** require immediate care; condition is severe, and threat to life or limb is present.
  - **Urgent patients** require care as soon as possible; condition is acute, and condition presents danger if not treated.
  - **Nonurgent patients** can safely wait for care.
- In many EDs, the **Emergency Severity Index (ESI)** is used as a triage algorithm to assign each patient with a level of acuity to assist with treatment priority decisions. The ESI has five levels of acuity.
  - Level 5: This patient arrives at the department stable, and requires no resources as defined by ESI in order to address their chief complaint.
  - Level 4: This patient arrives in stable condition and may require one resource to address the chief complaint.

- ✧ Level 3: This patient arrives in stable condition; however, two or more resources may be needed to care for the patient. This patient has the potential to deteriorate into a more acute state.

- ✧ Level 2: This patient is unstable and requires many resources to address care needs. The patient may deteriorate into needing immediate lifesaving intervention but does not require it immediately upon arrival.

- ✧ Level 1: This patient requires immediate life- or limb-saving intervention upon arrival.

+ The **triage nurse** in the ED requires a high level of skill and experience to determine, with limited information, the acuity of patients in an often chaotic and challenging environment.

+ Triage nursing generally requires a formal orientation with clinical and didactic training.

QUICK REVIEW QUESTION

22. A patient approaches the triage desk to ask why patients who arrived later than him are being seen earlier. What is the best answer for this patient?

ANSWER KEY

1. Gather resources for the agency CISM, encourage her to use the resources, and assist her in a debriefing of the pediatric code if it was not already done.

2. Consider asking family if there is a living will or advance directive. If it is feasible, suggest an emergency meeting of the agency ethics committee if the two providers are unable to make a decision. Ultimately, the attending on record is responsible for the decision.

3. The nurse should not change practice or introduce new nursing interventions without a formal literature review and EBP change project. One article is not enough to support change in practice, and it should be a collaborative decision among the multidisciplinary team to make such changes.

4. Participate in any journal clubs available, meet with research coordinators, and join professional associations.

5. The nurse can produce a record of continuing education activities in the form of certificates or letters to credentialing offices or boards of nursing.

6. Emergency nurses can identify patient needs or gaps in care and can help the patient find resources to bridge the gap. In adult patients, the responsibility of the nurse ends once the resources are provided, presuming that the patient has the capacity to access the resources if they choose to.

7. The nurse should review the wishes of the patient and family regarding organ donation, contact the local procurement agency, and maintain the hemodynamic stability of the patient in preparation for organ procurement.

8. Continue to resuscitate the patient, and ask the daughter to procure the DNR paperwork, if it is available. Explain that the ED team cannot act on the request until it has been verified as a valid, legal document.

9. The nurse should describe the postmortem care procedures to the family in a sensitive manner. The nurse should take the opportunity to discuss things such as organ procurement (if appropriate) and give the family an opportunity to see the patient again. Offering CISM or grief support services to the family is appropriate.

10. The nurse should stop the technician in a professional manner and demonstrate proper evidence removal and collection to him. The nurse should not delay immediate life-saving measures but instead debrief with the technician after the incident to follow up on the feedback.

11. The nurse, in collaboration with the physician, can explain to the mother that general anesthesia is not needed to reduce her son's fractured arm, and doing it in the ED under moderate sedation greatly reduces both risks and time spent in the hospital.

12. The nurse manager should assist the nurse with reporting the incident through a patient safety reporting system, or the nurse manager should report it directly to the risk manager or quality management division of the agency. The nurse should anticipate the incident being investigated for formal root-cause analysis and provide as much detail as possible.

13. Patient satisfaction scores are the first step in identifying ways to improve the patient care experience and can also affect practice decisions. Patients often report issues they experience or witness that would otherwise go unreported. Measuring patient satisfaction contributes significantly to patient safety data.

14. The emergency nurse should make sure that the patient has adequate peripheral access and a catheter if appropriate, and should prepare the patient for flight, if applicable. The nurse should ensure that all consents for transfers are signed and in the patient's medical record.

15. The nurse can respectfully ask the patient if there is any religious consideration that he should be aware of as he begins to care for the patient. He should document these considerations in the medical record.

16. The nurse may ask the technician directly, ask the charge nurse, refer to local nursing policy, or ask the immediate supervisor or manager. She should not delegate the task without a definitive answer.

17. ED nurses must have a concrete understanding of their assigned role in a disaster, which may be different from their everyday role. Disaster management roles may involve START triage (at times outside of the actual department, at the casualty collection/delivery point), delayed treatment (management of patient

triaged as yellow), patient movement and transport, decontamination (if trained), and palliative care for expectant patients.

18. The nurse should immediately report it to the HIPAA compliance office or to their immediate supervisor.

19. Due to the nature of the complaint, in some states it may be appropriate to take express consent. This patient is a pediatric patient by definition; however, the sensitivity of the complaint may preclude the need for parental consent.

20. The ED manager should consider the reasons patients are leaving, if that information is available. She should also monitor and assess other throughput metrics to determine if wait times are longer than normal or if there are other contributing factors. A process improvement project may be appropriate to address these issues.

21. He should communicate with the senior medical officer in the department or the public health representative to share these observations. He should not keep this information to himself, because it could quickly develop into a large public health concern.

22. The triage nurse should inform the patient of the triage system and explain that some patients may require rapid or immediate care, while others may not. The nurse should not lessen the importance of the patient's chief complaint but should instead explain that emergency care is not always provided on a first-come, first-served basis.

SEVENTEEN: Practice Test

1. The ED nurse is caring for a patient with a subdural hematoma sustained in an automobile accident. The patient currently has an ICP of 22 mmHg. Which of the following would NOT be an appropriate intervention?

   A. BMP and CBC

   B. lumbar puncture

   C. mechanical ventilation

   D. Foley catheter placement

2. Which of the following substances is contraindicated for an 80-year-old patient with acute heart failure?

   A. dopamine

   B. adrenaline

   C. digoxin

   D. dobutamine

3. Which observation in a patient with abdominal aortic aneurysm indicates the need for immediate treatment?

   A. complaints of yellow-tinted vision

   B. hemoptysis

   C. urinary output of 75 mL/hr per urinary catheter

   D. complaints of sudden and severe back pain and dyspnea

4. The nurse is evaluating patients for risk of heparin-induced thrombocytopenia (HIT). Which patient is at greatest risk for HIT, based on the nurse's assessment?

    A. a male patient who just completed a 1-week course of heparin

    B. a male patient taking enoxaparin for management of unstable angina

    C. a female patient receiving heparin for postsurgical thromboprophylaxis

    D. a female patient taking enoxaparin to prevent clots following a mild myocardial infarction

5. During cardiac assessment of a patient with pericarditis, the nurse should expect to hear

    A. mitral regurgitation.

    B. S3 gallop.

    C. S4 gallop.

    D. pericardial friction rub.

6. Complications resulting from an untreated/undertreated high-velocity injection injury may be minimized by

    A. educating the patient to return if signs of infection appear.

    B. administering prophylactic antibiotics.

    C. obtaining a surgical consultation and exploration.

    D. immobilizing the extremity involved.

7. A patient arrives in the ED with midsternal chest pain radiating down the left arm and left jaw. He slumps to the floor and is unresponsive, pulseless, and apneic. High-quality compressions are started, and the patient's ECG shows the following rhythm. What is the priority nursing intervention?

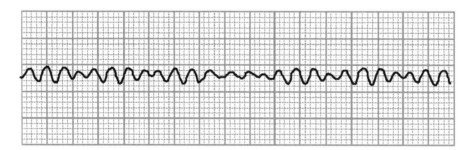

    A. administer a fluid bolus of 1 L normal saline

    B. defibrillate with 200 J

    C. administer 1 mg epinephrine IV

    D. insert an advanced airway

8. A patient comes to the ED complaining of intermittent nausea and vomiting for the past month. She states that she has pain in the abdomen that is relieved by eating. She began having diarrhea the day before. Medical history shows that the patient takes naproxen daily for arthritis. The nurse should assess for

    A. obesity.

    B. appendicitis.

    C. hypertension.

    D. gastritis.

9. An infant's parents bring him to the ED because of bloody, mucous stools. The child cries constantly and pulls his knees up to his chest. Which of the following findings would be the most critical?

    A. vomiting

    B. diarrhea

    C. abdominal swelling

    D. a lump in the abdomen

10. A patient with abdominal pain and possible appendicitis wants to leave the ED. What should the nurse do next?

    A. Inform the patient he will be involuntarily committed to the hospital if he tries to leave.

    B. Inform the physician of the patient's wish to leave.

    C. Warn the patient he will die if he leaves the department.

    D. Give the patient directions to the exit.

11. The current American Heart Association (AHA) guidelines for CPR on an adult patient with 2 rescuers is

    A. 30 compressions : 2 ventilations.

    B. 15 compressions : 2 ventilations.

    C. 30 compressions : 1 ventilation.

    D. 15 compressions : 1 ventilation.

12. A patient in the ED is diagnosed with a right ventricular infarction with hypotension. The nurse should prepare to administer which of the following to treat the hypotension?

    A. normal saline fluid boluses 1 to 2 L

    B. dopamine (Intropine) at 10 mcg/kg/min

    C. D5W fluid boluses titrate 3 L

    D. furosemide drip at 20 mg/hr

13. Which lab results confirm a diagnosis of carbon monoxide toxicity in a nonsmoking adult?

    A. COHb 0.8%

    B. COHb 8%

    C. $PaCO_2$ 38

    D. $PaCO_2$ 41

14. A 43-year-old female patient comes to the ED with complaints of vaginal discharge with itching and burning. The nurse notes a non-odorous white discharge that resembles cottage cheese. The nurse should prepare to treat the patient for which of the following?

    A. bacterial vaginosis

    B. trichomoniasis vaginitis

    C. Candida vulvovaginitis

    D. Neisseria gonorrhoeae

15. An 82-year-old patient presents to triage with a complaint of diarrhea for the past 3 days. She tells the triage nurse that she is on her third day of antibiotics. Which precautions should the nurse implement?

    A. airborne precautions

    B. contact precautions

    C. droplet precautions

    D. contact and droplet precautions

16. A 20-year-old female patient comes to the ED complaining of a green-gray frothy malodorous vaginal discharge and vaginal itching. The wet prep shows only WBCs. The nurse should prepare to assess for

    A. trichomoniasis.

    B. bacterial vaginosis.

    C. herpes simplex virus.

    D. chlamydia.

17. The nurse is performing an abdominal assessment on a patient with suspected heart failure. The patient asks the nurse the reason for assessing the abdomen. Which of the following would be the best response from the nurse?

    A. "Sometimes the medications used in heart failure will cause stomach upset."

    B. "Hepatomegaly, or an enlarged liver, is common in heart failure."

    C. "I am checking to see if you are constipated."

    D. "Heart failure can lead to appendicitis."

18. When trying to find a piece of glass in the soft tissue of the lateral thigh, which assessment technique should the nurse avoid?

    A. deep tissue palpation

    B. visual inspection

    C. palpation of distal pulses

    D. CSM of extremity

19. A patient's cardiac monitor shows the rhythm below. He is awake and alert but is pale and confused. His blood pressure reads 64/40 mm Hg. What is the priority nursing intervention for this patient?

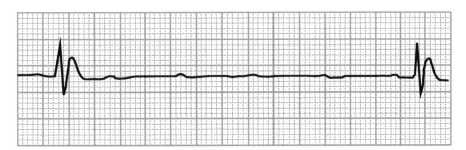

    A. defibrillate at 200 J

    B. prepare for transcutaneous pacing

    C. administer epinephrine 1 mg

    D. begin CPR

20. A patient who is 28 weeks pregnant presents to the ED with a malodorous vaginal discharge, a temperature of 102.3°F (39°C), and no complaints of uterine contractions. These signs and symptoms are most indicative of which of the following?

    A. septic spontaneous abortion

    B. ectopic pregnancy

    C. missed abortion

    D. abdominal trauma

21. Which of the following lab values should the nurse expect to order for a patient receiving IV heparin therapy for a pulmonary embolism?

    A. hematocrit

    B. HDL and LDL

    C. PT and PTT

    D. troponin level

22. A patient is being treated for rapidly evolving disseminated intravascular coagulation (DIC) in the ED. Which of the following lab values would the nurse expect?

    A. increased hemoglobin

    B. decreased D-dimer

    C. increased platelets

    D. decreased fibrinogen

23. The nurse is caring for a patient with Guillain–Barré syndrome who is at risk for autonomic dysfunction. The nurse should monitor the patient for

    A. trigeminy.

    B. heart block.

    C. atrial flutter.

    D. tachycardia.

24. Which of the following procedures can be performed under procedural sedation in the ED?

    A. perimortem cesarean section

    B. synchronized cardioversion

    C. dilatation and curettage

    D. open fracture reduction

25. A nurse notes crackles while assessing lung sounds in a child with pneumonia. How would the nurse classify this respiratory disorder?

    A. upper airway disorder

    B. lower airway disorder

    C. lung tissue disorder

    D. disordered control of breathing

26. The ECG in the exhibit supports the diagnosis of

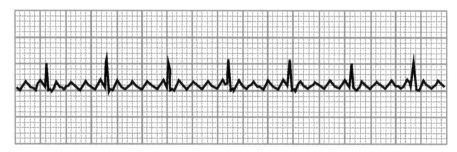

    A. atrial flutter.

    B. atrial fibrillation.

    C. torsades de pointes.

    D. ventricular fibrillation.

27. A patient who was playing basketball outside all day has been drinking only water to stay hydrated. He suddenly became confused, complained of a headache, and collapsed. The nurse should suspect

   A. hyperkalemia.

   B. hyponatremia.

   C. hypernatremia.

   D. hypokalemia.

28. Which of the following medications should a nurse anticipate administering to an 18-month-old patient with a barking cough first?

   A. epinephrine 0.01 mg/kg IV stat

   B. nebulized epinephrine breathing treatment

   C. albuterol breathing treatment

   D. dexamethasone PO or IV

29. Classic signs of Bell's palsy include

   A. facial droop, dysphagia, dysarthria.

   B. facial droop, confusion, ataxia.

   C. hemiparalysis, photophobia, headache.

   D. tinnitus, nausea, vertigo.

30. Which of the following is most likely to be found in a patient with left-sided heart failure?

   A. jugular vein distention

   B. crackles

   C. hepatomegaly

   D. ascites

31. Localized pain and edema associated with systemic fever and left shift differential may be indicative of

   A. foreign body infection of surgical hardware.

   B. superficial foreign body.

   C. buckle fracture.

   D. Achilles tendon rupture.

32. The most common site of injection injuries is

   A. the second digit of the nondominant hand.

   B. the first digit of the nondominant hand.

   C. the second digit of the dominant hand.

   D. the first digit of the dominant hand.

33. A 12-year-old patient is brought to the ED after falling 15 feet out of a tree. She is complaining of severe pain in the right side of the chest and severe dyspnea. Upon auscultation, the nurse notes absent breath sounds on the right and should suspect

    A. pneumothorax.

    B. foreign body lodged in the right side of the chest.

    C. hematoma.

    D. pleural effusion.

34. A patient with a subarachnoid hemorrhage from a fall at home arrives at the ED. When reviewing the medical orders, which medication order should prompt the nurse to notify the health care provider?

    A. warfarin

    B. morphine

    C. nimodipine

    D. a stool softener

35. Which symptom, identified by the patient, is the most common and consistent with a myocardial infarction?

    A. palpitations

    B. lower extremity edema

    C. feeling of pressure in the chest

    D. nausea

36. A patient arrives to the ED with a grossly deformed shoulder injury obtained while surfing. Suspecting a dislocation, which nursing intervention should the nurse initiate immediately?

    A. elevate the extremity

    B. put patient on NPO status

    C. apply ice

    D. provide ice chips

37. Which of the following statements should be included in the discharge instructions for a patient who has been prescribed carbamazepine to control seizures?

    A. Avoid exposure to sunlight.

    B. Limit foods high in vitamin K.

    C. Do not take on an empty stomach.

    D. Use caution when driving or operating machinery.

38. The nurse is caring for a patient with a traumatic brain injury who has a Glasgow Coma Scale (GCS) of 7. The nurse should anticipate the need to

   A. bolus with NS via IV.

   B. assist patient to chair.

   C. assist with intubation.

   D. apply 2L O_2 via nasal cannula.

39. The nurse is caring for a patient who just had a lumbar puncture to rule out meningitis. Which assessment finding would prompt the nurse to notify the health care provider?

   A. The patient is drinking fluids.

   B. The patient is lying flat in the bed.

   C. The patient's pain scale is 3 out of 10.

   D. The patient complains of severe headache.

40. A patient presents with signs and symptoms characteristic of myocardial infarction (MI). Which of the following diagnostic tools should the nurse anticipate will be used to determine the location of the myocardial damage?

   A. electrocardiogram

   B. echocardiogram

   C. cardiac enzymes

   D. cardiac catheterization

41. The ED nurse is waiting for a bed for a 72-year-old patient with Alzheimer's disease who has episodes of confusion. Which of the following will be included in the plan of care for this patient?

   A. prescribe haloperidol to prevent agitation

   B. provide toileting every 2 hours

   C. use restraints at night to prevent wandering

   D. allow choices when possible to promote feelings of respect

42. A 16-year-old patient arrives to the ED after ingesting an entire bottle of acetaminophen 4 hours before. The most appropriate intervention is

   A. administration of N-acetylcysteine.

   B. endotracheal intubation.

   C. administration of naloxone.

   D. gastric lavage.

43. A patient with emphysema comes to the ED complaining of dyspnea. The nurse should assist the patient into which of the following positions?

    A. lying flat on the back

    B. in a prone position

    C. sitting up and leaning forward

    D. lying on the side with feet elevated

44. A patient with severe dementia is brought to the ED for urinary retention. The patient repeatedly asks for her mother, who passed away many years ago. Which technique should the nurse use when the patient asks for her mother?

    A. confrontation

    B. reality orientation

    C. validation therapy

    D. seeking clarification

45. The nurse sees a bedbug on the personal linens of a child transported from the home setting to the ED via ambulance. What is the most appropriate action?

    A. Place the patient on airborne precautions.

    B. File a report with the local child welfare agency.

    C. Wash the patient thoroughly and replace all linens and clothing items with hospital-provided materials.

    D. Ask the parents to provide new clothing and linen from the home.

46. The nurse is caring for a patient with suspected diverticulitis. The nurse should anticipate all of the following findings EXCEPT

    A. fever.

    B. anorexia.

    C. lower abdominal pain.

    D. low WBC count.

47. A patient presents to the ED with abdominal pain and is found to have an incarcerated hernia. The patient is prepared for surgery. Which assessment finding by the nurse should be reported immediately to the health care provider?

    A. a burning sensation at the site of the hernia

    B. sudden nausea and vomiting with increased pain since arrival

    C. a palpable mass in the abdomen

    D. pain that occurs when bending over or coughing

48. EMS arrives to the ED with a stable adult patient who has a clear developmental delay. Emergent intervention is not needed upon arrival. What should the ED nurse do before treating the patient?

   A. Call the legal guardian of the patient to obtain consent for care.

   B. Continue to care for the patient.

   C. Obtain consent for care from the patient.

   D. Obtain permission from the hospital legal department to care for the patient.

49. A patient arrives at the ED complaining of severe pain to the right lower abdominal quadrant. The patient states that the pain is worse with coughing. The nursing assessment reveals that pain is relieved by bending the right hip. The patient has not had a bowel movement in three days. The nurse should anticipate all of the following interventions EXCEPT

   A. IV fluids.

   B. morphine 2mg IV.

   C. STAT MRI of abdomen.

   D. maintain NPO status.

50. A patient is admitted to the ED with an acute myocardial infarction (MI). The nurse is preparing the patient for transport to the cardiac catheterization laboratory. An alarm sounds on the cardiac monitor, and the patient becomes unresponsive. V-fib is noted. The nurse should anticipate doing which of the following first?

   A. beginning high-quality CPR

   B. defibrillation at 200 J

   C. administering epinephrine 1 mg

   D. placing an IV

51. A nursing home patient with an enterocutaneous fistula caused by an acute exacerbation of Crohn's disease arrives at the ED. The nursing priority is to

   A. administer antibiotics.

   B. preserve and protect the skin.

   C. apply a wound VAC to the area.

   D. provide quiet times for relaxation.

52. A patient with cardiogenic shock is expected to have

   A. hypertension; dyspnea.

   B. decreased urine output; warm, pink skin.

   C. increased urine output; cool, clammy skin.

   D. hypotension; weak pulse; cool, clammy skin.

53. A patient in the ED with chronic pain is requesting more intravenous pain medication for reported 10/10 pain. The physician will not give any more medication. How should the nurse approach this patient?

   A. Inform the patient that it is the physician's decision.

   B. Discuss chronic pain relief and realistic expectations with the patient.

   C. Ignore the patient's pain complaint.

   D. Discuss drug-seeking concerns with the patient.

54. Which appearance is most consistent with an avulsion?

   A. open wound with presence of sloughing and eschar tissue

   B. skin tear with approximated edges

   C. shearing of the top epidermal layers

   D. separation of skin from the underlying structures that cannot be approximated

55. The ED nurse receives a patient with blunt-force abdominal injury due to a knife wound. On inspection, a common kitchen knife is found in the patient's abdomen in the upper right quadrant. The patient is rapidly placed on a non-rebreather mask, two large-bore IVs are started, and labs are drawn. No evisceration is noted. Which should the nurse do next?

   A. Notify next of kin.

   B. Estimate blood loss.

   C. Stabilize the knife with bulky dressings.

   D. Attempt to gently pull the knife straight out.

56. In a hypothermic patient, hypovolemia occurs as the result of

   A. diuresis and third spacing.

   B. shivering and vasoconstriction.

   C. diaphoresis and dehydration.

   D. tachycardia and tachypnea.

57. A 14-year-old male patient is brought to the ED, stating he woke up in the middle of the night with sudden, severe groin pain and nausea. The pain persists despite elevation of the testes. These findings most likely indicate

   A. testicular torsion.

   B. epididymitis.

   C. UTI.

   D. orchitis.

58. A 16-year-old patient is brought to the ED complaining of abdominal pain, nausea, and sharp constant pain on both sides of the pelvis. She has a history of pelvic inflammatory disease and is not sexually active. The nurse notes a purulent vaginal discharge. These signs and symptoms are most indicative of which condition?

   A. ectopic pregnancy

   B. tubo-ovarian abscess

   C. diverticulitis

   D. ruptured appendix

59. A patient who is 9 weeks pregnant comes to the ED with complaints of abdominal cramping. During the physical assessment the nurse notes slight vaginal bleeding and a large, solid tissue clot. These findings most likely indicate

   A. septic spontaneous abortion.

   B. incomplete spontaneous abortion

   C. threatened abortion.

   D. complete spontaneous abortion.

60. A 4-month-old infant is brought to the ED with croup. Which of the following medications will the nurse administer in order to decrease inflammation?

   A. ipratropium

   B. albuterol

   C. corticosteroids

   D. antibiotics

61. A 21-year-old male patient reports to the ED with complaints of burning on urination and urethral itching. During the assessment, the nurse notes a mucopurulent discharge and no lesions. These signs and symptoms are most indicative of which of the following?

   A. chlamydia

   B. syphilis

   C. HPV

   D. herpes simplex virus

62. The mother of a 3-year-old patient diagnosed with varicella asks for the best at-home treatment. Which of the following treatments is NOT appropriate for the nurse to suggest?

   A. oral antihistamines

   B. colloidal oatmeal baths

   C. acetaminophen

   D. aspirin

63. A full-term neonate is delivered in the ED. After stimulation and suctioning, the infant is apneic with strong palpable pulses at 126/minute. The nursing priority is to

   A. rescue breaths at 12 – 20 breaths per minute.

   B. rescue breaths at 40 – 60 breaths per minute.

   C. insert endotracheal intubation.

   D. insert an LMA.

64. A pediatric patient in cardiopulmonary arrest has had a 40-minute resuscitation attempt in the ED. The ED nurse feels that the resuscitation is reaching the point of concern for medical futility. What is the nurse's responsibility at this time?

   A. Tell the parents to order the resuscitation attempt to be stopped.

   B. Suggest that the team leader consider ending the resuscitation.

   C. Order the team to stop the resuscitation.

   D. Continue with the resuscitation and allow the team leader to decide when to stop.

65. After an emergent delivery, a full-term infant is apneic with a pulse rate of 48 bpm. The infant has not responded to chest compressions. The nurse should prepare to administer

   A. atropine 0.5 mg/kg.

   B. epinephrine 0.01 – 0.03 mg/kg.

   C. sodium bicarbonate 1 to 2 mEq/mL.

   D. dobutamine drip.

66. Which treatment is appropriate for a minor blunt injury resulting in intact skin, ecchymosis, edema, and localized pain and tenderness?

   A. fasciotomy and opioid pain medications

   B. rest, ice, compression, elevation, and opioid pain medications

   C. rest, ice, compression, elevation, and use of NSAIDs

   D. immobilization and use of NSAIDs

67. A patient with depression and Alzheimer's disease presents to the ED complaining of abdominal pain. In reviewing the patient's health care orders, which medication should prompt the nurse to notify the health care provider?

   A. sertraline

   B. paroxetine

   C. memantine

   D. amitriptyline

68. A 14-year-old patient arrives to the ED with delirium, respiratory distress, and headache. Upon examination of the airway, the nurse notes a burn to the roof of the patient's mouth. What does the nurse suspect?

   A. ingestion of a hot beverage

   B. inhalation of chemicals from a compressed gas can

   C. ingestion of dry ice

   D. marijuana use

69. The nurse is caring for a patient who was brought to the ED with seizures. The patient begins having a seizure. The nursing priority is

   A. padding the bed rails.

   B. inserting a tongue blade.

   C. administering IV diazepam.

   D. turning the patient to his side.

70. A patient who is 32 weeks pregnant is having profuse bright red painless vaginal bleeding after being in a motor vehicle crash (MVC). The nurse should prepare to treat her for

   A. abruptio placentae.

   B. placenta previa.

   C. ectopic pregnancy.

   D. complete abortion.

71. A 30-week pregnant patient comes to the ED after falling down a flight of steps. She complains of uterine tenderness, and a small amount of dark bloody vaginal drainage is noted. The nurse should suspect

   A. abruptio placenta.

   B. placenta previa.

   C. incomplete spontaneous abortion.

   D. complete spontaneous abortion.

72. The ED nurse is caring for a patient with schizophrenia. The patient appears to be looking at someone and asks the nurse, "Aren't you going to speak to Martha?" No one else is in the room. Which response by the nurse is appropriate?

   A. "There's nobody there."

   B. "I will find a blanket for Martha."

   C. "Is Martha going to stay a while?"

   D. "Does Martha ever tell you to hurt yourself or others?"

73. A patient in the ED is having difficulty breathing and is diagnosed with a large plural effusion. The nurse prepares her for which of the following procedures?

    A.   pericardiocentesis

    B.   chest tube insertion

    C.   thoracentesis

    D.   pericardial window

74. When caring for a patient with esophageal varices, the nurse should first prepare to administer

    A.   phenytoin

    B.   octreotide

    C.   levofloxacin

    D.   pantoprazole

75. The ED nurse is caring for a patient who is deeply depressed following the death of her mother. She tells the nurse, "I just lost my world when Mom died. She was my anchor, and now I have no one." Which response by the nurse is the most appropriate?

    A.   "You will feel better in time."

    B.   "You should join a grief support group."

    C.   "I felt the same way when my mother died."

    D.   "You're feeling lost since your mother died."

76. A patient is admitted to the ED with chest pain. A 12-lead ECG is performed with ST elevations noted in leads II, III and aVF. The nurse should prepare to administer

    A.   nitrates.

    B.   diuretics.

    C.   morphine.

    D.   IV fluids.

77. A 20-year-old male college student arrives to the ED during spring break complaining of a headache, fever, nausea, and vomiting. He shows the ED nurse a petechial rash on his trunk and chest. Which of the following should the nurse suspect?

    A.   influenza

    B.   pertussis

    C.   meningitis

    D.   scabies

78. A patient comes to the ED with complaints of nausea and vomiting for 3 days. His ECG reading is shown in the exhibit. The nurse should suspect

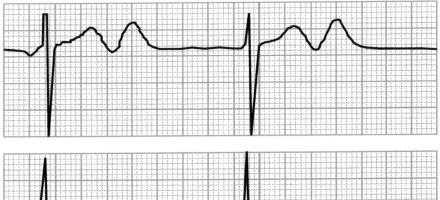
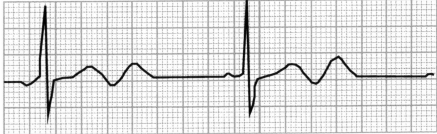

- **A.** hyperkalemia.
- **B.** hypokalemia.
- **C.** hypercalcemia.
- **D.** hypocalcemia.

79. An ED nurse is caring for a patient who was injured during a violent crime. Which of the following is a priority in evidence collection and care?

- **A.** chain of custody
- **B.** chain of evidence
- **C.** photographing of evidence
- **D.** documenting of evidence

80. A patient is brought to the ED following a motor vehicle crash. He was driving without a seat belt and was hit with the steering wheel on the left side of his chest. He complains of severe chest pain and dyspnea. During assessment, the nurse is unable to hear breath sounds on the left. The nurse should prepare to assist with immediate

- **A.** endotracheal intubation.
- **B.** chest compressions.
- **C.** chest tube insertion.
- **D.** thoracotomy.

81. Epistaxis occurring from Kiesselbach's plexus is controlled by all methods EXCEPT

   A. cauterization of a visualized vessel.

   B. high Fowler's position leaning forward and applying continuous pressure to the midline septum.

   C. nasal packing with hemostatic material.

   D. endoscopic litigation.

82. Which of the following interventions is NOT appropriate for a patient with adrenal hypofunction?

   A. peripheral blood draws

   B. low-sodium diet

   C. blood glucose monitoring

   D. hydrocortisone therapy

83. A patient is brought to the ED with dyspnea, headache, light-headedness, and diaphoresis. A diagnosis of hyperventilation syndrome is made. The nurse is aware that hyperventilation syndrome can present with signs and symptoms similar to which of the following?

   A. pneumonia

   B. bronchitis

   C. pulmonary embolism

   D. pneumothorax

84. Which test should a nurse expect before a health care provider prescribes risperidone to manage psychotic symptoms?

   A. a cardiac workup

   B. comprehensive metabolic panel (CMP)

   C. creatinine clearance

   D. complete blood count (CBC)

85. The nurse is caring for a patient who says he wants to commit suicide. He has a detailed, concrete plan. The nurse places the patient on suicide precautions, which include a 24-hour sitter. The patient becomes angry and refuses the sitter. Which action is the most appropriate?

   A. place the patient in soft wrist restraints

   B. have security sit outside the patient's door

   C. assign a sitter despite the patient's refusal

   D. allow the patient to leave against medical advice (AMA)

86. Which laboratory finding indicates that a 62-year-old male patient is at risk for ventricular dysrhythmia?

    A. magnesium 0.8 mEq/L

    B. potassium 4.2 mmol/L

    C. creatinine 1.3 mg/dL

    D. total calcium 2.8 mmol/L

87. A patient presents to the ED with chest pain, dyspnea, and diaphoresis. The nurse finds a narrow complex tachycardia with a HR of 210 bpm, BP of 70/42 mm Hg, and a RR of 18. The nurse should anticipate which priority intervention?

    A. administer adenosine 6 mg IV

    B. defibrillate at 200 J

    C. administer amiodarone 300 mg IV

    D. prepare for synchronized cardioversion

88. A patient is brought to the ED in supraventricular tachycardia (SVT) with a rate of 220. EMS has administered 6 mg of adenosine, but the patient remains in SVT. What is the next intervention the nurse should anticipate?

    A. administer 12 mg adenosine IV

    B. administer 1 mg epinephrine IV

    C. administer 300 mg amiodarone IV

    D. administer 0.5 atropine IV

89. A 6-year-old child is admitted to the ED with an acute asthma attack. A pulse oximetry is attached with a reading of 91%. The nursing priority is to

    A. administer dexamethasone.

    B. provide supplemental oxygen.

    C. prepare for immediate endotracheal intubation.

    D. administer a nebulized albuterol treatment.

90. A patient is admitted to the ED with a sickle cell crisis. The nurse should prepare to administer which of the following blood products?

    A. warm packed RBCs

    B. whole blood

    C. fresh frozen plasma (FFP)

    D. cryoprecipitate

91. Which complication of compartment syndrome would the nurse suspect if urinalysis reveals myoglobinuria?

   A. disseminated intravascular coagulation (DIC)

   B. rhabdomyolysis

   C. Volkmann's contracture

   D. sepsis

92. A patient presents to the ED with complaints of substernal sharp, tearing knifelike chest pain radiating to the neck, jaw, and face. Morphine sulfate is given with no relief of the pain. These signs and symptoms are most indicative of which of the following?

   A. myocardial infarction (MI)

   B. pericarditis

   C. pneumonia

   D. acute aortic dissection

93. A patient is admitted to the ED with a potassium level of 6.9. Which of the following medications could have caused her electrolyte imbalance?

   A. bumetanide

   B. captopril

   C. furosemide

   D. digoxin

94. A patient presents to the ED with a bleeding laceration to the arm and a history of idiopathic thrombocytopenic purpura (ITP). The nurse should anticipate which treatment to be ordered?

   A. cryoprecipitate

   B. fresh frozen plasma (FFP)

   C. platelets

   D. protamine sulfate

95. Which of the following is usually associated with variant (Prinzmetal's) angina?

   A. cyanide poisoning

   B. gastroesophageal reflux

   C. Raynaud's phenomena

   D. beta-blocker toxicity

96. Hyperglycemic hyperosmolar state (HHS) is most often caused by

   A. inadequate glucose monitoring.

   B. dehydration.

   C. noncompliance with insulin therapy.

   D. a breakdown of ketones.

97. Fluoxetine for moderate depression is contraindicated in patients with

    A. arthritis.

    B. migraines.

    C. glaucoma.

    D. appendicitis.

98. A patient presents to the ED with severe throbbing fingers after coming home from the gym. Upon observing thin, shiny skin, pallor, and thick fingernails, the nurse should suspect

    A. acute arterial injury.

    B. acute arterial occlusion.

    C. peripheral venous thrombosis.

    D. peripheral vascular disease.

99. Which of the following IV solutions should be administered to a patient with diabetic ketoacidosis (DKA) who is placed on an insulin drip?

    A. lactated Ringer's

    B. normal saline

    C. normal saline with potassium

    D. normal saline with dextrose

100. EMS brings in a patient with a history of alcohol abuse, homelessness, and poor adherence to antiseizure medications. The patient has experienced 3 seizures in 30 minutes. These findings support the diagnosis of

    A. atonic seizure.

    B. tonic–clonic seizure.

    C. status epilepticus.

    D. simple partial seizure.

101. When taking the history of a patient with suspected pancreatitis, the nurse should expect to find

    A. the patient feels better when lying supine.

    B. the patient has a history of alcohol abuse and peptic ulcer disease.

    C. the pain is described as a sharp, burning sensation.

    D. the pain began gradually and radiated to the right lower abdomen.

102. A pediatric patient is being resuscitated in a trauma bay, and his father wants to be in the room. What should the nurse do?

    A. Tell the father he may not be in the trauma room during resuscitation.

    B. Allow the father in the trauma room with a knowledgeable staff member for support.

    C. Ask the father to stand just outside the trauma room.

    D. Call the legal department for advice.

103. A patient arrives to the ED after an attempted suicide by a self-inflicted gunshot wound. He is determined to be brain dead, but his life can be sustained for organ procurement. The patient is identified as an organ donor. Which of the following is the next step for the ED nurse?

   A. notify local organ procurement organization

   B. remove all life-supporting interventions

   C. perform postmortem care on the patient

   D. complete the death certificate

104. When caring for a patient with thyroid storm, the nurse should first prepare to administer which medication?

   A. propylthiouracil (PTU)

   B. epinephrine

   C. levothyroxine

   D. atropine

105. A patient arrives to the ED with a sheriff escort after being found in a street acting erratically and shouting. She is unkempt and not appropriately dressed for the weather. She states that she wants to commit suicide. What can the ED nurse expect to happen to the patient?

   A. She will be given benzodiazepines for anxiety and discharged.

   B. She will be medically cleared and brought to jail.

   C. She will be involuntarily committed.

   D. She will be voluntarily admitted to the hospital.

106. A patient with a blood glucose reading of 475 mg/dL presents to the ED with Kussmaul respirations, nausea, and vomiting, and a pH of 7.3. The nurse should expect to treat which condition?

   A. myxedema coma

   B. hyperosmolar hyperglycemic state (HHS)

   C. pheochromocytoma

   D. diabetic ketoacidosis (DKA)

107. The nurse is using the Glasgow Coma Scale (GCS) to assess a patient who fell in a parking lot. The patient opens his eyes to sound, localizes pain, and makes incoherent sounds when spoken to. Which GCS score will the nurse document?

   A. 9

   B. 10

   C. 11

   D. 12

108. A patient arrives to the ED with a complaint of sore throat and fever. Which of the following findings is the most immediate concern?

   A. visualized white abscess on the soft palate

   B. patchy tonsillar exudate

   C. petechiae on the hard palate

   D. lymphedema

109. A patient in the ED is diagnosed with ulcerative colitis (UC). Which dietary changes can the nurse recommend to help manage symptoms?

   A. Eat a high-fiber diet.

   B. Limit coffee to two cups daily.

   C. Avoid lactose-containing foods.

   D. Consume dried fruit several times a week.

110. A 32-year-old female patient comes to the ED with complaints of abdominal pain. She describes the pain as sharp and states it began suddenly during intercourse. The pain is worse with movement, and there is no vaginal discharge noted. These findings support the diagnosis of

   A. ectopic pregnancy.

   B. ruptured appendix.

   C. ruptured ovarian cyst.

   D. STD.

111. Which of the following signs or symptoms should lead a nurse to suspect septic shock?

   A. WBC of 2,500

   B. serum lactate level of 2.6

   C. decrease in neutrophils

   D. increase in RBCs

112. A patient is admitted to the ED with nausea, vomiting, and diarrhea for 3 days and signs of severe dehydration. The nurse starts an IV and prepares to administer which fluid replacement?

   A. hypertonic solution

   B. isotonic crystalloid

   C. hypotonic solution

   D. colloid solution

113. The nurse is reviewing the history of a patient with heart failure. Which of the following coexisting health problems will cause an increase in the patient's afterload?

    A. diabetes

    B. endocrine disorders

    C. hypertension

    D. Marfan syndrome

114. The nurse is caring for a patient who presented to the ED with a subarachnoid hemorrhage. While taking the patient's history, what symptoms would the nurse expect to see with this patient?

    A. sudden food cravings

    B. rash on the lower trunk

    C. Battle's sign

    D. a severe, sudden headache

115. The nurse is discharging a patient who has been prescribed medications to control progressive MS. Which statement by the patient indicates a need for further teaching by the nurse?

    A. "I will wear an eye patch on alternating eyes if I have double vision."

    B. "I will clear rugs and extra furniture from my walking paths at home."

    C. "I hope I feel like going to Disney World this summer with my grandchildren."

    D. "I will call my doctor if I have any signs or symptoms of infection, such as fever."

116. Lower abdominal pain that is worsened with movement, a non-malodorous vaginal discharge, a fever, and tachycardia are usually associated with

    A. appendicitis.

    B. pelvic inflammatory disease.

    C. ectopic pregnancy.

    D. STI.

117. Which prescription would the nurse anticipate administering to a patient with no known medication allergies who presents with orofacial edema, halitosis, and a complaint of tasting pus in the mouth?

    A. nystatin

    B. sodium fluoride drops

    C. penicillin V potassium

    D. saliva substitute

118. A patient with a myocardial infarction (MI). The patient has received nitroglycerin sublingual and is still experiencing chest pain. The nurse should prepare to administer

   A. hydromorphone.

   B. meperidine.

   C. morphine sulfate.

   D. acetaminophen.

119. A patient presents to the ED with complaints of dizziness and fatigue and a past medical history of HIV. She states she is noncompliant with her antiviral medications. Her temperature is 101.2°F (38.4°C), BP 100/72 mm Hg, HR 130 bpm, RR 22, and O$_2$ 96%.

   Which of the following orders would be the priority intervention?

   A. administering an antibiotic

   B. administering acetaminophen

   C. administering prescribed antivirals

   D. administering 2 units of packed RBCs

120. The nurse is caring for a patient who suffered a head injury following a fall off a ladder. The nurse assesses the patient for signs of increased intracranial pressure (ICP). Which finding by the nurse is a LATE sign of increased ICP?

   A. headache

   B. restlessness

   C. dilated pupils

   D. decreasing LOC

121. An 11-month-old infant is brought to the ED with a barking cough, a respiratory rate of 66, substernal retractions, and copious nasal secretions. Which of the following positions will best facilitate the child's breathing?

   A. sitting upright in a parent's lap

   B. on a stretcher in a prone position

   C. reverse Trendelenburg

   D. semi-Fowler's

122. Which of the following statements would be included in the discharge teaching for a patient with ulcerative colitis (UC)?

   A. "Hemorrhage is a potential complication."

   B. "Patients may have 5 – 6 loose stools per day."

   C. "Patients with UC are more likely to have fistulas."

   D. "Many times, surgery is needed to treat symptoms."

123. Which pain characteristics are associated with inflammation of the fifth cranial nerve?

    A. progressive onset, bilateral, throbbing

    B. abrupt onset, unilateral, hemifacial spasm

    C. intermittent, circumoral, shooting

    D. paroxysmal, bilateral, paresthesia

124. Two weeks post–left-sided myocardial infarction (MI) a patient presents to the ED with dyspnea and cough with hemoptysis. The nurse should suspect the patient has developed

    A. pneumonia.

    B. over-coagulation.

    C. pulmonary edema.

    D. ruptured ventricle.

125. A patient arrives to the ED with altered mental status, blood pressure of 70/40, and declining vital signs. Her husband states that she does not wish to be resuscitated. What should the ED nurse do?

    A. Tell the patient that the physician will decide her advance directive status.

    B. Ask the spouse for the advanced directive paperwork.

    C. Document the patient's advanced directive wishes and honor the request in case resuscitation is needed.

    D. Inform the patient that advanced directives are not used in EDs.

126. A family in the ED must decide whether to withdraw care for a family member with no advance directive. Which person would NOT be consulted as a part of a multidisciplinary team to make this decision?

    A. chair of ethics committee

    B. legal department

    C. critical care physician

    D. pharmacist

127. A 2-year-old child presents to the ED with septal deviation and a visualized foreign body in the right naris. Which nursing intervention is most appropriate?

    A. instructing the parent to perform nasal positive pressure

    B. instructing the child to blow his nose

    C. instructing the parent to perform oral positive pressure

    D. restraining the child for forceps retraction

128. Which treatment is contraindicated for a corneal abrasion?

    A. application of ophthalmic lubricating solution

    B. application of topical anesthetics

    C. patching the affected eye

    D. wearing glasses instead of contact lenses

129. The ED nurse is caring for a patient with delirium who tells the nurse, "There are snakes crawling up on my bed." How should the nurse respond?

    A. "That's just the wrinkles in your blanket."

    B. "I will see if I can move you to another room."

    C. "I will call maintenance to come and remove them."

    D. "I know you're scared, but I don't see any snakes on your bed."

130. The nurse is caring for a patient who has been prescribed rasagiline mesylate for Parkinson's disease. Which medication on the patient's current record should prompt the nurse to notify the health care provider?

    A. baclofen

    B. amantadine

    C. benztropine

    D. isocarboxazid

131. Which medication would the nurse anticipate administering to a patient with a periorbital vesicular rash along the trigeminal nerve?

    A. acyclovir

    B. erythromycin

    C. ketorolac

    D. ciprofloxacin

132. The nurse is caring for a patient who presents to the ED with the following arterial blood gas (ABG) results:

> pH 7.32
> $PaCO_2$ 47 mm Hg
> HCO_3 24 mEq/L
> PaO_2 91 mm Hg

The nurse should expect the patient to present with

    A. chest pain.

    B. nausea and vomiting.

    C. deep, rapid respirations.

    D. hypoventilation with hypoxia.

133. Management of acute iritis includes
   A. topical mydriatic ophthalmic drops and topical corticosteroids.
   B. copious irrigation.
   C. IV mannitol and acetazolamide.
   D. topical anesthetics and topical antibiotics.

134. Discharge teaching for a patient diagnosed with ulcerative keratitis is effective if she states which of the following?
   A. "There is no need to follow up with an ophthalmologist."
   B. "I will stop the antibiotic drops tomorrow if the pain is better."
   C. "I will wear glasses and not contacts for at least two weeks."
   D. "I need to stay home from work until the infection clears because I am highly contagious."

135. The nurse is caring for a patient with a history of cirrhosis who arrived at the ED with a new onset of confusion. The patient's skin is jaundiced. Labs are as follows:

   Ammonia 130 mcg/dL
   ALT 98 U/L
   Blood glucose 128

   The nurse should prepare to administer
   A. lactulose.
   B. bisacodyl.
   C. mesalamine.
   D. insulin 2 units.

136. Which of the following is a clinical feature of an open globe rupture?
   A. cherry red macula
   B. rust ring
   C. pale optic disc
   D. afferent pupillary defect

137. Dopamine (Intropin) is ordered for a patient with heart failure because the drug
   A. lowers the heart rate.
   B. opens blocked arteries.
   C. prevents plaque from building up.
   D. increases the amount of oxygen delivered to the heart.

138. Which statement regarding tourniquet use to control hemorrhagic bleeding for a partial limb amputation is correct?

   A. A commercially available tourniquet that is at least 2 inches wide with a windlass, a ratcheting device to occlude arterial flow, is recommended.

   B. Tourniquet application is never recommended even when direct pressure does not control blood loss from an extremity.

   C. Tourniquets properly applied in the prehospital setting should always be removed upon arrival to the ED, regardless if there is adequate team support to manage bleeding.

   D. Time of tourniquet application should be noted clearly on the device and should not exceed 4-hour intervals before reassessment of bleeding.

139. Which of the following will confirm the diagnosis of a pulmonary embolism?

   A. chest X-ray

   B. D-dimer

   C. fibrin split products

   D. CT angiography

140. The nurse is caring for a patient with a history of schizophrenia, alcohol abuse, bipolar disorder, and noncompliance with treatment and medications. The patient has also been arrested in the past for violent behavior. Which action by the nurse is the most important when caring for a potentially violent patient?

   A. treat the patient with courtesy and respect

   B. always maintain an open pathway to the door

   C. be sure the patient swallows his pills and does not "cheek" them

   D. ask permission from the patient before drawing blood or performing other invasive procedures

141. A 13-year-old female arrives to the ED complaining of chest pain. A physical exam reveals tenderness along the fourth, fifth, and sixth ribs. Which diagnosis does the nurse suspect?

   A. myocardial infarction

   B. Ludwig's angina

   C. pleurisy

   D. costochondritis

142. Which of the following describes the characteristics of a flail chest?

   A. The chest sinks in with inspiration and out with expiration.

   B. Only the right side of the chest has movement.

   C. Movement is noted on the left side of the chest only.

   D. There is no movement noted on either side of the chest.

143. The ED nurse is providing discharge teaching to a patient newly diagnosed with migraines who has been given a prescription for sumatriptan. Which of the following statements indicates the patient understands the discharge teaching?

   A.   "This medication is safe to take while pregnant."

   B.   "I will report chest pain immediately to my physician."

   C.   "I will take my blood pressure medicine before I take sumatriptan."

   D.   "I will take this medication 15 minutes after I feel a migraine starting."

144. A 4-year-old child was in a bicycle accident and presents with oral lacerations and complete dental avulsions to the 2 top front teeth. The best initial management by the health care provider is

   A.   immediate replantation of the avulsed teeth.

   B.   laceration repair.

   C.   replantation of the avulsed tooth after soaking for 30 minutes in Hank's solution.

   D.   dental consult.

145. Diagnostic findings common with gouty arthritis include

   A.   hyperammonemia.

   B.   hyperbilirubinemia.

   C.   hyperuricemia.

   D.   hyperhomocysteinemia.

146. Which dressing would be most appropriate for a patient with a partial thickness wound to the epidermis?

   A.   transparent dressing

   B.   occlusive dressing

   C.   nonstick adherent dressing

   D.   bulky dressing

147. A patient arrives to the ED from a house fire. The nurse notes soot at the opening of her mouth and both nares. What is the primary concern for this patient?

   A.   total body surface areas covered in burns

   B.   airway edema related to inhalation injury

   C.   foreign body ingestion during the fire

   D.   trauma as a result of rescue from the fire

148. Which intervention is contraindicated for a patient with acute angle glaucoma?

    A. administration of ophthalmic beta blocker

    B. maintaining patient in a supine position

    C. dimming lights in the room or providing a blindfold for comfort

    D. administration of IV mannitol

149. Which of the following chest X-ray readings is consistent with acute respiratory distress syndrome (ARDS)?

    A. bilateral, diffuse white infiltrates without cardiomegaly

    B. bilateral, diffuse infiltrates with cardiomegaly

    C. tapering vascular shadows with hyperlucency and right ventricular enlargement

    D. prominent hilar vascular shadows with left ventricular enlargement

150. Which positive toxicology result would the nurse suspect in a patient with a MRSA-positive infectious abscess of the right antecubital space?

    A. alcohol

    B. opioid

    C. benzodiazepine

    D. tetrahydrocannabinol (THC)

151. A patient arrives to the ED after taking a sedative and subsequently becoming confused and disoriented. His temperature is 96.2°F (35.6°C), pulse is 47 bpm with distant heart tones, and BP is 82/65 mm Hg. He states that he is currently receiving thyroid replacement therapy. The nurse should suspect

    A. allergic reaction to the sedative.

    B. thyroid storm.

    C. myxedema coma.

    D. acute stroke.

152. The health care provider orders xylocaine with epinephrine to be prepared for a patient with a

    A. 2 cm laceration to the penile shaft.

    B. 2 cm laceration above the right eyebrow.

    C. 3 cm laceration to the left index finger.

    D. 7 cm laceration to the left forearm.

153. Which is the most appropriate post-exposure rabies prophylaxis treatment for an animal bite in a patient not previously vaccinated?

    A.   rabies vaccine on days 0, 3, 7, and 14

    B.   human rabies immune globulin injected into the wound bed

    C.   human rabies immune globulin injected into the wound bed and rabies vaccine on days 0, 3, 7, and 14

    D.   tetanus 0.5 mL via intramuscular injection

154. A child is admitted to the ED with wheezing on exhalation, use of accessory muscles, using 1-word sentences, and tripod positioning. The nurse should suspect

    A.   pneumonia.

    B.   pneumonitis.

    C.   foreign body aspiration.

    D.   asthma.

155. Which of the following IV medications should a nurse anticipate administering to a patient experiencing a severe anaphylactic reaction to a bee sting?

    A.   epinephrine 1:1000 0.3 – 0.5 mL

    B.   diphenhydramine 25 – 50 mg

    C.   Solu-Medrol 125 mg

    D.   theophylline 6mg/kg

156. The best medical management for carbon monoxide toxicity is

    A.   hydroxocobalamin

    B.   hyperbaric oxygen

    C.   N-acetylcysteine

    D.   sodium bicarbonate

157. A patient presents to the ED with complaints of severe headache, irritability, confusion, and lethargy. During triage he mentions that he has spent the last several days in his shop with a wood-burning stove. The ED nurse should be concerned for which of the following?

    A.   migraine headache

    B.   stroke

    C.   carbon monoxide poisoning

    D.   allergic reaction

158. The nurse is reviewing the laboratory results of a patient with renal failure and notes a serum potassium level of 7.2. The nurse should prepare to administer which of the following medications to protect cardiac status?

   A. aspirin

   B. insulin

   C. calcium gluconate

   D. digoxin

159. A college student arrived at the ED with suspected meningitis, and a positive diagnosis was confirmed via lumbar puncture. Which of the following findings suggests that she may have developed hydrocephalus?

   A. sluggish pupillary response

   B. inability to wrinkle the forehead

   C. inability to move the eyes laterally

   D. inability to move the eyes downward

160. Appropriate discharge teaching for a patient with diverticular disease includes instructions to

   A. avoid foods high in sodium.

   B. consume clear liquids until pain subsides.

   C. limit alcohol to one glass per day.

   D. include strawberries to get enough vitamin C.

161. Which neurological assessment finding commonly occurs in a patient struck by lightning?

   A. tic douloureux

   B. ascending paralysis

   C. Bell's palsy

   D. keraunoparalysis

162. A patient presents to the ED with confusion, anxiety, irritability, and a slight tremor. During assessment, she states she drinks two or more bottles of wine per day. Which of the following questions is important to ask?

   A. Do you drink any other alcoholic drinks on a regular basis?

   B. When was your last drink?

   C. When was your first drink?

   D. Have you ever experienced alcohol withdrawal?

163. A 34-year-old patient attempted suicide by consuming his grandmother's oral antidiabetic agent. Administration of glucose has been unsuccessful in reversing the effect of the medication. Which antidote should the nurse expect to administer next?

A. flumazenil

B. acetylcysteine

C. octreotide

D. methylene blue

164. A patient presents to triage with a complaint of cough lasting three weeks without improvement. The patient confirms recent travel to a developing country, and states she has had fevers and chills for the last three days. The nurse should suspect

A. herpes zoster.

B. tuberculosis.

C. influenza.

D. hepatitis C.

165. A woman arrives to the ED with her 5-year-old child, whom she discovered eating her nifedipine. She does not know how many pills the child consumed. The nursing priority is to

A. place a referral to child protective services.

B. obtain a 12-lead ECG.

C. place the child on oxygen.

D. ask the child how many she took.

166. A 10-year-old child presents to triage with conjunctivitis, cough, and a rash in the back of his mouth. During the assessment, the patient's father indicates that the child is not vaccinated. These findings most likely indicate

A. varicella.

B. mumps.

C. measles.

D. pertussis.

167. Which of the following medications should the nurse expect to administer to a patient who chronically abuses alcohol?

A. naloxone

B. thiamine

C. flumazenil

D. vitamin K

168. A 35-year-old patient in the ED has been diagnosed with herpes zoster. Which of the following statements should the nurse include in her discharge teaching?

    A. Herpes zoster occurs any time after an initial varicella infection and may recur several times.

    B. The varicella vaccine is known to cause latent herpes zoster when administered to children.

    C. Herpes zoster outbreaks are caused by a latent virus, so it is not contagious.

    D. The zoster vaccine should not be given to patients who have had a herpes zoster outbreak.

169. A 7-year-old unvaccinated child arrives to the ED. The nurse suspects diphtheria, based on which of the following symptoms?

    A. thick gray membrane covering the tonsils and pharynx

    B. temperature of 104°F (40°C) or greater

    C. macular rash on the thorax and back, along the dermatomes

    D. cluster headache with nausea and symptoms of an aura

170. Which of the following statements from a nurse demonstrates that his participation in a Critical Incident Stress Debriefing (CISD) session was effective?

    A. He agrees to meet with the manager regarding the incident.

    B. He agrees to attend future debriefing sessions as needed.

    C. He agrees to schedule an appointment for further counseling.

    D. He provides the incident details before departing the debrief.

171. The ED nurse's responsibility to practice quality nursing care is achieved through which of the following?

    A. reading research articles

    B. participating in Evidence-Based Practice (EBP) projects

    C. participating in research studies

    D. participating in grand rounds

172. Nurses managing patient transitions of care in the ED should consider all of the following characteristics EXCEPT

    A. accessibility of services.

    B. safety.

    C. community partnerships.

    D. patient income.

173. What is the appropriate ratio of compressions to ventilations for a full-term neonate who is apneic with a pulse rate of 50 bpm?

    A. 30:2

    B. 15:1

    C. 15:2

    D. 3:1

174. Which of the following interventions is NOT necessary for a patient who has died in the ED and is not in a vegetative state?

    A. maintaining the head of the bed at 20 degrees

    B. instilling artificial tears in eyes to preserve tissue

    C. taping eyes closed with paper tape

    D. inserting Foley catheter to decompress the bladder

175. A 24-year-old male patient arrives at the ED with a complaint of a 1-month history of a rash that is annular, with raised margins and centralized clearing. Which of the following dermal infections does the nurse expect?

    A. scabies

    B. ringworm

    C. impetigo

    D. cellulitis

ANSWER KEY

1. B

Rationale: Lumbar punctures are contraindicated for patients with increased ICP because of the risk of brain shift caused by the sudden release of CSF pressure. Severe brain shift can result in permanent damage. BMP and CBC labs are routinely monitored in patients with increased ICP. Mechanical ventilation and Foley catheter placement are commonly ordered for patients with increased ICP.

Objective: Neurological Emergencies

Subobjective: Increased Intracranial Pressure (ICP)

2. C

Rationale: Adrenaline, dopamine, digoxin, and dobutamine are all positive inotropes and can be helpful in the management of heart failure. However, digoxin is not recommended in the treatment of acute heart failure in an 80-year-old patient as elderly patients are more susceptible to digoxin toxicity.

Objective: Cardiovascular Emergencies

Subobjective: Heart Failure

3. D

Rationale: Sudden back pain and dyspnea indicate rupture of the aneurysm, which is an emergency. The nurse should notify the health care provider, monitor neurological and vital signs, and remain with the patient. Yellow-tinted vision is a finding of digitalis toxicity. Hemoptysis a sign of pulmonary edema. Urinary output of 75 mL/hr is normal.

Objective: Cardiovascular Emergencies

Subobjective: Aneurysm/Dissection

4. C

Rationale: Increased risk factors for heparin-induced thrombocytopenia (HIT) include being female and heparin use for postsurgical thromboprophylaxis. HIT is more common in patients who have been on unfractionated heparin or who have used heparin for longer than 1 week. Enoxaparin is a low-molecular-weight heparin, which carries a lower risk of causing HIT. It is often prescribed for patients with unstable angina to help increase blood flow through the heart.

Objective: Cardiovascular Emergencies

Subobjective: Thromboembolic Disease

5. D

Rationale: A pericardial friction rub is heard in pericarditis due to the inflammation of the pericardial layers rubbing together. Mitral regurgitation does not occur in pericarditis. An S3 gallop is heard in heart failure. S4 gallop is heard in cardiomyopathies and congenital heart disease.

Objective: Cardiovascular Emergencies

Subobjective: Pericarditis

6. C

Rationale: High-velocity injection injuries damage underlying tissue and often result in necrosis and compartment syndrome and may require amputation. Obtaining a surgical consultation and exploration minimizes the risk of long-term complications. While administering prophylactic antibiotics, providing patient education, and immobilizing the affected extremity are correct nursing interventions, they alone will not minimize the risk for complications.

Objective: Wound

Subobjective: Injection Injuries

7. B

Rationale: The patient is in V-fib and is pulseless. After CPR is started, the next priority intervention is defibrillation. Epinephrine should not be administered until after defibrillation. Inserting an advanced airway may be indicated but is not the priority. A fluid bolus is not a priority for a patient in V-fib.

Objective: Cardiovascular Emergencies

Subobjective: Cardiopulmonary Arrest

8. D

Rationale: The patient has signs and symptoms of gastritis. Pain relievers such as naproxen can inflame the lining of the stomach and lead to gastritis. Tobacco use, radiation, and viral or bacterial infection are also risk factors. Obesity, appendicitis, and hypertension are not associated with naproxen.

Objective: Gastrointestinal Emergencies

Subobjective: Gastritis

9. **C**

   Rationale: The infant has signs of intussusception, in which part of the intestine telescopes into another area of the intestine. Abdominal swelling in a child with intussusception is a sign of peritonitis, which can be life-threatening. Vomiting, diarrhea, and a lump in the abdomen are expected findings in a child with intussusception.

   Objective: Gastrointestinal Emergencies

   Subobjective: Intussusception

10. **B**

   Rationale: The physician will counsel the patient on the risks associated with leaving against medical advice (AMA). Whenever possible, the patient should be counseled by the physician, sign AMA paperwork, and then leave the department. A patient with appendicitis will not be involuntarily committed. It is not appropriate to tell a patient he will die if he leaves, although he should be informed of possible negative consequences. The patient should speak with the physician before he tries to leave.

   Objective: Professional Issues

   Subobjective: Patient (Discharge Planning)

11. **A**

   Rationale: Current 2015 guidelines for CPR from the AHA is 30 compressions to 2 ventilations for adult patients with 2 rescuers.

   Objective: Cardiovascular Emergencies

   Subobjective: Cardiopulmonary Arrest

12. **A**

   Rationale: Fluid boluses of 1 to 2 L normal saline should be used to treat hypotension. The patient is dehydrated at the cellular level and needs fluid resuscitation. Furosemide is used

as a diuretic and would further dehydrate the patient, exacerbating the issue. Inotropes such as dopamine are used to promote cardiac contractility and will not hydrate the patient. D5W is not indicated because it is not an isotonic solution that will add to the systemic fluid volume.

Objective: Cardiac Emergencies

Subobjective: Acute Coronary Syndromes

13. **B**

   Rationale: An elevated carboxyhemoglobin (COHb) level of 2% or higher for nonsmokers and 10% or higher for smokers strongly supports a diagnosis of carbon monoxide poisoning. COHb may be measured with a fingertip pulse CO-oximeter or by serum lab values. $PaCO_2$ measurements remain normal (38 – 42).

   Objective: Environmental

   Subobjective: Chemical Exposure

14. **C**

   Rationale: A non-odorous white "cottage cheese"–appearing vaginal discharge describes *Candida* vulvovaginitis. Bacterial vaginosis presents with thin white, gray, or green discharge and a fishy odor. *Trichomoniasis* vaginitis typically presents with thin discharge and itching or burning of the genital area. *Neisseria gonorrhoeae* usually does not cause any symptoms but may have dysuria and thin discharge.

   Objective: Gynecological

   Subobjective: Infection

15. **B**

   Rationale: The nurse should place the patient on contact precautions with concern for C. difficile. The other levels of precautions are not appropriate based on the information presented.

   Objective: Communicable Diseases

   Subobjective: C. Difficile

16. **A**

   Rationale: A greenish-gray frothy malodorous vaginal discharge and itching are signs and symptoms of *trichomoniasis.*

Bacterial vaginosis would present with a thin discharge and presence of clue cells on the wet prep. Herpes would most likely present with lesions upon inspection. Chlamydia would not cause frothy discharge.

Objective: Gynecological

Subobjective: Infection

17. B

Rationale: Hepatomegaly is seen in patients with right-sided heart failure due to vascular engorgement. Heart failure does not lead to appendicitis. Constipation is not directly a result of heart failure and therefore is not a priority assessment consideration. Stomach upset is a common side effect of many medications but is not a cause for focused or priority assessment.

Objective: Cardiac Emergencies

Subobjective: Heart Failure

18. A

Rationale: Deep tissue palpation should be avoided to minimize the risk of injury to the nurse and to prevent advancement of the foreign body deeper into the tissue structure.

Objective: Wound

Subobjective: Foreign Bodies

19. B

Rationale: The patient is unstable in a third-degree or complete heart block, so transcutaneous pacing is indicated.

Objective: Cardiovascular Emergencies

Subobjective: Dysrhythmias

20. A

Rationale: The patient's symptoms are signs of a septic abortion. An ectopic pregnancy typically presents with vaginal bleeding and pain without fever. A missed abortion may have no other symptoms except a brown discharge. The symptoms are not indicative of abdominal trauma.

Objective: Obstetrical

Subobjective: Threatened/Spontaneous Abortion

21. C

Rationale: PT (prothrombin time) and PTT (partial thromboplastin time) are blood tests that monitor effectiveness of anticoagulant therapy. Hematocrit measures packed RBCs and is not a specific study of anticoagulant effectiveness. HDL and LDL are components of cholesterol measurement. Troponin levels measure myocardial muscle injury.

Objective: Respiratory Emergencies

Subobjective: Pulmonary Embolism

22. D

Rationale: The patient who is diagnosed with disseminated intravascular coagulation (DIC) has both a clotting and bleeding problem. Increased PT/PTT, elevated D-dimer levels, decreased platelets, decreased hemoglobin, and a decreased fibrinogen level are all expected lab values for this patient.

Objective: Medical Emergencies

Subobjective: Blood Dyscrasias

23. B

Rationale: Symptoms of autonomic dysfunction include heart block, bradycardia, hypertension, hypotension, and orthostatic hypotension. Deficits in CN X (vagus nerve) contribute to the development of autonomic dysfunction. Trigeminy, atrial flutter, and tachycardia are not symptoms of autonomic dysfunction.

Objective: Neurological Emergencies

Subobjective: Guillain–Barré Syndrome

24. B

Rationale: Procedural sedation is appropriate for synchronized cardioversion. A perimortem cesarean section typically is done emergently. Open fracture reductions should occur in the operating room, as should dilatation and curettage.

Objective: Professional Issues

Subobjective: Patient (Pain Management and Procedural Sedation)

25. C

Rationale: Lung tissue disorders include pneumonia and pulmonary edema. Examples of lower airway disorders are bronchiolitis and asthma. An upper airway disorder would be croup, anaphylaxis, or foreign body obstruction. Disordered control of breathing means an irregular, slow breathing pattern with a neurological component, such as a seizure.

Objective: Respiratory Emergencies

Subobjective: Infections

26. **A**

Rationale: In atrial flutter, there are no discernible P waves, and a distinct sawtooth wave pattern is present. The atrial rate is regular, and the PR interval is not measurable. In atrial fibrillation, the rhythm would be very irregular with coarse, asynchronous waves. Torasades de pointes, or "twisting of the points," is characterized by QRS complexes that twist around the baseline and is a form of polymorphic ventricular tachycardia. It may resolve spontaneously or progress to ventricular fibrillation, which is emergent, as the ventricles are unable to pump any blood due to disorganized electrical activity. Untreated, it quickly leads to cardiac arrest.

Objective: Cardiovascular Emergencies

Subobjective: Dysrhythmias

27. **B**

Rationale: The patient has been playing sports, sweating and replacing lost fluid with only water, which can cause hyponatremia. A loss of sodium will cause neurological effects such as confusion, seizures, and coma. The symptoms are not indicative of a potassium imbalance. Hyperkalemia would cause thirst and nausea/vomiting.

Objective: Medical Emergencies

Subobjective: Electrolyte/Fluid Imbalance

28. **B**

Rationale: A barking cough is a symptom of croup, and nebulized epinephrine is the treatment of choice. IV epinephrine is not indicated in croup; it is more often used in anaphylaxis and resuscitation efforts. Albuterol has a primary effect on lower lung structures and will not improve symptoms of croup. Dexamethasone is indicated for croup but is not the priority intervention.

Objective: Respiratory Emergencies

Subobjective: Infections

29. **A**

Rationale: Bell's palsy is caused by an inflammation of the seventh cranial nerve and presents with facial paralysis and weakness.

Objective: Maxillofacial

Subobjective: Facial Nerve Disorders

30. **B**

Rationale: Left-sided heart failure manifestations include pulmonary symptoms such as crackles and dyspnea. Right-sided heart failure causes systemic congestion, leading to hepatomegaly, dependent edema, jugular vein distention, and ascites.

Objective: Cardiovascular Emergencies

Subobjective: Heart Failure

31. **A**

Rationale: Foreign body infections and cellulitis of surgical hardware sites present with local pain and systemic infectious indicators such as fever, edema, warmth, and elevated WBCs with left shift in neutrophils.

Objective: Orthopedic

Subobjective: Foreign Bodies

32. **A**

Rationale: The second digit of the nondominant hand is the most common site, as these types of injuries are usually self-inflicted.

Objective: Wound

Subobjective: Injection Injuries

33. **A**

Rationale: Absent or decreased breath sounds are present in a pneumothorax. A nurse would be able to visualize a foreign body on the right side of chest while doing the initial assessment. Hematoma and pleural effusion are both associated with decreased breath sounds, not with absent sounds.

Objective: Respiratory Emergencies

Subobjective: Pneumothorax

34. A

Rationale: Warfarin is an anticoagulant commonly prescribed for patients with A-fib. Any anticoagulant must be given cautiously to patients with subarachnoid hemorrhage due to the increased risk of bleeding. Morphine is commonly prescribed for pain, and nimodipine is given to treat or prevent cerebral vasospasm. Stool softeners are given to reduce the need to strain during a bowel movement.

Objective: Neurological Emergencies

Subobjective: Trauma

35. C

Rationale: An uncomfortable feeling of pressure, squeezing, fullness, or pain in the center of the chest is the predominant symptom of a myocardial infarction (MI), particularly in women. Palpitations indicate a dysrhythmia. Edema in the lower extremities is a later sign of cardiac failure. A feeling of nausea is not common with MI.

Objective: Cardiovascular Emergencies

Subobjective: Acute Coronary Syndrome

36. B

Rationale: NPO status is essential for all suspected surgical cases. Elevation is limited with regard to injury. Ice, while therapeutic, would not be a priority intervention.

Objective: Orthopedic

Subobjective: Fractures/Dislocations

37. D

Rationale: Carbamazepine may cause dizziness or drowsiness. The patient should use caution while driving or operating machinery until he understands how the medication will affect him. There is no contraindication to sunlight exposure with this medication. Dietary concerns with carbamazepine are limited to consulting the health care provider before taking with grapefruit juice.

Objective: Neurological Emergencies

Subobjective: Seizure Disorders

38. C

Rationale: A Glasgow Coma Scale (GCS) of 7 indicates that the patient is experiencing deficits in eye opening, motor response, and verbal response. As the GCS drops, the patient is less alert and able to follow commands. Patients with a GCS of 7 will require intubation to maintain oxygenation. The lower the GCS, the less likely the patient is to fully recover without permanent deficits. An IV bolus will not negate the need for assisted breathing. This patient will be unable to get up to a chair. As the GCS drops, a nasal cannula becomes ineffective at providing oxygenation.

Objective: Neurological Emergencies

Subobjective: Trauma

39. D

Rationale: A severe headache indicates increased intracranial pressure (ICP), a complication of lumbar puncture. The health care provider should be notified immediately. Other indications of increased ICP are nausea, vomiting, photophobia, and changes in LOC. The patient should be encouraged to increase fluid intake unless contraindicated. The patient will remain flat and on bed rest following the procedure, per agency and health care provider guidelines. Minor pain controlled with analgesics is not a concern but should be monitored for changes.

Objective: Neurological Emergencies

Subobjective: Meningitis

40. A

Rationale: The electrocardiogram (ECG) is most commonly used to initially determine the location of myocardial damage. An echocardiogram is used to view myocardial wall function after a myocardial infarction (MI) has been diagnosed. Cardiac enzymes will aid in diagnosing an MI but will not determine the location. While not performed initially, cardiac catheterization determines coronary artery disease and would suggest the location of myocardial damage.

Objective: Cardiovascular Emergencies

Subobjective: Acute Coronary Syndrome

41. B

Rationale: As Alzheimer's disease progresses, confusion increases. Providing regular toileting can prevent possible falls that result when to hurrying to the bathroom to maintain continence. Haloperidol should be used with extreme caution in geriatric patients with Alzheimer's. Restraints can increase confusion in these patients and should be used only per facility guidelines. Offering too many choices can overwhelm the patient and lead to increased confusion and frustration.

Objective: Neurological Emergencies

Subobjective: Alzheimer's Disease/Dementia

42. **A**

Rationale: N-acetylcysteine is the antidote for acetaminophen toxicity and is administered to patients with hepatotoxic levels of serum acetaminophen levels. Intubation is not indicated, and naloxone is not the correct antidote. Gastric lavage is not indicated in this circumstance.

Objective: Communicable Diseases

Subobjective: Overdose and Ingestion

43. **C**

Rationale: The patient with emphysema can gain optimal lung expansion by sitting up and leaning forward. Lying in a prone position, flat on the back, or on the side with feet elevated will further potentiate any airway obstruction and effort, exacerbating the problem.

Objective: Respiratory Emergencies

Subobjective: Chronic Obstructive Pulmonary Disease

44. **C**

Rationale: Validation therapy is used with patients with severe dementia when reality orientation is not appropriate. The nurse may ask the patient what her mother looks like or what she is wearing but does not argue about whether her mother is living. This allows the nurse to acknowledge the patient's concerns while avoiding confrontation or encouraging further belief that her mother is alive. Confrontation may cause the patient with dementia to react inappropriately and is used only when the nurse has established patient trust. Reality orientation works best with patients in the early stages of dementia. Seeking clarification will only cause more confusion because the nurse is asking the

patient to explain something, which can lead to patient frustration.

Objective: Neurological Emergencies

Subobjective: Alzheimer's Disease/Dementia

45. **C**

Rationale: The patient should be thoroughly washed, and all linens and clothing items should be replaced with hospital-provided materials to prevent spread of bedbugs. All home-provided clothing and linens must be double-bagged and either disposed of or placed in a dryer on hot setting for 30 minutes. The presence of bedbugs is not necessarily a sign of abuse or neglect and therefore does not warrant a call to child welfare services. Contact precautions would be most appropriate.

Objective: Environmental

Subobjective: Parasite and Fungal Infestations

46. **D**

Rationale: A patient with diverticulitis would be expected to have lower abdominal pain with anorexia and fever in addition to an elevated WBC count.

Objective: Gastrointestinal Emergencies

Subobjective: Diverticulitis

47. **B**

Rationale: An increase in pain with nausea and vomiting are signs that an incarcerated hernia may be causing a bowel obstruction and should be reported immediately. The other findings are expected in a patient with a hernia and do not need to be immediately reported to the health care provider.

Objective: Gastrointestinal Emergencies

Subobjective: Hernia

48. **A**

Rationale: If the patient has diminished decisional capacity due to a developmental delay, the legal guardian must consent to any intervention for the patient unless there is an emergent issue.

Objective: Professional Issues

Subobjective: System (Patient Consent for Treatment)

49. C

Rationale: This patient is experiencing appendicitis. Pain that is relieved by bending the right hip suggests perforation and peritonitis. The patient would not need an abdominal MRI based on her symptoms. The patient will need surgery, so maintaining NPO status and administering IV fluids are a priority. Morphine will be given for pain.

Objective: Gastrointestinal Emergencies

Subobjective: Acute Abdomen

50. A

Rationale: The first priority for an unresponsive patient in V-fib is performing high-quality CPR. The patient should then be prepared to be defibrillated. Epinephrine should be administered after the patient has been defibrillated at least twice. IV access is not the initial priority.

Objective: Cardiovascular Emergencies

Subobjective: Dysrhythmias

51. B

Rationale: The nursing priority for patients with fistulas is preserving and protecting the skin. The nurse should inspect the skin frequently and assess for any redness, irritation, or broken areas. The skin should remain dry and intact. Antibiotics may be given but are not the first priority. Wound VACs should not be used simply to manage drainage or in patients with increased bleeding risk. Providing a quiet environment is important, but skin integrity is the first priority with this patient.

Objective: Gastrointestinal Emergencies

Subobjective: Inflammatory Bowel Disease

52. D

Rationale: Classic signs of cardiogenic shock include a rapid pulse that weakens; cool, clammy skin; and decreased urine output. Hypotension is another classic sign.

Objective: Cardiovascular Emergencies

Subobjective: Shock

53. B

Rationale: Having a frank, professional conversation regarding chronic pain relief is the nurse's priority. The nurse should not immediately assume the patient is drug-seeking, nor should the nurse ignore the patient's pain complaint.

Objective: Professional Issues

Subobjective:

Patient (Pain Management and Procedural Sedation)

54. D

Rationale: An avulsion is characterized by the separation of skin from the underlying structures that cannot be approximated.

Objective: Wound

Subobjective: Avulsions

55. C

Rationale: The priority for this patient is to prepare for surgical removal of the knife, so it should be stabilized with bulky dressings to avoid shifting as the patient is transported. The nurse should never attempt to remove an embedded object in a patient, as this is beyond the scope of practice for nursing. Blood loss may be estimated based on how many dressings or towels are saturated. Next of kin should be notified only after the patient is stabilized.

Objective: Gastrointestinal Emergencies

Subobjective: Abdominal Trauma

56. A

Rationale: Dysfunction of the renal cells and decreased levels of ADH hormone/vasopressin lead to diuresis, and fluid leakage into the interstitial spaces further contributes to hypovolemia. Shivering and vasoconstriction mask the symptoms of hypovolemia rather than contribute to it. Diaphoresis, dehydration, tachycardia, and tachypnea are all common symptoms of hyperthermia.

Objective: Environmental

Subobjective: Temperature-Related Emergencies

57. A

Rationale: A sudden, severe onset of testicular pain indicates the possibility of testicular torsion and a stat ultrasound should be ordered to confirm. Epididymitis typically presents gradually with unilateral pain and discharge, and pain is relieved with elevation of the testes. Sudden, severe pain is not an indication of UTI or orchitis.

Objective: Genitourinary

Subobjective: Testicular Torsion

58. B

Rationale: A purulent vaginal discharge with bilateral pelvic pain and nausea are symptoms of a tubo-ovarian abscess. An ectopic pregnancy would most commonly present with vaginal bleeding, not purulent discharge. A ruptured appendix would typically present as RLQ pain. Diverticulitis may cause abdominal pain and nausea but not purulent vaginal discharge.

Objective: Gynecological

Subobjective: Infection

59. D

Rationale: Abdominal cramping with vaginal bleeding and expulsion of tissue are signs of a complete spontaneous abortion. An incomplete spontaneous abortion would have retained tissue. Septic abortions are typically febrile. A threatened abortion may progress to a spontaneous abortion but would not result in passing a large solid tissue clot.

Objective: Obstetrical

Subobjective: Threatened/Spontaneous Abortion

60. C

Rationale: Corticosteroids will be administered to decrease inflammation of the airways. Albuterol and ipratropium are bronchodilators and do not address the swelling and inflammation caused by croup. Antibiotics are not indicated for croup.

Objective: Respiratory Emergencies

Subobjective: Infections

61. A

Rationale: Mucopurulent discharge, burning, and itching are symptoms of chlamydia. A herpes infection would have lesions. Syphilis typically presents with a small, painless sore. HPV typically presents asymptomatically but may also have warts.

Objective: Gynecological

Subobjective: Infection

62. D

Rationale: Aspirin is contraindicated for children with varicella because it can lead to Reye syndrome, a rare form of encephalopathy. Antihistamines, colloidal oatmeal baths, and non-aspirin antipyretics such as acetaminophen are all recommended in-home therapies to relieve symptoms.

Objective: Communicable Diseases

Subobjective: Childhood Diseases

63. B

Rationale: Current NRP guidelines (2015) recommend 40 – 60 breaths per minute for rescue breathing in the newborn. Rescue breaths at a rate of 12 – 20 are not adequate to provide enough ventilation for the neonate. Inserting an LMA or intubation may be indicated but is not the immediate nursing priority.

Objective: Obstetrical

Subobjective: Neonatal Resuscitation

64. B

Rationale: As a member of the team the nurse can suggest to the team leader to consider the futility of the resuscitation at that point. The nurse does not have the authority to end the resuscitation and should not advise the patient's parents to make that decision. Ethically, the nurse should speak up if he or she feels that the efforts are futile.

Objective: Professional Issues

Subobjective: Patient (End-of-Life Issues)

65. B

Rationale: The current (2015) guidelines for neonatal resuscitation recommend epinephrine to be administered at 0.01 – 0.03mg/kg. The other medication dosages are not appropriate as a first-line medication to be administered to a neonate with bradycardia.

Objective: Obstetrical

Subobjective: Neonatal Resuscitation

66. C

Rationale: Contusions accompanied by the symptoms mentioned should be treated with rest, ice, compression, and elevation. NSAIDs will provide appropriate pain relief; opioid therapy is not indicated for minor contusions.

Objective: Orthopedic

Subobjective: Trauma

67. D

Rationale: Amitriptyline is a tricyclic antidepressant. This class of drugs has anticholinergic effects, which frequently cause serious side effects. In older, confused patients such as those with Alzheimer's disease, amitriptyline can cause increased confusion, constipation, and urinary retention. Paroxetine and sertraline are SSRIs and may be given to patients with Alzheimer's. Memantine is an NMDA receptor antagonist prescribed to slow the progression of Alzheimer's.

Objective: Neurological Emergencies

Subobjective: Alzheimer's Disease/Dementia

68. B

Rationale: Adolescent patients presenting with frostbite burns to the roof of the mouth are most likely abusing inhalants, typically in the form of aerosols, glues, paints, and solvents. A hot beverage would not cause the other symptoms, nor would marijuana use. Dry ice would cause tissue injury to the entire mouth.

Objective: Communicable Diseases

Subobjective: Substance Abuse

69. D

Rationale: The patient should be turned on his side because he may lose consciousness and aspirate. The side-lying position facilitates the drainage of any oral secretions. Padded side rails may be used as part of seizure protocols, but turning the patient on his side is the priority. Tongue blades should never be left at the bedside, as their use can chip teeth, which can be aspirated. Administering IV diazepam should be done only after the patient is turned to his side to avoid aspiration.

Objective: Neurological Emergencies

Subobjective: Seizure Disorders

70. B

Rationale: The patient has suffered trauma in the motor vehicle crash (MVC). The bright red painless vaginal bleeding is a sign of placenta previa. Abruptio placentae results in painful bleeding that is typically dark red. An ectopic pregnancy and complete abortion would not occur due to an MVC.

Objective: Obstetrical

Subobjective: Placenta Previa

71. A

Rationale: Abdominal tenderness and dark red vaginal bleeding are signs of abruptio placenta. Placenta previa would present with bright red painless bleeding. Spontaneous abortions typically do not occur after 20 weeks.

Objective: Obstetrical

Subjective: Abruptio Placenta

72. D

Rationale: Safety is the priority for patients with altered mental status. The nurse should ask if the patient is hearing voices telling him to harm himself or others. Simply saying that no one is there dismisses the patient's feelings. Offering to find a blanket validates the delusion that someone is there. Asking if Martha is staying also prevents reality orientation and may worsen the patient's confusion.

Objective: Psychosocial Emergencies

Subobjective: Psychosis

73. C

Rationale: A thoracentesis is performed to remove the fluid. A chest tube is used to decompress a hemothorax or pneumothorax and is not indicated in the presence of pleural effusion. A pericardial window is used to drain excess fluid from the pericardium, not the pleural space.

Objective: Respiratory Emergencies

Subobjective: Plural Effusion

74. **B**

Rationale: Esophageal varices can lead to death via hemorrhage. Octreotide is a vasoconstrictor used to control bleeding before performing endoscopy. Phenytoin is an anticonvulsant, levofloxacin is an antibiotic, and pantoprazole is a proton pump inhibitor; none of these are indicated at this time.

Objective: Gastrointestinal Emergencies

Subobjective: Esophageal Varices

75. **D**

Rationale: "You're feeling lost since your mother died," uses the therapeutic technique of restating. The nurse repeats the patient's words back to her. This therapeutic communication technique allows the patient to verify that the nurse understood the patient and allows for clarification if needed. It also encourages the patient to continue. Telling the patient that she will feel better in time minimizes the patient's feelings and sounds uncaring. Telling the patient to join a grief support group forces the nurse's decision onto the patient. Stating shared feelings takes the focus from the patient to the nurse.

Objective: Psychosocial Emergencies

Subobjective: Depression

76. **D**

Rationale: The symptoms indicate right-sided myocardial infarction (MI), so IV fluids are the priority treatment for this patient. When treating patients with right ventricular infarction, nitrates, diuretics, and morphine are to be avoided due to their pre-load-reducing effects.

Objective: Cardiac Emergencies

Subobjective: Acute Coronary Syndromes

77. **C**

Rationale: The symptoms are characteristic of meningococcal meningitis, which is commonly contracted in crowded living

spaces such as college dorms. Influenza is characterized by upper-respiratory symptoms; scabies is a dermal infection; and pertussis is a respiratory illness.

Objective: Communicable Diseases

Subobjective: Childhood Diseases

78. **B**

Rationale: The patient has had nausea and vomiting, which can cause hypokalemia. A U wave can be noted on an ECG or cardiac monitor. Hyperkalemia would show peaked T waves. Hypercalcemia may produce a shortened QT interval, and hypocalcemia may show QT prolongation.

Objective: Medical Emergencies

Subobjective: Electrolyte/Fluid Imbalance

79. **A**

Rationale: Chain of custody is the concept of limiting the number of people handling and collecting evidence after a crime is committed. Nurses caring for patients and handling evidence should use local official documents to demonstrate the chain of custody for evidence and to document when it is given to authorities.

Objective: Professional Issues

Subobjective: Patient (Forensic Evidence Collection)

80. **C**

Rationale: The patient has a pneumothorax and will need a chest tube. Chest compressions are indicated only for cardiac arrest. Thoracotomy is done when there is severe trauma and impending or present cardiac arrest and is the final effort made to sustain life; it is associated with a low rate of successful outcomes. Endotracheal intubation is not indicated if the patient is able to protect his own airway, as is evidenced by his ability to communicate verbally.

Objective: Respiratory Emergencies

Subobjective: Pneumothorax

81. **D**

Rationale: Endoscopic litigation is indicated for *posterior* epistaxis stemming from the ethmoid or sphenopalatine arteries. Kiesselbach's plexus is the most common site of *anterior* epistaxis that responds to conventional treatments.

Objective: Maxillofacial

Subobjective: Epistaxis

82. B

Rationale: The patient with adrenal hypofunction should not be on a sodium-restrictive diet, as it may lead to an adrenal crisis. Peripheral blood draws, glucose monitoring, and hydrocortisone therapy are all appropriate for adrenal insufficiency.

Objective: Medical Emergencies

Subobjective: Endocrine Conditions

83. C

Rationale: Patients with hyperventilation syndrome will present with similar signs and symptoms as pulmonary emboli. Patients with a pneumothorax will present with absent breath sounds on the side of the injury, anxiety, and pain on inspiration. Pneumonia is characterized by fever, malaise, and crackles at the base of the lungs.

Objective: Respiratory Emergencies

Subobjective: Pulmonary Embolus

84. A

Rationale: Antipsychotics are used to treat psychotic symptoms such as hallucinations, paranoia, and delusions. They carry an increased risk of mortality, primarily from cardiovascular complications. A cardiac workup identifies any risk factors that would be a contraindication to antipsychotics. A comprehensive metabolic panel (CMP), creatinine clearance, and a CBC do not address the underlying risk of cardiovascular complications.

Objective: Psychosocial Emergencies

Subobjective: Psychosis

85. C

Rationale: The nurse should assign a sitter because the patient's safety is more important than his right to refuse care. Placing the patient in restraints does not guarantee his

safety and may escalate the situation. If the patient manages to get out of the restraints, he might hang himself with them. Having security sit outside the door does not provide direct observation of the patient and uses up a limited resource of the facility. Allowing the patient to leave against medical advice (AMA) leaves the nurse and the facility vulnerable to legal action if he commits suicide after leaving.

Objective: Psychosocial Emergencies

Subobjective: Suicidal Ideation

86. A

Rationale: Abnormalities in magnesium levels may put the patient at risk for ventricular dysrhythmia. A hypomagnesemia level of 0.8 mEq/L would be of concern (normal range is 1.5 – 2.5 mEq/L). The other values are within normal ranges.

Objective: Cardiovascular Emergencies

Subobjective: Dysrhythmias

87. D

Rationale: The patient is experiencing an unstable supraventricular tachycardia (SVT) with BP of 70/42 mm Hg and requires immediate synchronized cardioversion. Defibrillation is not indicated because the patient is awake and has an organized heart rhythm. Adenosine can be used in patients with stable SVT; however, this patient is not stable. Amiodarone is not indicated for unstable patients in SVT.

Objective: Cardiovascular Emergencies

Subobjective: Dysrhythmias

88. A

Rationale: The drug of choice for supraventricular tachycardia (SVT) is adenosine. The first dose of 6 mg has already been given, so the next appropriate dose would be 12 mg. The other options are not the next appropriate intervention for a patient in SVT.

Objective: Cardiovascular Emergencies

Subobjective: Dysrhythmias

89. B

Rationale: The goal for pulse oximetry readings is 94% – 99%. The nurse should apply supplemental oxygen for an SpO_2 below 94%. Albuterol and dexamethasone are appropriate for asthma but are not the priority intervention. Endotracheal intubation is needed only if a patient is unable to maintain their airway.

Objective: Respiratory Emergencies

Subobjective: Asthma

90. A

Rationale: The patient experiencing a sickle cell crisis needs fluid resuscitation with crystalloid solutions and the administration of warmed RBCs. Whole blood contains additional components such as plasma or platelets, which are not needed. Fresh frozen plasma and cryoprecipitate are not indicated for sickle cell crisis.

Objective: Medical Emergencies

Subobjective: Blood Dyscrasias

91. B

Rationale: Rhabdomyolysis is characterized by the breakdown of skeletal muscle with the release of myoglobin and other intercellular proteins and electrolytes into the circulation. The presence of myoglobin produces heme-positive results in the urinalysis.

Objective: Orthopedic

Subobjective: Trauma

92. D

Rationale: The sharp, tearing knifelike substernal chest pain with no relief from morphine is a hallmark sign of an aortic dissection. Pneumonia presents with pain related to coughing. Pain from a myocardial infarction (MI) or pericarditis would likely be relieved with doses of morphine sulfate.

Objective: Cardiovascular Emergencies

Subobjective: Aneurysm/Dissection

93. B

Rationale: Captopril is an ACE inhibitor, which can cause hyperkalemia. Bumetanide and furosemide are diuretics, which would cause hypokalemia. Digoxin is an antidysrhythmic and can also cause hypokalemia.

Objective: Medical Emergencies

Subobjective: Electrolyte/Fluid Imbalance

94. C

Rationale: Patients with idiopathic thrombocytopenic purpura (ITP) have decreased platelet production, so platelets are the expected treatment. The other options are not indicated for this condition.

Objective: Medical Emergencies

Subobjective: Blood Dyscrasias

95. C

Rationale: Vasospastic disorders such as Raynaud's phenomena and migraine headaches are associated with variant (Prinzmetal's) angina.

Objective: Cardiac Emergencies

Subobjective: Chronic Stable Angina Pectoris

96. B

Rationale: Hyperosmolar hyperglycemic state (HHS) is often caused by dehydration, especially in patients over 65. Inadequate glucose monitoring and medication noncompliance are not the most common causes of HHS. A breakdown of ketones causing ketoacidosis would be found in diabetic ketoacidosis (DKA).

Objective: Medical Emergencies

Subobjective: Endocrine Conditions

97. C

Rationale: Fluoxetine is given cautiously to patients with glaucoma, due to the anticholinergic side effects. There are no current indications that this medication causes side effects with arthritis, migraines, or appendicitis.

Objective: Psychosocial Emergencies

Subobjective: Depression

98. D

Rationale: Throbbing fingers or toes after exercise accompanied with thin, shiny skin and thick fingernails are symptoms of peripheral vascular disease. Acute occlusion would present with pain and cyanosis distal to the occlusion. Venous thrombosis occurs more often in the lower extremities, and there is no information suggesting arterial injury.

Objective: Cardiovascular Emergencies

Subobjective: Peripheral Vascular Disease

99. **C**

   Rationale: Insulin administration shifts potassium into the cells causing hypokalemia, so fluids with potassium are indicated for this patient. The other fluids are not indicated for this patient.

   Objective: Medical Emergencies

   Subobjective: Endocrine Conditions

100. **C**

   Rationale: Status epilepticus occurs when a person experiences a seizure that lasts more than 5 minutes or has repeated episodes over 30 minutes. This is a medical emergency, as death can result if seizures last more than 10 minutes. Causes of status epilepticus include alcohol or drug withdrawal, suddenly stopping antiseizure medications, head trauma, and infection. Atonic seizures occur when the patient has a sudden loss of muscle tone for a few seconds, followed by postictal confusion. Tonic–clonic (grand mal) seizures last for only a few minutes. With a simple partial seizure, the patient remains conscious during the episode, which may be preceded by auras. Autonomic changes may occur, such as heart rate changes and epigastric discomfort.

   Objective: Neurological Emergencies

   Subobjective: Seizure Disorders

101. **B**

   Rationale: Risk factors for pancreatitis include alcohol abuse, peptic ulcer disease, renal failure, vascular disorders, hyperlipidemia, and hyperparathyroidism. Patients often find relief in the fetal position, while the supine position worsens pain. The pain is severe and sudden and feels intense and boring, as if it is going through the body. Pain occurs in the mid-epigastric area or left upper quadrant. Pain can radiate to the left flank, the left shoulder, or the back.

   Objective: Gastrointestinal Emergencies

   Subobjective: Pancreatitis

102. **B**

   Rationale: Family member at the bedside for resuscitation has been demonstrated in the evidence as a preference for patients and families and should be offered when possible and appropriate. Family members should be present only if they are not disruptive to patient care.

103. **A**

   Rationale: When an organ donor patient dies in the ED the nurse should first contact the organ procurement organization because of time sensitivity. Life-supporting interventions such as ventilators and medications should be continued until the organ procurement agency arrives. Postmortem care and completing the death certificate can be performed after organ procurement has taken place.

   Objective: Professional Issues

   Subobjective: Patient (End-of-Life Issues)

104. **A**

   Rationale: Propylthiouracil (PTU) is the drug of choice in treating thyroid storm, as it inhibits the synthesis of thyroxine. Epinephrine and atropine are contraindicated for thyroid storm, as these patients already have a dangerously high heart rate. Levothyroxine would be indicated for myxedema coma.

   Objective: Medical Emergencies

   Subobjective: Endocrine Conditions

105. **C**

   Rationale: The patient will be involuntarily committed because she is a threat to her own safety. She has not committed a crime. She will not be admitted voluntarily because she did not come to the hospital of her own volition.

   Objective: Professional Issues

   Subobjective: Patient (Transitions of Care)

106. D

Rationale: The patient is in acidosis and has Kussmaul respirations, which are indicative of diabetic ketoacidosis (DKA). Myxedema coma and pheochromocytoma would not cause these symptoms. Hyperosmolar hyperglycemic state (HHS) normally causes higher blood sugar levels and does not present in acidosis.

Objective: Medical Emergencies

Subobjective: Endocrine Conditions

107. B

Rationale: The Glasgow Coma Scale (GCS) is calculated as follows: opening eyes to sound (3), localizing pain (5), and making incoherent sounds (2) gives a GCS score of 10.

Objective: Neurological Emergencies

Subobjective: Trauma

108. A

Rationale: The patient is showing signs of peritonsillar abscess. Peritonsillar abscess is an emergent condition that occurs from the accumulation of purulent exudate between the tonsillar capsule and the pharyngeal constrictor muscle. Patchy tonsillar exudate, petechiae, and lymphedema are common findings with viral and bacterial strep throat infections.

Objective: Maxillofacial

Subobjective: Peritonsillar Abscess

109. C

Rationale: Foods high in lactose may be poorly tolerated by patients with ulcerative colitis (UC) and should be limited or avoided. High-fiber foods can aggravate GI symptoms in some patients and should be avoided. Caffeine is a stimulant that can increase cramping and diarrhea. Dried fruit stimulates the GI tract and can exacerbate symptoms.

Objective: Gastrointestinal Emergencies

Subobjective: Inflammatory Bowel Disease

110. C

Rationale: A sudden sharp pain in the pelvic region associated with sexual intercourse and no vaginal discharge is common with an ovarian cyst rupture. An ectopic pregnancy does not typically present with sudden pain, and there is usually vaginal bleeding. A ruptured appendix will cause constant pain to the RLQ and commonly causes a fever. The symptoms are not indicative of an STD.

Objective: Gynecological

Subobjective: Ovarian Cyst

111. B

Rationale: An elevation in serum lactate level will conclude the diagnosis of sepsis. The WBC count and neutrophil count would be increased. RBCs do not give adequate information to suspect sepsis.

Objective: Medical Emergencies

Subobjective: Sepsis and Septic Shock

112. B

Rationale: Dehydration requires an isotonic crystalloid solution, such as normal saline or lactated Ringer's, which will evenly distribute between the intravascular space and cells. Hypertonic solutions pull water from cells into the intravascular space, and hypotonic solutions move fluid from the intravascular space into the cells. Colloid solutions, such as albumin, draw fluid into intravascular compartments and would not be appropriate for this patient.

Objective: Medical Emergencies

Subobjective: Electrolyte/Fluid Imbalance

113. C

Rationale: A history of hypertension will cause an increase in afterload. Diabetes will cause complications with microvascular disease, leading to poor cardiac function. Endocrine disorders will cause an increase in cardiac workload. Marfan syndrome causes the cardiac muscle to stretch and weaken.

Objective: Cardiac Emergencies

Subobjective: Heart Failure

114. D

Rationale: Patients with subarachnoid hemorrhage commonly describe having the "worst headache of my life." Nausea and vomiting, not food cravings, may occur. There is no rash associated with subarachnoid hemorrhage. Battle's sign is a characteristic symptom of basilar skull fracture.

Objective: Neurological Emergencies

Subobjective: Trauma

115. C

Rationale: Several of the medications used to treat MS are immunosuppressants; therefore, the patient is more susceptible to infection while taking them. Patients should avoid crowds and anyone who appears to have an infection, such as the flu. Alternating an eye patch from one eye to the other every few hours can relieve diplopia. Patients with MS have alterations in mobility, and clearing walking paths in the home makes it safer to ambulate, especially with a walker or cane. If the patient suspects infection, he or she should notify the health care provider immediately.

Objective: Neurological Emergencies

Subobjective: Chronic Neurological Disorders

116. B

Rationale: The signs and symptoms of pelvic inflammatory disease are lower abdominal pain that worsens with movement, a temperature greater than 101.3°F (38.5°C), tachycardia, and non-malodorous vaginal discharge. Appendicitis does not cause vaginal discharge. Ectopic pregnancy typically causes vaginal bleeding. Most STIs present with malodorous discharge and do not cause fever and tachycardia.

Objective: Gynecological

Subobjective: Infection

117. C

Rationale: Penicillin V potassium for antibiotic therapy is indicated for the treatment of dental abscesses, a condition indicated by this patient's symptoms. Sodium fluoride drops are a supplement for children, nystatin is used to treat oral candida albicans infections, and saliva substitute is a rinse for dry mouth.

Objective: Maxillofacial

Subobjective: Dental Conditions

118. C

Rationale: Morphine sulfate is the analgesic of choice in acute coronary syndrome (ACS): it provides analgesic and sedation and also decreases preload and afterload. Morphine is administered to relieve pain as well as to decrease pain-related anxiety that can further exacerbate the symptoms of the myocardial infarction (MI). Meperidine is not indicated for use in MI. Hydromorphone is more appropriate for patients with no cardiac compromise, and acetaminophen is not indicated in MI.

Objective: Cardiovascular Emergencies

Subobjective: Acute Coronary Syndrome

119. A

Rationale: HIV patients with a fever are considered emergent, and a septic workup is expected. After drawing blood cultures, antibiotics should be the priority intervention. Acetaminophen may be administered but is not the priority. Taking the patient's antivirals after she has been noncompliant is not a priority. She does not need a blood transfusion.

Objective: Medical Emergencies

Subobjective: Immunocompromised

120. C

Rationale: Late signs of increased intracranial pressure (ICP) include dilated or pinpoint pupils that are sluggish or nonreactive to light. Headache, restlessness, and decreasing LOC are early signs of increased ICP.

Objective: Neurological Emergencies

Subobjective: Increased Intracranial Pressure (ICP)

121. A

Rationale: The child should remain with the parent in an upright position. Taking the child from the parent could cause anxiety and crying and worsen the respiratory distress.

Objective: Respiratory Emergencies

Subobjective: Infections

122. A

Rationale: Complications of ulcerative colitis (UC) include hemorrhage and nutritional deficiencies. Patients may have up to 10 – 20 bloody, liquid stools per day. Loose, non-bloody stools and fistulas are more common in patients with Crohn's disease. Surgery is rarely required for these symptoms.

Objective: Gastrointestinal Emergencies

Subobjective: Inflammatory Bowel Disease

123. B

Rationale: Trigeminal neuralgia pain has an abrupt onset, is unilateral along the branch of the fifth cranial nerve, and causes hemifacial spasms.

Objective: Maxillofacial

Subobjective: Facial Nerve Disorders

124. C

Rationale: The patient is experiencing symptoms of pulmonary edema, a complication of left-sided heart failure. Coagulation is not a secondary effect of myocardial infarction (MI). Pneumonia is not generally related to post–MI concerns. A ruptured ventricle would present symptoms closer to the time of injury.

Objective: Cardiovascular Emergencies

Subobjective: Heart Failure and Cardiogenic Pulmonary Edema

125. B

Rationale: Advance directives must be valid, up to date, and documented before they can be honored in the ED. The nurse can document the patient's wishes, but it is not official until the paperwork is present. The physician does not make that decision, and with the correct documentation, EDs will honor advance directives.

Objective: Professional Issues

Subobjective: Patient (End-of-Life Issues)

126. D

Rationale: A pharmacist would not be consulted in this situation. Other members of the team may include ED physicians, social workers, and hospital religious team members.

Objective: Professional Issues

Subobjective: Patient (End-of-Life Issues)

127. C

Rationale: Instruct the parent to perform oral positive pressure by sealing his or her mouth securely over the child's mouth and providing a short, sharp puff of air while simultaneously occluding the unaffected nostril.

Objective: Maxillofacial

Subobjective: Foreign Bodies

128. C

Rationale: Patching the affected eye decreases oxygen delivery to the cornea, delays wound healing, and creates an environment that increases the risk for infection.

Objective: Ocular

Subobjective: Abrasions

129. D

Rationale: When a patient is experiencing hallucinations, the nurse should acknowledge the patient's fear but reinforce reality. Telling the patient that it is the wrinkles in the blanket dismisses the patient's fear and does not reorient the patient. Offering to move the patient to another room accepts the snakes as real and does not help the patient with reality. Offering to call maintenance reinforces the patient's belief that the snakes are real.

Objective: Psychosocial Emergencies

Subobjective: Psychosis

130. D

Rationale: Isocarboxazid and other MAOI inhibitors should not be taken with rasagiline mesylate due to the risk of increased blood pressure and hypertensive crisis. The other medications are not contraindicated for this patient: baclofen relieves muscle spasms, benztropine is an older drug that treats severe motor symptoms such as rigidity and tremors, and amantadine is an antiviral drug often prescribed with carbidopa and levodopa to reduce dyskinesias.

Objective: Neurological Emergencies

Subobjective: Chronic Neurological Disorders

131. A

Rationale: Herpes zoster infection of the facial nerves commonly involves the eyelid and surrounding structures. Treatment is palliative, using antiviral medications such as acyclovir.

Objective: Ocular

Subobjective: Infections

132. D

Rationale: These ABGs indicate acute respiratory acidosis. Common signs of respiratory acidosis include hypoventilation with hypoxia, disorientation, and dizziness. Untreated respiratory acidosis can progress to ventricular fibrillation, hypotension, seizures, and coma. Deep, rapid respirations and nausea and vomiting are signs of metabolic acidosis. Chest pain is not a symptom of respiratory acidosis.

Objective: Respiratory Emergencies

Subobjective: Chronic Obstructive Pulmonary Disorder

133. A

Rationale: Iritis is treated with topical mydriatic ophthalmic drops to dilate the pupil, topical corticosteroids to reduce inflammation, and referral to ophthalmology within 24 hours.

Objective: Ocular

Subobjective: Infections

134. C

Rationale: Patients with ulcerative keratitis MUST NOT use contact lenses until the infection has resolved and been cleared by an ophthalmologist. The patient should complete the full course of prescribed antibiotics. Not all ulcers are contagious, so she could safely return to work after 24 hours of antibiotic use.

Objective: Ocular

Subobjective: Ulcerations/Keratitis

135. A

Rationale: The patient's ammonia level and ALT are elevated, which is expected with cirrhosis. Lactulose is given to lower ammonia levels in patients with cirrhosis. Bisacodyl is a laxative and is not indicated for this patient.

Mesalamine is an anti-inflammatory given for ulcerative colitis. The patient's blood glucose is not elevated enough to require 2 units of insulin.

Objective: Gastrointestinal Emergencies

Subobjective: Cirrhosis

136. D

Rationale: Clinical open globe rupture features include afferent pupillary defect, impaired visual acuity, gross deformity of the eye, and prolapsing uvea.

Objective: Ocular

Subobjective: Trauma

137. D

Rationale: Dopamine (Intropin) is a positive inotrope, which will increase cardiac contractility and cardiac output, decrease the myocardial workload, and improve myocardial oxygen delivery.

Objective: Cardiovascular Emergencies

Subobjective: Heart Failure

138. A

Rationale: A commercially available tourniquet at least 2 inches wide with a windlass or ratcheting device is recommended for both prehospital and in-hospital use. The nurse should never remove a tourniquet without team support to control hemorrhagic bleeding. Assessment occurs in 2-hour intervals.

Objective: Orthopedic

Subobjective: Amputation

139. D

Rationale: Only the CT angiography will confirm the diagnosis. D-dimer may be increased in the presence of pulmonary embolism (PE) but is not a stand-alone indicator for definitive diagnosis. A chest X-ray will rule out other disease processes but does not rule in a PE. Fibrin split products are measured in the presence of disseminated intravascular coagulation and are not relevant for the concern of PE.

Objective: Respiratory Emergencies

Subobjective: Pulmonary Embolism

140. B

Rationale: When caring for mentally unstable or possibly violent patients, staff safety is the primary concern. The nurse should avoid getting blocked into a corner between the patient and the door. If possible, the patient should be in a room near the nurses' station, and the nurse should notify someone before entering the room. Bringing another nurse or patient care technician can also maintain safety. All patients should be treated with courtesy and respect, especially someone who may be prone to paranoia. It may be necessary to observe the patient closely for "cheeking" pills instead of swallowing them. Some medications may be ordered in IV form to ensure that the patient receives the medication if he has surreptitiously avoided swallowing pills in the past. Always ask permission before touching or approaching the patient to avoid startling him. If the patient refuses medications or blood draws, do not argue. Chart the refusal in the medical record and notify the health care provider.

Objective: Psychosocial Emergencies

Subobjective: Aggressive/Violent Behavior

141. D

Rationale: Costochondritis occurs from localized inflammation of the joints attaching the ribs to the sternum and most commonly presents in females ages 12 to 14.

Objective: Orthopedic

Subobjective: Costochondritis

142. A

Rationale: In a flail chest there is asymmetrical movement of the chest wall. Ribs are completely broken and cause abnormal movement of the chest wall. As the patient breathes in, the flail segment will sink in; as the patient breathes out, the segment will bulge outward.

Objective: Respiratory Emergencies

Subobjective: Trauma

143. B

Rationale: Chest pain can occur with the first dose of sumatriptan and should be reported immediately. Sumatriptan may not be safe for pregnant women, so the patient should be coached on using an effective birth control method while taking it. Most triptans are contraindicated with hypertension and would not be prescribed if the patient is taking antihypertensives due to the risk of coronary vasospasm. The medication should be taken as soon as the first symptoms of migraine appear.

Objective: Neurological Emergencies

Subobjective: Headache

144. B

Rationale: Avulsed primary teeth are not replanted because of the potential for subsequent damage to the developing permanent tooth and the increased frequency of pulpal necrosis. Best initial management would be to repair the lacerations.

Objective: Maxillofacial

Subobjective: Dental Conditions

145. C

Rationale: Gouty arthritis characteristically occurs in patients with hyperuricemia, which causes high levels of uric acid in the blood from breakdown of purines. Hyperammonemia is the presence of an excess of ammonia in the blood. Hyperbilirubinemia is too much bilirubin in the blood. Hyperhomocysteinemia is a marker for the development of heart disease.

Objective: Orthopedic

Subobjective: Inflammatory Conditions

146. C

Rationale: Nonstick adherent dressing such as a Band-Aid or Telfa pad is the appropriate choice.

Objective: Wound

Subobjective: Abrasions

147. B

Rationale: There should be a high index of suspicion that the patient experienced an inhalation injury, and measures should be taken to protect her airway. Burns and trauma are secondary concerns to airway compromise. Soot at the mouth opening suggests smoke inhalation, not foreign body ingestion.

Objective: Respiratory Emergencies

Subobjective: Inhalation Injuries

148. C

Rationale: Dimming lights or providing a blindfold are contraindicated, as low lighting will increase pupillary size, creating an increase in intraocular pressure. Pupil size should remain constricted through use of bright lighting and miotic ophthalmic drops.

Objective: Ocular

Subobjective: Glaucoma

149. A

Rationale: The typical chest radiography for a patient with adult respiratory distress syndrome (ARDS) is bilateral, diffuse white infiltrates without cardiomegaly. Options C and D show results for abnormal heart tissue but not for lung tissue and do not give any information about infiltrates.

Objective: Respiratory Emergencies

Subobjective: Respiratory Distress Syndrome

150. B

Rationale: Many opioid substances are commonly injected, resulting in abscess formation from use of non-sterile equipment and aseptic technique. Cocaine, amphetamines, and other substances may also be injected. Alcohol, benzodiazepine, and tetrahydrocannabinol use may be co-occurring in the patient, but these substances are not commonly injected.

Objective: Wound

Subobjective: Infections

151. C

Rationale: The patient is hypotensive, hypothermic, and bradycardic. He has ingested thyroid replacement medications and sedatives, which can lead to a myxedema coma. The symptoms are not indicative of an allergic reaction or an acute stroke. A thyroid storm would show increased heart rate, temperature, and blood pressure.

Objective: Medical Emergencies

Subobjective: Endocrine Conditions

152. D

Rationale: Epinephrine is never used for lacerations of the fingers, toes, face, or penis.

Objective: Wound

Subobjective: Lacerations

153. C

Rationale: Post-exposure prophylaxis in a patient who has not been vaccinated must consist of both immunoglobin and vaccine therapy. While up-to-date tetanus immunization should be considered, it is a targeted vaccine against infection by *Clostridium tetani*.

Objective: Environmental

Subobjective: Vector-Borne Illnesses

154. D

Rationale: The child is presenting with signs of asthma exacerbation. Symptoms of foreign body aspiration are consistent with acute airway obstruction to include respiratory distress and drooling. Pneumonitis would present with chest pain and dyspnea but not these acute symptoms. Pneumonia is characterized with crackles in the lower lobes and decreased oxygen saturation.

Objective: Respiratory Emergencies

Subobjective: Asthma

155. A

Rationale: The patient will need epinephrine administered immediately. Most anaphylactic deaths occur due to a delay in epinephrine administration. Diphenhydramine and Solu-Medrol are indicated for minor allergic reactions. Theophylline is typically used to treat asthma and is not indicated for anaphylaxis.

Objective: Medical Emergencies

Subobjective: Allergic Reactions and Anaphylaxis

156. B

Rationale: Hyperbaric oxygen is used to treat severe carbon monoxide toxicity.

Hydroxocobalamin is a cyanide-binding agent. N-acetylcysteine restores depleted hepatic glutathione, reversing effects of acetaminophen toxicity. Sodium bicarbonate is standard treatment for salicylate toxicity.

Objective: Environmental

Subobjective: Chemical Exposure

157. C

Rationale: Patients presenting with vague neurological symptoms may be difficult to diagnose. The history and information leading up to presentation in the department is vital in determining differential diagnoses. This patient is not presenting with stroke-like symptoms. The symptoms are similar to those of a migraine; however, the history makes carbon monoxide poisoning more likely. The patient is not demonstrating stroke or allergic reaction symptoms.

Objective: Toxicology

Subobjective: Carbon Monoxide

158. C

Rationale: Calcium gluconate is administered to the patient with hyperkalemia for cardiac and neuromuscular protection. Aspirin is used for acute coronary syndrome but would not be a first-line drug for this condition. Insulin and dextrose may be given to lower potassium levels but do not function to protect cardiac status. Digoxin is an antidysrhythmic and is not indicated for hyperkalemia.

Objective: Medical Emergencies

Subobjective: Renal Failure

159. C

Rationale: Monitoring neurological status is the most important nursing intervention for patients with meningitis. Deficits of cranial nerve VI prevent lateral eye movement, which is an indicator of hydrocephalus. Other indicators of hydrocephalus include urinary incontinence and signs of increased intracranial pressure (ICP). Declining LOC is the first sign of increased ICP, and the nurse must be sensitive to even small changes in LOC. The other findings do not indicate increasing ICP.

Objective: Neurological Emergencies

Subobjective: Increased Intracranial Pressure (ICP)

160. B

Rationale: Patients with diverticular disease should remain on clear liquids until pain has subsided. For maintenance, they will need to eat 25 to 35 grams of fiber daily to provide bulk to the stool. Patients should avoid high-sodium foods and alcohol, which irritates the bowel. Strawberries contain seeds that may block a diverticulum and should be avoided, along with nuts, corn, popcorn, and tomatoes.

Objective: Gastrointestinal Emergencies

Subobjective: Diverticulitis

161. D

Rationale: Keraunoparalysis is a condition specific to lightning strikes, resulting from vasoconstriction in the tissues surrounding entry and exit points. Ascending paralysis is a common finding in Guillain–Barré syndrome. Bell's palsy and tic douloureux are both facial nerve disorders.

Objective: Environmental

Subobjective: Electrical Injuries

162. B

Rationale: The patient's last drink is important to determine the possibility of withdrawal or delirium tremens. The other questions are relevant but are not the priority based on the patient's presentation.

Objective: Communicable Diseases

Subobjective: Withdrawal Syndrome

163. C

Rationale: Octreotide is used for overdoses refractory to glucose administration. It stimulates the release of insulin from the beta islet cells of the pancreas. Flumazenil is the antidote for benzodiazepine overdose. Acetylcysteine is used for acetaminophen overdose, and methylene blue is used for nitrites and anesthetics overdose.

Objective: Communicable Diseases

Subobjective: Overdose and Ingestion

164. B

Rationale: Tuberculosis is characterized by a cough lasting 2 – 3 weeks or more, fever, chills, night sweats, and fatigue. The recent travel to a developing country is a concern for potential infectious disease. The other conditions have similar symptoms, but the travel and chronic cough indicate strong concern for pulmonary tuberculosis.

Objective: Communicable Diseases

Subobjective: Tuberculosis

165. B

Rationale: Calcium channel blockers can cause symptoms in children with doses as low as 1 tablet. Rapid deterioration may occur if the tablets are short acting. A 5-year-old may not accurately count or recollect the number of tablets consumed. A referral to child protective services should be made if there is a reasonable suspicion for the need but is not a priority intervention. Oxygen should be provided only if pulse oximetry is less than 92%.

Objective: Communicable Diseases

Subobjective: Overdose and Ingestion

166. C

Rationale: The rash, conjunctivitis, and cough are indicative of measles, and the patient's vaccination status makes this diagnosis even more likely. Varicella is characterized by vesicular rash on the trunk and face; mumps, by nonspecific respiratory symptoms and edema in the parotid gland; and pertussis is a respiratory disease with a specific "whoop"-sounding cough.

Objective: Communicable Diseases

Subobjective: Childhood Diseases

167. B

Rationale: People who chronically abuse alcohol are deficient in thiamine and are given IV thiamine. Naloxone blocks opioid receptors and is given for opioid overdose. Flumazenil is a benzodiazepine receptor antagonist and is given for benzodiazepine overdose. Vitamin K is given for warfarin overdose.

Objective: Communicable Diseases

Subobjective: Substance Abuse

168. A

Rationale: Herpes zoster, also known as shingles, is caused by the reactivation of dormant varicella virus. It can occur several times over the lifetime of a patient who has had an initial varicella infection. The varicella vaccine is not known to cause herpes zoster. Herpes zoster can be spread by contact with the rash; someone who has never had varicella may contract it from contact with a herpes zoster rash. The zoster vaccine may prevent a second or third outbreak in patients who have had active herpes zoster.

Objective: Communicable Diseases

Subobjective: Herpes Zoster

169. A

Rationale: A pseudomembrane, or thick gray membrane, covering the tonsils, the pharynx, and sometimes the larynx is characteristic of diphtheria infection. Patients with diphtheria may have a low-grade fever; they will not have a macular rash or headache.

Objective: Communicable Diseases

Subobjective: Childhood Diseases

170. C

Rationale: The nurse demonstrates personal insight that further help is needed via the Critical Incident Stress Management (CISM) system. CISM does not require or recommend that nurses needing debriefing or assistance meet with managers specifically about the event or experience. The nurse should not depart the debriefing before it is complete, and future debrief sessions may or may not occur. Scheduling appointments is a concrete action that demonstrates the nurse's effective participation.

Objective: Professional Issues

Subobjective: Nurse (Critical Incident Stress Management)

171. B

Rationale: Participation and engagement in Evidence-Based Practice (EBP) projects supports an environment of quality and safe care using up-to-date evidence and practices that have been thoroughly researched. Reading research articles is important, but the data must be synthesized through formal processes to implement evidence into practice.

Objective: Professional Issues

Subobjective: Nurse (Evidence-Based Practice)

172. D

Rationale: Patient income is not directly relevant to transitions of care and is not appropriate for ED nurses to ask about when managing care transitions. Safety, community partnerships, and accessibility of services are all appropriate considerations.

Objective: Professional Issues

Subobjective: Patient (Transitions of Care)

173. D

Rationale: The current (2015) AHA and NRP guidelines for newborn resuscitation is 3 compressions to 1 ventilation. A ratio of 30:2 is appropriate for all adults or a single rescuer infant/child; a ratio of 15:2 is appropriate for 2 rescuers with children and infants. A ratio of 15:1 is not recommended for anyone.

Objective: Obstetrical

Subobjective: Neonatal Resuscitation

174. D

Rationale: A Foley catheter is not necessary to decompress the bladder in this patient. Typically, these patients are eligible for eye donation, and the head should be at 20 degrees, with artificial tears or saline in the eyes to preserve the tissue. Tape should be used if eyes do not close after death.

Objective: Professional Issues

Subobjective: Patient (End-of-Life Issues)

175. B

Rationale: Annular lesions with raised borders and cleared central areas of the rash indicate ringworm. Scabies are characterized by red pruritic rashes, and cellulitis and impetigo do not present in this way.

Objective: Environmental

Subobjective: Parasite and Fungal Infestations

Follow the link below to take your SECOND CEN practice test:

www.ascenciatestprep.com/cen-online-resources

APPENDIX: SIGNS & SYMPTOMS GLOSSARY

abdominal guarding: involuntary contraction of the abdominal muscles to prevent pain caused by pressure

agonal respiration: breathing pattern characterized by labored breathing, gasping, and myoclonus

amenorrhea: abnormal absence of menstruation

anisocoria: unequal pupil size

anosmia: inability to smell

anuria (anuresis): inability to urinate or production of < 100 mL of urine a day

aphasia: impairment in ability to speak, write, and understand others

apnea: temporary cessation of breathing

ascites: abdominal swelling caused by fluid in the peritoneal cavity

asterixis: bilateral tremor or "flapping" of the wrist or fingers

ataxia: abnormal, uncoordinated movements

aura: unusual sensations (e.g., flashing lights, odors) that precede a migraine

blepharospasm: involuntary contractions of the eyelids

bradycardia: slow heart rate

bradypnea: slow respiration rate

chemosis: edema of the conjunctiva

clonus: rhythmic, involuntary muscular spasms

crepitus: abnormal cracking sounds heard in fractures, joints, or the lungs or in subcutaneous emphysema

cyanosis: blueish skin

decerebrate posturing: arms and legs extended and the head arched back

decorticate posturing: arms flexed onto chest, fists clenched, and legs extended

diaphoresis: excessive sweating

diplopia: double vision

dysarthria: slurred speech caused by muscle weakness

dysesthesia: uncomfortable or painful sensation caused by nerve damage

dyspareunia: painful sexual intercourse

dysphagia: difficulty swallowing

dyspnea: difficulty breathing

dysuria: difficult or painful urination

ecchymosis: bruising

edema: swelling caused by excess fluid

edentulous: without teeth

effusion: accumulation of fluid

emesis: the act of vomiting

enophthalmos: posterior displacement of the eyeball

epistaxis: bleeding from the nose

erythema: redness of the skin

exophthalmos: bulging of the eyeball out of the orbit

febrile: related to fever

halitosis: foul-smelling breath

hematemesis: blood in vomit

hematochezia: bright red blood in stool

hematuria: blood in urine

hemiplegia: unilateral paralysis

hemoptysis: blood in expectorate from respiratory tract

hemotympanum: blood in the middle ear

hepatomegaly: enlargement of liver

herniation: protrusion of tissue from a cavity

hydrophobia: fear of water

hypercapnia: high levels of CO_2 in blood

hyperpyrexia: body temperature > 106.7°F (41.5°C)

hyperreflexia: overreactive reflexes

hypertension: high blood pressure

hypertonia: tightness of muscles due to nerve damage

hypotension: low blood pressure

hypoxemia: low levels of oxygen in the blood

hypoxia: lack of oxygen supplied to tissues

ileus: lack of movement in the intestines

ischemia: restricted blood flow to tissue

jaundice: yellowing of the skin or sclera

Kussmaul respirations: deep, labored breathing

lacrimation: excessive secretion of tears

laryngospasm: spasm of the vocal cords

lymphadenopathy (adenopathy): swollen lymph nodes

lymphopenia: low levels of lymphocytes

malocclusion: misalignment of the upper and lower teeth

melena: dark, sticky digested blood in the stool

menorrhagia: heavy bleeding during menstruation

myoclonus: twitches or jerks of muscles

nocturia: excessive urination at night

nystagmus: repetitive, uncontrolled movement of the eyes

oliguria: low urine output

orthopnea: dyspnea that occurs while lying flat

orthostatic (postural) hypotension: decrease in blood pressure after standing

otalgia: ear pain

otorrhea: drainage from the ear

pallor: pale appearance

pancytopenia: low levels of RBCs, WBCs, and platelets

papilledema: swelling of the optic disk

paresthesia: abnormal dermal sensation such as burning or "pins and needles"

parotitis: inflammation of the parotid glands

periorbital ecchymosis: bruising under and around the eyes ("raccoon eyes")

petechiae: tiny red or brown spots on the skin caused by subcutaneous bleeding

photophobia: sensitivity to light

photopsia: perceived flashes of light

photosensitivity: immune system response to UV light

pleurisy: inflammation of the pleura

poikilothermia: inability to regulate body temperature

polydipsia: excessive thirst

polyphagia: excessive hunger

polyuria: abnormally high urine output

presyncope: feeling of weakness and light-headedness

pruritus: severely itchy skin

ptosis: drooping of upper eyelid

pulsus alternans: alternating strong and weak pulse

pulsus paradoxus: abnormally large drop in blood pressure during inspiration

rhinorrhea: drainage from the nose

scotoma: loss of vision restricted to part of the visual field ("blind spot")

steatorrhea: excretion of excess fat in the stool

stenosis: narrowing of a passage

strangury: blockage at the base of the bladder causing a painful need to urinate

stridor: high-pitched wheezing sound caused by a disruption in airflow

syncope: temporary loss of consciousness

tachycardia: fast heart rate

tachypnea: fast respiratory rate

tetany: muscle spasms and cramps usually caused by hypocalcemia

tinnitus: perception of sounds that are not present ("ringing in the ears")

trismus: restricted movement of mandible ("lockjaw")

urticaria: hives

vertigo: sensation of dizziness and loss of balance

APPENDIX B: MEDICAL SIGNS

Babinski sign (reflex): dorsiflexion of big toe when bottom of foot is stroked (normal in infants; sign of disease in adults)

Battle's sign: ecchymosis over the mastoid process

Chvostek's sign: twitching of facial muscles caused by tapping the facial nerve (CN VII) near the tragus

Cullen's sign: a bluish discoloration to the umbilical area

Grey Turner's sign: ecchymosis in the flank area

Homan's sign: discomfort behind the knee or increased resistance in response to dorsiflexion of the foot

Kehr's sign: pain in the tip of the shoulder caused by blood in the peritoneal cavity

Kussmaul's sign: rise in jugular venous pressure during inspiration

Levine's sign: a clenched fist held over the chest in response to ischemic chest pain

Markle test (heel drop): pain caused when patient stands on tiptoes and drops heels down quickly or when patient hops on one leg

McBurney's point: RLQ pain at point halfway between umbilicus and iliac spine

Murphy's sign: cessation of inspiration when RUQ is palpated

Prehn's sign: lack of pain relief after scrotal elevation

Psoas sign: abdominal pain when right hip is hyperextended

Rovsing's sign: pain in the RLQ with palpation of LLQ

Schafer's sign: presence of pigmented cells in the anterior vitreous

Trousseau sign: flexing of wrist and adduction of fingers when brachial artery is obstructed for > 3 minutes

APPENDIX: DIAGNOSTIC TESTS & CRITICAL VALUES

Test	Description	Normal Range
Basic Metabolic Panel		
Potassium (K^+)	electrolyte that helps with muscle contraction and regulates water and acid-base balance	3.5 – 5.2 mEq/L
Sodium (Na^+)	maintains fluid balance and plays a major role in muscle and nerve function	135 – 145 mEq/L
Calcium (Ca^+)	plays an important role in skeletal function and structure, nerve function, muscle contraction, and cell communication	8.5 – 10.3 mg/dL
Chloride (Cl^-)	electrolyte that plays a major role in muscle and nerve function	98 – 107 mEq/L
Blood urea nitrogen (BUN)	filtered by the kidneys; high levels can indicate insufficient kidney function	7 – 20 mg/dL
Creatinine	filtered by the kidneys; high levels can indicate insufficient kidney function	0.6 – 1.2 mg/dL
BUN to creatinine ratio	increased ratio indicates dehydration, AKI, or GI bleeding; decreased ratio indicates renal damage	10:1 – 20:1
Glucose	tests for hyper- and hypoglycemia	non-fasting: < 140 mg/dL fasting: 70 – 99 mg/dL
Bicarbonate (HCO_3 or CO_2)	measures amount of CO_2 in the blood; decreased levels indicate acidosis or kidney damage; increased levels indicate alkalosis or lung damage	23 – 29 mEq/L
Other Serum Tests		
Magnesium	electrolyte that regulates muscle, nerve, and cardiac function	1.8 – 2.5 mg/dL
Glomerular filtration rate (GFR)	volume of fluid filtered by the renal glomerular capillaries per unit of time; decreased GFR rate indicates decreased renal function	men: 100 – 130 mL/min/1.73m^2 women: 90 – 120 mL/min/1.73m^2 GFR < 60 mL/min/1.73m^2 is common in adults > 70 years

Test	Description	Normal Range
Other Serum Tests (continued)		
Total cholesterol (LDL and HDL)	a steroid produced by the liver that is needed to build and maintain animal cell membranes and that has protective properties for the heart; goals for low-density lipoprotein (LDL) and high-density lipoprotein (HDL) levels are based on the patient's risk factors for cardiovascular disease	< 200 mg/dL LDL: < 100 mg/dL HDL (men): 40 – 50 mg/dL HDL (women): 50 – 59 mg/dL
Triglycerides	stores fat	< 150 mg/dL
B-type natriuretic peptide (BNP)	protein produced by the heart; high levels can indicate heart failure	< 100 pg/ml
Highly selective CRP test for C-reactive protein	marker for inflammation used to determine a patient's risk for heart disease	low risk: < 1.0 mg/L average risk: 1.0 – 3.0 mg/L high risk: > 3.0 mg/L
Homocysteine	an amino acid used as a marker for heart disease and vitamin deficiency (B_6, B_{12}, and folate)	4 – 14 μmol/L
Prostate-specific antigen (PSA)	enzyme produced by prostate gland; high levels can indicate prostate cancer, prostatitis, or BPH	< 4 ng/mL
Erythrocyte sedimentation rate (ESR or sed rate)	measures rate at which RBCs sediment (fall); increased ESR may indicate inflammation, anemia, or infection; decreased ESR may indicate heart failure or liver or kidney disease; ESR increases with age	men: 12 – 14 mm/h women: 18 – 21 mm/h
Ammonia	produced by bacteria in the intestines during the breakdown of proteins; increased levels may indicate liver or kidney damage; decreased levels are associated with hypertension	15 – 45 mcg/dL
Serum lipase (LPS)	protein secreted by the pancreas that helps break down fats; increased levels can indicate damage to the pancreas	0 – 160 U/L
Amylase	enzyme produced by pancreas and salivary glands; increased levels may indicate damage to the pancreas	23 – 85 U/L
Complete Blood Count (CBC)		
White blood cells (WBCs)	number of WBCs in blood; an increased number of WBCs can be an indication of inflammation or infection	4,500 – 10,000 cells/mcL
Red blood cells (RBCs)	carry oxygen throughout the body and filter carbon dioxide	men: 5 – 6 million cells/mcL women: 4 – 5 million cells/mcL
Hemoglobin (HgB)	protein that holds oxygen in the blood	men: 13.8 – 17.2 g/dL women: 12.1 – 15.1 g/dL
Hematocrit (Hct)	percentage of the blood composed of red blood cells	men: 41% – 50% women: 36% – 44%

Complete Blood Count (CBC) (continued)

Red blood cell indices	mean corpuscular volume (MCV): average size of the red blood cells mean corpuscular hemoglobin (MCH): average amount of hemoglobin per RBC mean corpuscular hemoglobin concentration (MCHC): average concentration of hemoglobin in RBCs	MCV: 80 – 95 fL MCH: 27.5 – 33.2 pg MCHC: 334 – 355 g/L
Platelets	play a role in the body's clotting process	150,000 – 450,000 cells/mcL

Coagulation Studies

Prothrombin time (PT)	tests how long it takes blood to clot	10 – 13 seconds
International normalized ratio (INR)	determines the effectiveness of an anticoagulant in thinning blood	healthy adults: < 1.1 patients receiving anticoagulants: 2.0 – 3.0
Partial thromboplastin time (PTT)	assess the body's ability to form blood clots	60 – 70 sec
Activated partial thromboplastin time (aPTT)	measures the body's ability to form blood clots using an activator to speed up the clotting process	20 – 35 sec

Cardiac Biomarkers

Troponin I (cTnI) and troponin T (cTnT)	proteins released when the heart muscle is damaged; high levels can indicate a myocardial infarction but may also be due to other conditions that stress the heart (e.g., renal failure, heart failure, PE); levels peak 24 hours post MI and can remain elevated for up to 2 weeks	cTnI: cutoff values for MI vary widely between assays cTnT: possible MI: > 0.01 ng/mL
Creatine kinase (CK)	responsible for muscle cell function; an increased amount indicates cardiac or skeletal muscle damage	22 – 198 U/L
Creatine kinase–muscle/brain (CK-MB or CPK-MB)	cardiac marker for damaged heart muscle; often used to diagnose a second MI or ongoing cardiovascular conditions; a high ratio of CK-MB to CK indicates damage to heart muscle (as opposed to skeletal muscle)	5 – 25 IU/L possible MI: ratio of CK-MB to CK is 2.5 – 3

Urinalysis

Leukocytes	presence of WBCs in urine indicates infection	negative
Nitrate	presence of nitrates in urine indicates infection by gram-negative bacteria	negative
Urobilinogen	produced during bilirubin reduction; presence in urine indicates liver disease, bilinear obstruction, or hepatitis	0.2 – 1 mg
Protein	presence of protein in the urine may indicate nephritis or eclampsia	negative

Test	Description	Normal Range
Urinalysis (continued)		
pH	decreased (acidic) pH may indicate systemic acidosis or diabetes mellitus; increased (alkali) pH may indicate systemic alkalosis or UTI	4.5 – 8
Blood	blood in urine may indicate infection, renal calculi, neoplasm, or coagulation disorders	negative
Specific gravity	concentration of urine; decreased may indicate diabetes insipidus or pyelonephritis; increased may indicate dehydration or SIADH	1.010 – 1.025
Ketone	ketones are produced during fat metabolism; presence in urine may indicate diabetes, hyperglycemia, starvation, alcoholism, or eclampsia	negative
Bilirubin	produced during the breakdown of heme; presence in urine may indicate liver disease, biliary obstruction, or hepatitis	negative
Glucose	presence of glucose in urine indicates hyperglycemia	0 – 15 mg/dL
Urine hCG	determination of pregnancy	N/A
Urine culture and sensitivity	study of urine with growth on a culture medium to determine which pathogenic bacteria is present and which antibiotic the pathogen is sensitive to	N/A
Liver Function Tests		
Albumin	a protein made in the liver; low levels may indicate liver damage	3.5 – 5.0 g/dL
Alkaline phosphatase (ALP)	an enzyme found in the liver and bones; increased levels indicate liver damage	45 – 147 U/L
Alanine transaminase (ALT)	an enzyme in the liver that helps metabolize protein; increased levels indicate liver damage	7 – 55 U/L
Aspartate transaminase (AST)	an enzyme in the liver that helps metabolize alanine; increased levels indicate liver or muscle damage	8 – 48 U/L
Total protein	low levels of total protein may indicate liver damage	6.3 – 7.9 g/dL
Total bilirubin	produced during the breakdown of heme; increased levels indicate liver damage or anemia	0.1 – 1.2 mg/dL
Gamma-glutamyl-transferase (GGT)	an enzyme that plays a role in antioxidant metabolism; increased levels indicate liver damage	9 – 48 U/L
L-lactate dehydrogenase (LD or LDH)	an enzyme found in most cells in the body; high levels may indicate liver damage, cancer, or tissue breakdown	adult: 122 – 222 U/L

Arterial Blood Gas (ABG)

pH	measure of blood pH	7.35 – 7.45
Partial pressure of oxygen (PaO$_2$)	amount of oxygen gas in the blood	75 – 100 mm Hg
Partial pressure of carbon dioxide (PaCO$_2$)	amount of carbon dioxide gas in the blood	35 – 45 mm Hg
Bicarbonate (HCO$_3$)	amount of bicarbonate in the blood	22 – 26 mEq/L
Oxygen (O$_2$) saturation	measurement of the amount of oxygen-saturated hemoglobin relative to unsaturated hemoglobin	94 – 100%
Lactate	molecule produced during anaerobic cellular respiration; high levels indicate lack of available oxygen in cells	4.5 – 14.4 mg/dL

APPENDIX: ABBREVIATIONS

A

ABC: A1c (hemoglobin), blood pressure, and cholesterol

ABG: arterial blood gas

ACE inhibitors: angiotensin-converting enzyme inhibitors

ACLS: advanced cardiovascular life support

ACS: acute coronary syndrome

ACTH: adrenocorticotropic hormone stimulation test

A-fib: atrial fibrillation

ALL: acute lymphocytic leukemia

ALP: alkaline phosphatase

ALS: amyotrophic lateral sclerosis

ALT: alanine aminotransferase

AMA: against medical advice *or* American Medical Association

AML: acute myeloid leukemia

AND: allow natural death

AOM: acute otitis media

aPTT: activated partial thromboplastin time

ARBs: angiotensin II receptor blockers

ARDS: acute respiratory distress syndrome

ARF: acute renal failure

AST: aspartate aminotransferase

AUB: abnormal uterine bleeding

aVF: augmented vector foot (ECG lead)

aVL: augmented vector left (ECG lead)

AVM: arteriovenous malformation

aVR: augmented vector right (ECG lead)

B

BBB: bundle branch block

BNP: B-type natriuretic peptide

BPH: benign prostatic hyperplasia

bpm: beats per minute

BPM: breaths per minute

BRAT: banana, rice, applesauce, toast (e.g., BRAT diet)

BUN: blood urea nitrogen

BZK: benzalkonium chloride (e.g., BZK wipes)

C

CAD: coronary artery disease

CA-MRSA: community-acquired methicillin-resistant *Staphylococcus aureus*

CAP: community-acquired pneumonia

CBC: complete blood count

CDC: Centers for Disease Control and Prevention

CISD: critical incident stress debriefing

CISM: critical incident stress management

CIWA-Ar: Clinical Institute Withdrawal Assessment for Alcohol

CK-MB: creatine kinase–muscle/brain

CLL: chronic lymphocytic leukemia

CML: chronic myelogenous leukemia

CMP: comprehensive metabolic panel

CO: cardiac output

COBRA: Consolidated Omnibus Budget Reconciliation Act

COCA: color, odor, clarity, amount (urinary assessment)

COWS: Clinical Opiate Withdrawal Scale

CPG: clinical practice guideline

CPP: cerebral perfusion pressure

CPR: cardiopulmonary resuscitation

CRF: chronic renal failure

CRI: cutaneous radiation injury

CRP: C-reactive protein

CRT: capillary refill time

CS: culture and sensitivity

CSF: cerebrospinal fluid

CSM: circulation, sensation, and movement

CT scan: computed tomography scan

CTPA: computed tomography pulmonary angiography

CVA: cerebrovascular accident

CVP: central venous pressure

D

D&C: dilation and curettage

D50: dextrose 50% solution

D5W: dextrose 5% in water

DAI: diffuse axonal injury

DBP: diastolic blood pressure

DIC: disseminated intravascular coagulation

DKA: diabetic ketoacidosis

DMARDs: disease-modifying antirheumatic drugs

DNI: do not intubate

DNR: do not resuscitate

DT: diphtheria and tetanus (vaccine)

DTaP: diphtheria, tetanus, and pertussis (vaccine)

DTI: deep tissue injury

DTPA: diethylenetriamine pentaacetate

DTs: delirium tremens

DUBB: dangerous underwater breath-holding behaviors

DVT: deep vein thrombosis

E

EAPs: Employee Assistance Programs

EBP: evidence-based practice

ECF: extracellular fluid

ECG: electrocardiogram

ECR: extracorporeal core rewarming

EEG: electroencephalogram

EGD: esophagogastroduodenoscopy

EIA: enzyme immunoassay

ELISA: enzyme-linked immunosorbent assay

EMB: ethambutol

EMTALA: Emergency Medical Treatment and Active Labor Act

ESI: Emergency Severity Index

ESR: erythrocyte sedimentation rate

ESWL: extracorporeal shock wave lithotripsy

ET tube: endotracheal tube

F

FAST ultrasound: focused assessment with sonography for trauma

FFP: fresh frozen plasma

FLT3: fms-related tyrosine kinase 3

FSH: follicle-stimulating hormone

G

GCS: Glasgow Coma Scale

GFR: glomerular filtration rate

GSW: gunshot wound

GU: genitourinary

H

H/H: hemoglobin and hematocrit

HA-MRSA: hospital-acquired methicillin-resistant *Staphylococcus aureus*

HAP: hospital-acquired pneumonia

HBSS: Hanks' Balanced Salt Solution

HCAHPS: Hospital Consumer Assessment of Healthcare Providers and Systems

hCG: human chorionic gonadotropin

HCS: Hazard Communication Standard

HELLP syndrome: hemolysis, elevated liver enzymes, low platelet count

HgB: hemoglobin

HHS: hyperosmolar hyperglycemic state

HIPAA: Health Insurance Portability and Accountability Act

HIT: heparin-induced thrombocytopenia

HR: heart rate

HSV: herpes simplex virus

I

IBS: irritable bowel syndrome

ICD: implantable cardioverter defibrillator

ICF: intracellular fluid

ICP: intracranial pressure

ICS: incident command system

IgM: immunoglobulin M

INH: isoniazid

INR: international normalized ratio

IO: intraosseous (infusion)

ITP: idiopathic thrombocytopenic purpura

IUD: intrauterine device

IV: intravenous

IVIG: intravenous immunoglobulin

IVP: intravenous pyelography

J

JVD: jugular vein distention

K

KUB: kidney, ureter, bladder

L

LFT: liver function test

LLQ: left lower quadrant

LMA: laryngeal mask airway

LOC: level of consciousness

LPN: licensed practical nurse

LUQ: left upper quadrant

LVN: licensed vocational nurse

M

MAP: mean arterial pressure

MCI: mass casualty incident

MD: muscular dystrophy

mEq: milliequivalent

MG: myasthenia gravis

MI: myocardial infarction

MMI: maximum medical improvement

MODS: multiple organ dysfunction syndrome

MRI: magnetic resonance imaging

MRSA: methicillin-resistant *Staphylococcus aureus*

MS: multiple sclerosis

MSDS: material safety data sheets

MVA: motor vehicle accident/motorized vehicle accident

MVC: motor vehicle crash/motorized vehicle crash

N

NAAT: nucleic acid amplification test

NG tube: nasogastric tube

NIH: National Institutes of Health

NIHSS: National Institutes of Health Stroke Scale

NPE: noncardiac pulmonary edema

NSAID: nonsteroidal anti-inflammatory drug

NSTEMI: non-ST-elevation myocardial infarction

O

OME: otitis media with effusion

P

PALM-COEIN: polyp, adenomyosis, leiomyoma, malignancy, coagulopathy, ovulatory disorder, endometrial, iatrogenic, not otherwise classified (risk factors for abdominal uterine bleeding)

PCI: percutaneous coronary intervention

PCR: polymerase chain reaction

PE: pulmonary embolism

PEA: pulseless electrical activity

PHI: protected health information

PID: pelvic inflammatory disease

PO: *per os* (by mouth)

PPE: personal protective equipment

PRN: *pro re nata* (as needed)

PSP: primary spontaneous pneumothorax

PT: prothrombin time

PTH: post-traumatic headaches

PTT: partial thromboplastin time

PTU: propylthiouracil

PVD: peripheral vascular disease

PZA: pyrazinamide

R

RhoGAM: Rho(D) immune globulin

RIF: rifampin

RIG: rabies immune globulin

RLQ: right lower quadrant

ROM: range of motion

ROSC: return of spontaneous circulation

RPR: rapid plasma reagent

RR: respiration rate

RSI: rapid sequence intubation

RSV: respiratory syncytial virus

RT–PCR: real-time polymerase chain reaction

RUQ: right upper quadrant

S

SANE: sexual assault nurse examiner

SARS: severe acute respiratory syndrome

SBP: systolic blood pressure

SDS: safety data sheets

SSP: secondary spontaneous pneumothorax

START: simple triage and rapid treatment

STEMI: ST-segment elevation myocardial infarction

STI: sexually transmitted infection

SV: stroke volume

SVT: supraventricular tachycardia

T

TBSA: total body surface area

TCP: transcutaneous pacing

Td: tetanus and diphtheria (vaccine)

Tdap: tetanus, diphtheria, and pertussis (booster DTaP vaccine)

TEE: transesophageal echocardiogram

TIA: transient ischemic attack

TMJ: temporomandibular joint

tPA: tissue plasminogen activator

TPN: total parenteral nutrition

TSH: thyroid stimulating hormone

TTM: targeted temperature management

U

U/L: units per liter

ULQ: upper left quadrant

URQ: upper right quadrant

UTI: urinary tract infection

V

VDLR: venereal disease research laboratories

V-fib: ventricular fibrillation

VRE: vancomycin-resistant enterococci

V-tach: ventricular tachycardia

W

WBC: white blood cell

WHO: World Health Organization

APPENDIX: COMMON ECG STRIPS

Sinus Rhythms

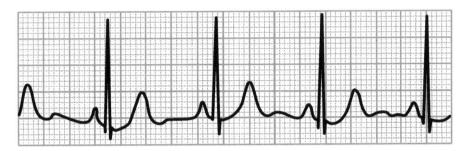

Normal sinus rhythm: Regular rhythm with a rate of 60-100 bpm. Every ORS is preceded by a P wave.

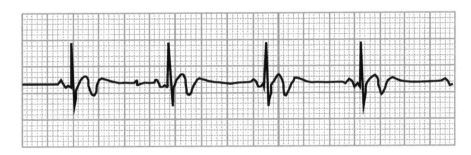

Sinus bradycardia: Regular rhythm with a slow rate <60. All other measurements are normal.

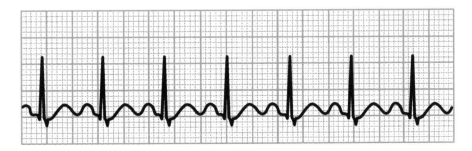

Sinus tachycardia: Regular rhythm with a fast rate >100 bpm. All other measurements are normal. Although P wave can merge with the T wave at very fast rates.

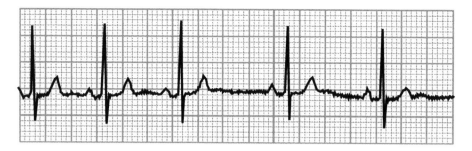

Sinus arrythmia: An irregular rhythm that can vary with respirations. All measurements are normal besides a varying R-R interval.

Atrial Rhythms

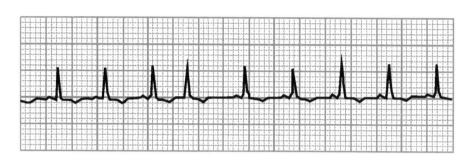

Premature atrial contractions: Irregular rhythm with premature, irregular P waves and QRS complexes.

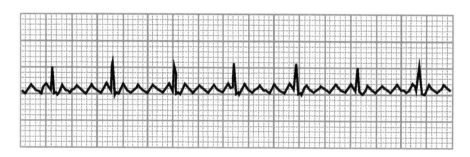

Atrial flutter: Rhythm can be regular or irregular with no observable P wave, but saw-toothed waves can be seen.

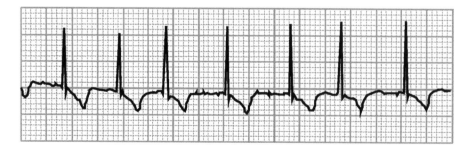

Atrial fibrillation: Irregular rhythm with absent P wave and PR interval.

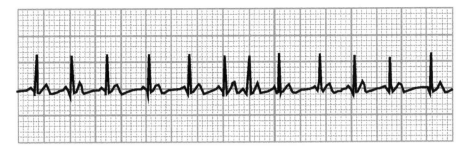

Atrial tachycardia: Irregular, fast rhythm (>100 bpm) with a variable PR interval and abnormal T wave.

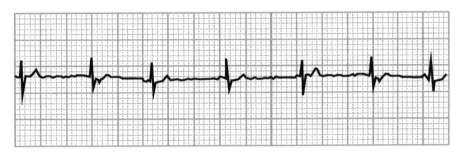

Wandering pacemaker: This rhythm can be regular or irregular and have a normal rate of 60-100 bpm. The P wave will change shape and size from one beat to another.

Junctional Rhythms

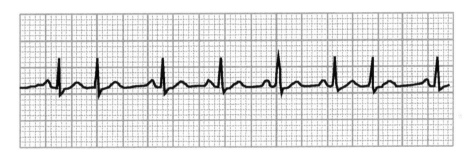

Premature junctional contractions: Regular rhythm with premature beats and a short or absent PR interval.

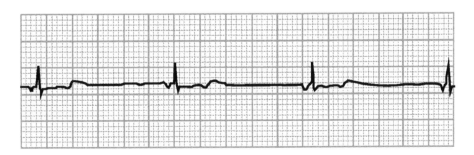

Junctional escape rhythm: A regular rhythm with a slow rate (40-60 bpm) and a PR interval that is unmeasurable. If a P wave can be seen it is inverted.

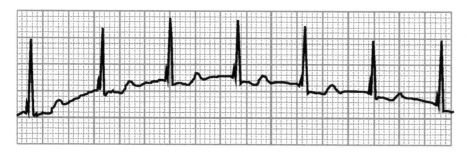

Accelerated junctional rhythm: A regular rhythm with a rate of 60-100 bpm and an unmeasurable PR interval.

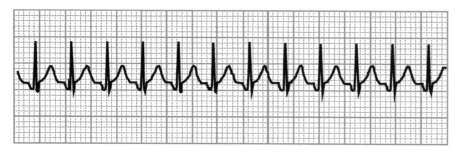

Junctional tachycardia: A regular rhythm with a rate of 100-180 bpm, with an absent or shorter PR interval. If a P wave is present it will be inverted.

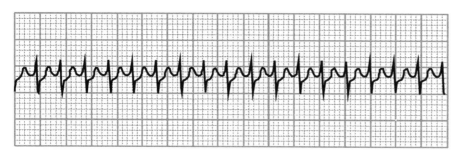

Supraventricular tachycardia: A regular rhythm with a rate of 150-250 bpm and T waves that are hidden in the QRS complex.

Heart Blocks

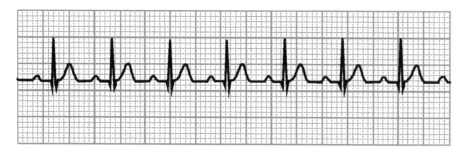

First degree block: A regular rhythm with a prolonged PR interval (>0.20 seconds).

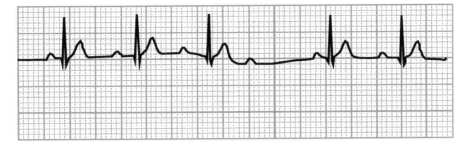

Second degree block type I Wenckebach: An irregular rhythm that has a PR interval that gets progressively longer until a QRS complex is dropped and then the cycle repeats itself.

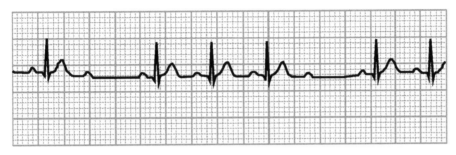

Second degree block type 2 Mobitz: An irregular rhythm with more P waves than QRS complexes.

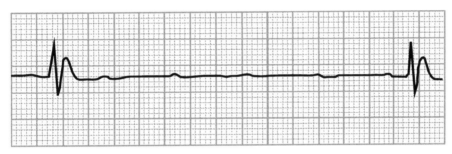

Third degree block/Complete heart block: An erratic rhythm that has no communication between the atria and ventricles.

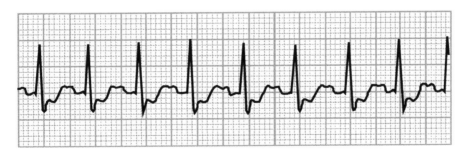

Bundle branch block: A regular rhythm with a wide QRS interval (>0.12 seconds).

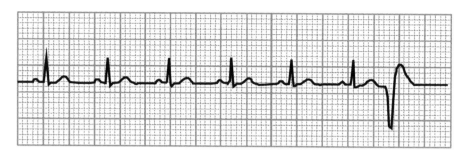

Premature ventricular contractions: A regular rhythm that possesses a wide and bizarre beat with a QRS interval greater than 0.10 seconds.

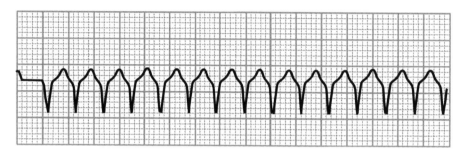

Ventricular tachycardia: A regular and fast rhythm (100-250 bpm) without P waves and wide bizarre QRS complexes.

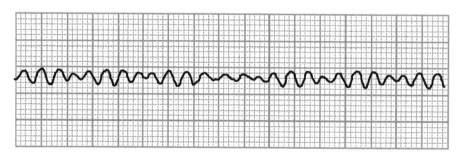

Ventricular fibrillation: An extremely irregular rhythm with an unmeasurable rate and no P waves. This rhythm does not have QRS complexes.

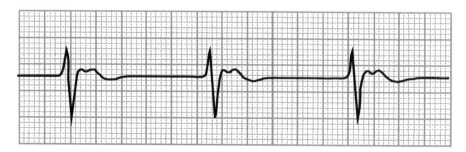

Idioventricular rhythm: A regular, but slow rhythm (20-40 bpm) without P waves and a wide bizarre QRS complex (>0.10 seconds).

Asystole

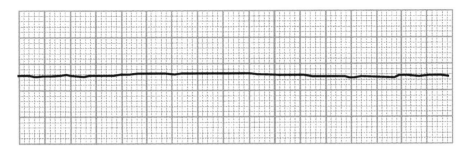

Asystole: This rhythm does not have a rate, P wave, or QRS complex.

APPENDIX E: MEDICATION PURPOSE & DOSAGE

Generic Name	Brand Name(s)	Dosage	Contraindications and Nursing Considerations
ACE Inhibitors			
benazepril	Lotensin	5 – 10 mg/day	+ not indicated for patients with history of angioedema + may cause a dry, hacking cough + patients with ascites or cirrhosis should avoid
captopril	Capoten	+ Initial: 6.25 mg 3×/day + Target: 50 mg 3×/day	+ neutropenia a risk for patients with renal impairment + symptomatic hypotension may occur to include syncope, may occur in first few doses
enalapril	Vasotec	+ Initial: 5 mg/day + Target: titrate up to 40 mg/day + Max: 40 mg/day	+ in patients with severe aortic stenosis, may reduce coronary perfusion resulting in ischemia + possible exaggerated response in patients > 65 to this and other ACE inhibitors
lisinopril	Zestril	5 – 10 mg/day; max dose: 40 mg/day	+ may cause a dry, hacking cough + increased BUN and serum creatinine and/or deteriorated renal function have been associated with it, especially in patients with low renal blood flow

Generic Name	Brand Name(s)	Dosage	Contraindications and Nursing Considerations
Analgesics			
acetaminophen	Tylenol	+ Regular strength: 650 mg every 4 – 6 hours + Extra strength: 1,000 mg every 6 hours + Max dose: 4 g/day	+ associated with acute liver failure, liver transplant, and death + associated with serious/fatal skin reactions, including Stevens–Johnson syndrome and toxic epidermal necrolysis + use with caution in patients with alcoholic liver disease
acetaminophen/ butalbital/ caffeine	Fioricet	+ 1 – 2 tablets every 4 hours + Max: 6 tablets	use may not be advised in patients with renal, hepatic, or respiratory impairment
Anesthetics			
capsaicin	Zostrix	Topical via cream or patch; ≤ 4 applications/ day	+ patients with uncontrolled hypertension or a history of cardiovascular events may experience increased blood pressure + may impair physical or mental abilities; inform patients mental alertness may be diminished
lidocaine	Xylocaine	Dosage dependent on method of application and concentration	+ use with caution in patients with known drug sensitivities + application to broken or inflamed skin may lead to increased systemic absorption + reduce dose for acutely ill patients
Antacids			
aluminum hydroxide	Alternagel	1.9 – 4.8 mg up to 4×/ day	+ anti-ulcer agent, also used as adjunct for treatment of high serum phosphate in kidney failure + avoid taking other medications within 2 hours of use
magnesium hydroxide	Maalox	400 – 1,200 mg/day	+ used for constipation + used for indigestion + not indicated for patients in acute severe renal failure

Antibiotics

amoxicillin	Augmentin	250 – 500 mg 2 – 3×/ day	+ dosage based on weight and clinical picture + patients should use alternate forms of birth control + indicated for use in otitis media, UTIs, skin infection
ampicillin	Principen	250 – 500 mg every 6 hours	+ used in respiratory infections, meningitis, UTIs, and GI infections + contraindicated in patients with PCN allergy
azithromycin	Zithromax	+ Dosing based on clinical picture + 250 – 600 mg 3x/ day	+ used for chancroid type infections, respiratory infections, and some STIs + may result in elongated QT interval on ECG
ceftriaxone	Rocephin	1 – 2 g every 12 – 24 hours	+ used in endocarditis, bite wounds, cholecystitis + may increase INR + serious hypersensitivity may occur
ciprofloxacin	Cipro	500 – 750 mg 2×/day	+ used for infections resulting from bite wounds, cat scratches, chancroids + used for anthrax exposure/infection + may cause photosensitivity
clindamycin	Cleocin	600 – 1,800 mg/day in 2 – 4 divided doses	+ used for anthrax infection, bacterial vaginosis, bite wounds + use with caution in patients with GI disease or hepatic impairment + risk of colitis with use
doxycycline	Acticlate	100 – 200 mg/day in 1 – 2 divided doses	+ broad spectrum use, used for acne vulgaris, cellulitis, bite infections, Lyme disease + may cause abdominal pain and discomfort + used as malaria prophylaxis
gentamicin	Gentak	3 – 5 mg/kg/day in divided doses every 8 hours	+ used in endocarditis, brucellosis, gonococcal infection, plague + use with caution in patients with electrolyte imbalance + do not use in pregnancy
isoniazid	Nydrazid	5 mg/kg/doses 1×/day	+ treatment of nontuberculous mycobacterium + may result in fatal hepatitis

Generic Name	Brand Name(s)	Dosage	Contraindications and Nursing Considerations
Antibiotics (continued)			
meropenem	Merrem	1.5 – 6 g/day divided every 8 hours	+ confusion, seizures, and other adverse CNS effects + use with caution in patients with renal impairment
metronidazole	Flagyl	500 mg 2×/day for 7 days	+ most frequently used for bacterial vaginosis + *Clostridioides* may be treated with this medication + possibly carcinogenic
penicillin	N/A	Oral: 125 – 500 mg every 6 – 8 hours	+ used in bite wounds, pneumococcal prophylaxis, streptococcal infections + use caution in patients with renal impairment and seizure disorders
piperacillin-tazobactam	Zosyn	3.375 g every 6 hours	+ used in bite wounds, sepsis, cystic fibrosis + may cause serious skin reactions + may cause electrolyte abnormalities
rifampin	Rifadin	10 mg/kg/day 1×/day (max: 600 mg/day)	+ used for treatment of active tuberculosis + may cause vitamin K–dependent coagulopathy
streptomycin	N/A	1 g every 12 hours for 1 week	+ used for Ménière's disease and mycobacterium infections + may cause neuromuscular blockade and respiratory paralysis
sulfamethoxazole	Bactrim	1 – 2 double-strength tablets every 12 – 24 hours	+ used for bite wounds, brain abscess, infectious diarrhea + may cause blood dyscrasias + may cause hyperkalemia + may cause hepatic necrosis
vancomycin	Vancocin	15 – 20 mg/kg/dose	+ used in catheter-related infections, endocarditis, community-acquired pneumonia + may cause nephrotoxicity, neutropenia, and ototoxicity

Antiemetics

ondansetron	Zofran	4 – 8 mg every 8 hours	+ used for nausea + may cause prolonged QT interval + may cause serotonin syndrome
promethazine	Phenergan	12.5 – 25 mg/dose	+ used for persistent nausea + may cause respiratory depression + extravasation may cause severe tissue injury, including gangrene

Anti-Inflammatories

ibuprofen	Motrin	200 – 800 mg 3 – 4×/day	+ used for analgesia and antipyretic properties + may have impact on liver enzymes and function + may cause skin reactions

Anticonvulsants

carbamazepine	Tegretol	400 mg/day in 2 divided doses or 4 divided doses	+ treatment for seizures, bipolar disorder + may cause blood dyscrasias + may cause hyponatremia + may cause psychiatric effects
fosphenytoin	Cerebyx	20 mg PE/kg as a single dose	+ used for status epilepticus + may cause cardiac events if infused too quickly + may cause hepatotoxicity
gabapentin	Neurontin	100 – 300 mg 1 – 3×/day	+ used for neuropathic pain, psychiatric disorder adjunct, and alcohol withdrawal + can be used for intractable hiccups + may cause anaphylaxis + neuropsychiatric effects may occur
levetiracetam	Keppra	+ 500 mg 2×/day + Increase every 2 weeks by 500 mg/dose based on response	+ used in status epilepticus, subarachnoid hemorrhage, and traumatic brain injury + may cause CNS depression + may cause hypertension + may cause increase in suicidal ideation
phenytoin	Dilantin	20 mg/kg at a max rate of 50 mg/minute	+ used in status epilepticus + can be used in seizures + chronic use may lead to decreased bone density

Generic Name	Brand Name(s)	Dosage	Contraindications and Nursing Considerations
Anticoagulants			
enoxaparin	Lovenox	40 – 60 mg every 12 hours	+ monitor patient closely for signs of bleeding + monitor for hyperkalemia; can cause hyperkalemia
heparin	N/A	+ 60 units/kg (max 4,000 units), then 12 units/kg/hour + Max: 1,000 units/hour	+ adjunct to fibrinolysis in the presence of STEMI + bleeding may occur, causing fatal events + high-alert medication
warfarin	Coumadin	2 – 5 mg 1×/day (may be higher; varies by patient age and physical status)	+ used for prophylaxis and treatment of thromboembolic disorders + may cause hypersensitivity reactions, including anaphylaxis
Anticholinergics			
dicyclomine	Bentyl	20 mg 4×/day for 7 days	+ gastrointestinal motility disorders/irritable bowel + use with caution in patients with coronary artery disease + use with caution in patients with autonomic neuropathy
Antidysrhythmics			
adenosine	Adenocard	Initial: 6 mg; if not effective within 1 – 2 minutes, another 6 mg may be given	+ used in the ED for supraventricular tachycardia for cardioversion + A-fib may occur + may cause conduction disturbances
amiodarone	Cordarone	150 mg over 10 minutes	+ used for A-fib + can cause life-threatening arrhythmias + pulmonary toxicity
digoxin/digitalis	Digox	+ 0.25 – 0.5 mg over several minutes + Maintenance dose: Oral: 0.125 – 0.25 mg 1×/day	used to control heart rate
lidocaine	Xylocaine	1 – 1.5 mg/kg bolus	+ can be used as an antidysrhythmic or in V-fib or V-tach + extreme caution in patients with severe hepatic dysfunction + risk of lidocaine toxicity

procainamide	Procan	10 – 17 mg/kg at a rate of 20 – 50 mg/minute or 100 mg every 5 minutes	+ used for hemodynamically stable ventricular arrhythmias + reduce dose if first-degree heart block occurs

Antidepressants

paroxetine	Paxil	20 mg 1×/day, preferably in the morning	+ may increase suicidal ideation or behavior + make cause extrapyramidal symptoms + may cause CNS depression
sertraline	Zoloft	50 mg 1×/day	+ may be used in a variety of depressive disorders, anxiety disorders, eating disorders + will not be initiated in ED + increased risk for suicidal ideation

Antihistamines

dimenhydrinate	Dramamine	50 – 100 mg every 4 – 6 hours	+ used for motion sickness and post-op vomiting + use with caution in patients with cardiovascular disease + some antibiotics can cause ototoxicity; if patient consumes, use dimenhydrinate with caution
diphenhydramine	Benadryl	25 – 50 mg every 4 – 8 hours	+ for use in allergic reactions, headaches, nausea + may cause CNS depression + use with caution in patients with asthma
meclizine	Antivert	Oral: 25 – 100 mg/day	+ used for symptoms caused by vertigo + use with caution in patients with narrow-angle glaucoma + use with caution in patients with hepatic disease

Antihypertensives

clonidine	Catapres	0.1 mg 2×/day; max dose: 2.4 mg/day	+ primary use for antihypertensive, secondary use for sedating side effects + may cause dose-dependent reductions in heart rate + symptomatic hypotension may occur with use
doxazosin	Cardura	Initial: 1 mg 1×/day	+ used for HTN and BPH + skin rash, urticaria, pruritus, angioedema, and respiratory symptoms may occur + use with caution in patients with heart failure, angina pectoris, or recent acute myocardial infarction

Generic Name	Brand Name(s)	Dosage	Contraindications and Nursing Considerations
Antihypertensives (continued)			
hydralazine	Apresoline	25 – 50 mg 3 or 4×/day	+ used for heart failure with reduced ejection fraction, hypertension emergency + may induce a lupus-like syndrome including glomerulonephritis + use with caution in patients with mitral valvular disease
nifedipine	Procardia	10 mg 3×/day; usual dose: 10 – 20 mg 3×/day	+ used for stable angina, hypertension, high-altitude pulmonary edema + possibility of increased angina and/or MI with initiation or dosage titration
Anthelmintic Agents			
albendazole	Albenza	800 mg/day in 2 divided doses for 8 – 30 days	+ used to treat infections with parasitic worms + in sensitized individuals, anaphylaxis may occur within minutes of exposure
Antifungals			
amphotericin B	Amphotec	3 – 4 mg/kg/day	+ used to treat invasive aspergillosis, candidiasis, and endocarditis + acute infusion reactions, sometimes severe, may occur 1 – 3 hours after starting infusion
fluconazole	Diflucan	Up to 1,600 mg/day	+ use in candidiasis infection + associated with QT prolongation and torsades de pointes + serious (sometimes fatal) hepatic toxicity
nystatin	Bio-Statin	400,000 – 600,000 units 4×/day	+ oral candidiasis and intestinal infections + in oral infections: patients who wear dentures must remove and clean them to prevent reinfection
terbinafine	Lamisil	250 mg 1×/day for 6 weeks	+ finger and toe infections and tinea capitis + use caution in patients sensitive to allylamine antifungals + patients should be alert to depressive symptoms/mood changes
Antiparasitics and Antimicrobials			
ivermectin	Stromectol, Soolantra	150 – 200 mcg/kg	+ parasitic infections + repeated treatment may be required in immunocompromised patients

nitazoxanide	Alinia	500 mg every 12 hours for 3 days	+ used in *C. difficile* infection or in giardiasis + possible hypersensitivity to nitazoxanide or inactive ingredients
Antiplatelets			
aspirin	Ecotrin, Bayer Aspirin	+ Primary preventative: 81 mg/day + Medical therapy (post-MI): 162 – 325 mg	+ increases risk of GI bleeding + should not be given to children or infants with viral infections (Reye syndrome)
clopidogrel	Plavix	Loading dose of 300 mg followed by 75 mg 1×/day	+ increased bleeding risk + patients with renal impairment should be closely monitored
Antipsychotics (Conventional and Atypical)			
chlorpromazine	Thorazine	30 – 800 mg/day in 2 – 4 divided doses	+ may alter cardiac conduction + chlorpromazine can suppress the cough reflex; aspiration of vomit is possible
droperidol	Inapsine	5 – 10 mg	+ used for undifferentiated agitation + can also be used for postoperative nausea and vomiting + possible impaired physical or mental abilities from CNS depression + black box warning due to arrhythmias
haloperidol	Haldol	0.5 – 10 mg depending on degree of agitation	+ used for acute agitation + patients > 65 with dementia-related psychosis exhibit increased mortality + possible impaired physical or mental abilities from CNS depression
olanzapine	Zyprexa	+ 5 – 10 mg 1×/day + Max: 60 mg/day	+ patients > 65 with dementia-related psychosis exhibit increased mortality + risk of post-injection delirium/sedation syndrome
ziprasidone	Geodon	10 mg every 2 hours or 20 mg every 4 hours	+ in the ED used for acute agitation + risk for leukopenia, neutropenia, and agranulocytosis + possible esophageal dysmotility and aspiration
ARBs			
telmisartan	Micardis	20 – 40 mg 1×/day	+ management of hypertension + salt- or volume-depleted patients may experience symptomatic hypotension

Generic Name	Brand Name(s)	Dosage	Contraindications and Nursing Considerations
ARBs (continued)			
valsartan	Diovan	80 mg or 160 mg 1×/day	+ used for management of hypertension or CHF + hyperkalemia possible in case of renal dysfunction, diabetes mellitus, use of potassium-sparing diuretics, potassium supplements
losartan	Cozaar	50 mg 1×/day; titrate as needed based on patient response up to 100 mg/day	+ unlikely to be newly prescribed in ED + management of hypertension + salt- or volume-depleted patients may experience symptomatic hypotension
Antitremors			
amantadine	Gocovri	137 mg 1×/day; after 1 week, increase to usual dose of 274 mg 1×/day	+ used for Parkinson's disease, extrapyramidal symptoms, and restless leg syndrome + risk of compulsive behaviors and/or loss of impulse control + suicidal ideation/attempt and depression in patients with and without a history of psychiatric illness
benztropine	Cogentin	1 – 2 mg 2 – 3×/day for reactions developing soon after initiation of antipsychotic medication	+ indicated for management of drug-induced extrapyramidal symptoms + used in parkinsonism + may be associated with confusion, visual hallucinations, or excitement + monitor patients with tachycardia
Antivirals			
acyclovir	Zovirax	400 mg 5×/day for 10 days	+ can be used for herpes simplex virus, cytomegalovirus, and new-onset Bell's palsy + neurotoxicity may be more common in patients with renal impairment + maintain adequate hydration during oral or IV therapy
valacyclovir	Valtrex	1 g 2×/day for 7 – 10 days	+ can be used for herpes simplex virus, cytomegalovirus, new-onset Bell's palsy, and shingles + risk for adverse CNS effects such as agitation, hallucinations, confusion, delirium, seizures, and encephalopathy

Benzodiazepines

alprazolam	Xanax	0.25 – 0.5 mg 3×/day	+ treatment of generalized anxiety disorder + associated with anterograde amnesia + possible impaired physical or mental abilities from CNS depression
diazepam	Valium	10 mg initially; may administer 5 – 10 mg 3 – 4 hours later	+ risks from concomitant use of opioids + used in anxiety and agitation or acute alcohol withdrawal
lorazepam	Ativan	2 – 3 mg/day	+ risks from concomitant use of opioids + used in anxiety and agitation or acute alcohol withdrawal
midazolam	Versed	2 – 3 mg	+ used for anxiety, sedation + used for status epilepticus + associated with anterograde amnesia + associated with respiratory depression and respiratory arrest

Beta-Blockers

atenolol	Tenormin	50 mg 1×/day	+ used for angina pectoris, A-fib, and ventricular arrhythmias + contraindicated in patients with bronchospastic disease + use caution in patients with conditions such as sick sinus syndrome
carvedilol	Coreg	6.25 mg 2×/day	+ used in heart failure and hypertension + measure apical heart rate before administering + hold for bradycardia
labetalol	Trandate	10 – 20 mg IV push over 2 minutes	+ indicated for hypertension or hypertensive urgency/emergency + monitor vitals (BP and pulse) throughout administration + symptomatic hypotension with or without syncope may occur
metoprolol	Lopressor	50 mg 2×/day	+ indicated for A-fib, atrial flutter, angina, and hypertension + monitor vitals (BP and pulse) throughout administration + symptomatic hypotension with or without syncope may occur

Generic Name	Brand Name(s)	Dosage	Contraindications and Nursing Considerations
Beta-Blockers (continued)			
propranolol	Hemangeol	10 – 30 mg/dose every 6 – 8 hours	+ used for A-fib, hypertension, migraine headache prophylaxis + contraindicated in patients with bronchospastic disease + monitor patients with myasthenia gravis closely
Bronchodilators			
albuterol	Proventil	2.5 mg 3 – 4×/day as needed	+ used for bronchospasm and asthma exacerbation + possibility of paradoxical bronchospasm
formoterol	Perforomist	12 mcg every 12 hours	+ used for treatment of asthma and COPD and exercise-induced bronchospasm + possibility of paradoxical, life-threatening bronchospasm
ipratropium	Atrovent HFA	2 inhalations (34 mcg) 4×/day	+ used in COPD and acute asthma exacerbations + often adjunct with albuterol + may cause dizziness and blurred vision
levalbuterol	Xopenex	1.25 – 2.5 mg every 20 minutes for 3 doses	+ indicated for bronchospasm or asthma exacerbation + use with caution in patients with cardiovascular disease + use with caution in hyperthyroidism; may stimulate thyroid activity
racemic epinephrine	Asthmanefrin	1 – 3 inhalations of 2.25%	+ for use in bronchospasm and croup as an upper airway instruction
Calcium Channel Blockers			
amlodipine	Norvasc	2.5 – 5 mg 1×/day	+ known to cause increased angina and/or MI with initiation + symptomatic hypotension can occur
diltiazem	Cardizem	120 mg 1×/day	+ transient dermatologic reactions have been observed + carefully consider use in patients with hepatic impairment
Diuretics			
bumetanide	Bumex	0.5 – 2 mg/dose 1 – 2×/day	+ in excess, can induce serious diuresis causing fluid and electrolyte loss + asymptomatic hyperuricemia has been reported with use

furosemide	Lasix	20 – 80 mg/dose	+ in excess, can induce serious diuresis causing fluid and electrolyte loss + fluid status renal function should be monitored to prevent oliguria
hydrochlorothi-azide	Microzide	25 – 100 mg/day	+ hypokalemia, hypochloremic alkalosis, hypomagnesemia, and hyponatremia may occur + hypersensitivity reactions may occur with hydrochlorothiazide
mannitol	Osmitrol	0.25 – 1 g/kg/dose	+ indicated for use in management of intracranial pressure + avoid extravasation of IV infusions of mannitol: vesicant

H$_2$ Blockers

ranitidine	Zantac	150 mg 2×/day	+ rare cases of reversible confusion have been associated with ranitidine + elevation in ALT levels has occurred with higher doses

Inotropes

milrinone	Primacor	50 mcg/kg administered over 10 minutes	+ indicated for use in inotropic support in heart failure + some cases of ventricular dysrhythmias (non-sustained V-tach and supraventricular dysrhythmias)

Immunosuppressants

methotrexate	Otrexup; Rasuvo; Rheumatrex	100 – 500 mg/m^2	+ indicated for use in the ED for ectopic pregnancy + black box warning for fetal toxicity, chemotherapeutic agent

Mood Stabilizers

lithium	Lithobid	600 – 900 mg/day	+ lithium toxicity is possible at doses close to therapeutic levels and is closely related to serum concentrations + may cause CNS depression + may cause behavior changes

Muscle Relaxants/Paralytics

rocuronium	Zemuron	8 – 12 mcg/kg/minute	+ resistance may occur in burn patients + carefully consider use in patients with cardiovascular disease
succinylcholine	Anectine	0.6 mg/kg	+ risk of bradycardia may be increased with second dose + may cause a transient increase in intracranial pressure

Generic Name	Brand Name(s)	Dosage	Contraindications and Nursing Considerations
Muscle Relaxants/Paralytics (continued)			
vecuronium bromide	Norcuron	0.08 – 0.1 mg/kg	+ severe anaphylactic reactions possible + carefully consider use in patients with hepatic impairment
Nitrates			
nitroglycerin	Nitro-Bid; Nitro-Dur	2.5 – 6.5 mg 3 – 4×/ day	+ indicated for use in angina, myocardial infarction + may cause headache + may lead to syncope or near syncope
Nonsteroidal Anti-Inflammatory Drugs (NSAIDs)			
naproxen	Aleve	500 – 1,000 mg/day	+ increased risk of serious (sometimes fatal) cardiovascular thrombotic events + increased risk of GI inflammation, ulceration, bleeding
Opioids			
codeine	N/A	15 – 60 mg every 4 hours as needed	+ may cause CNS depression + may cause or aggravate constipation
fentanyl	Duragesic; Fentora	0.35 – 0.5 mcg/kg every 30 – 60 minutes as needed	+ may cause severe hypotension + life-threatening or fatal respiratory depression possible
hydrocodone	Vicodin	10 – 20 mg/dose	+ possible impaired physical or mental abilities from CNS depression + life-threatening or fatal respiratory depression possible
hydromorphone	Dilaudid	2 – 4 mg every 4 – 6 hours	+ black box warning for high risk for addiction + possibility of severe hypotension (including orthostatic hypotension and syncope); patients with hypovolemia should be monitored
morphine sulfate	Duramorph	2.5 – 5 mg every 3 – 4 hours	+ possible impaired physical or mental abilities from CNS depression + life-threatening or fatal respiratory depression possible
oxycodone	OxyContin	5 – 15 mg every 4 – 6 hours as needed	+ high risk for addiction, should be used carefully + life-threatening respiratory depression possible

Potassium-Removing Agents

sodium polystyrene sulfonate	Kayexalate	15 g 1 – 4×/day	+ use for hyperkalemia + severe hypokalemia may occur + intestinal necrosis and other serious gastrointestinal events may occur

Proton-Pump Inhibitors

lansoprazole	Prevacid	15 mg 1×/day for up to 8 weeks	+ symptomatic GERD, erosive esophagitis, peptic ulcer disease + risk of fundic gland polyps; long-term use increases risk
pantoprazole	Protonix	20 – 40 mg 1×/day for 4 weeks	+ used for GERD and for erosive esophagitis + long-term use may result in C. difficile infection + increased risk of GI infection

Sedatives/Hypnotics

etomidate	Amidate	0.2 – 0.6 mg/kg	+ used in the ED for induction of anesthesia for rapid sequence intubation + may induce cardiac depression in elderly patients
ketamine	Ketalar	0.5 – 2 mg/kg (IV)	+ used for moderate sedation and for pain in the ED + ketamine increases the risk of laryngospasm in the presence of upper respiratory disease + may cause dependence
propofol	Diprivan	100 – 150 mcg/kg/minute	+ used for sedation in procedures or for sedation of patients with ET tubes + use with caution in patients with severe cardiac disease + use with caution in patients with increased intracranial pressure

Steroids

dexamethasone	Decadron	0.75 – 9 mg/day	+ has many indications + generally used to reduce inflammation + contraindicated in systemic fungal infections
fluticasone	Flovent Diskus	44 mg/actuation	+ indicated for use in prevention of asthma attacks + avoid use with concurrent infections + contraindicated in immunosuppressed patients

	Brand Name(s)	Dosage	Contraindications and Nursing Considerations
...eroids (continued)			
methylpredniso-lone	Medrol	4 – 48 mg orally, gradual taper off	+ has many uses, such as dermatologic concerns and endocrine disorders + may result in mild allergic reaction
prednisolone	Millipred	5 – 60 mg/day	+ acute myopathy has been reported with high-dose corticosteroids + psychiatric disturbances associated with corticosteroid use
prednisone	Deltasone	5 – 60 mg/day	+ may cause hypercortisolism + Kaposi's sarcoma associated with prolonged use of corticosteroids
Tricyclic Antidepressants			
amitriptyline	Elavil	75 – 100 mg/day	+ patients newly prescribed may have increased suicidal ideation + should not be given with MAOIs + may take up to 3 weeks to be effective
Triptans			
sumatriptan	Imitrex	+ 25 – 100 mg + Max dose: 200 mg/day	+ indicated for migraine headache + treats cluster headaches
Thrombolytics			
streptokinase	Streptase	+ MI: 1.5 million intl units + PE/DVT: 250,000 intl units	+ indicated in MI, DVT, and pulmonary embolism + may cause bleeding + may cause syncope
tenecteplase	TNKase	+ Dosage based on weight chart + Max dose: 50 mg	+ indicated for use in patients experiencing heart attack who cannot get to a cath lab in a reasonable period of time + increases risk of bleeding or hemorrhage + contraindicated in trauma patients
tPA (tissue plasminogen activator)	n/a	+ Dose is based on weight and time of infusion + 100 mg max dose	+ for use in patients with ischemic stroke + must be administered in specific window of time + window is measured from onset of symptoms + inclusion criteria is strict